The Specialist Registrar and New Consultant Handbook

Third edition

John Gatrell
BA(Hons) Chartered FCIPD MCIMgt
Leadership Development Consultant

and

Tony White
PhD FRCS MB BS AKC
Consultant Laryngologist (retired)

Foreword by
Mary Armitage

Radcliffe Publishing
Oxford • Seattle

Radcliffe Publishing Ltd
18 Marcham Road
Abingdon
Oxon OX14 1AA
United Kingdom

www.radcliffe-oxford.com

Electronic catalogue and worldwide online ordering facility.

_____

Reprinted 2008

British Library Cataloguing in Publication Data

A catalogue record for this book is available from the British Library.

ISBN-10 1 84619 047 9
ISBN-13 978 1 84619 047 6

Typeset by Advance Typesetting Ltd, Oxon
Printed and bound by TJI Digital, Padstow, Cornwall

Contents

Foreword

The subtitle of this new edition of *The Specialist Registrar and New Consultant Handbook* should surely be: Everything you ever wanted to know about the NHS, but never dared ask …

Once again John Gatrell and Tony White have come to the rescue of doctors in training. It is hard for any doctor to keep up to date with the constant changes in the NHS and to understand them in historical and political contexts. Management training and professional development have become increasingly important to all doctors, not just trainees. I suspect that there will be many others, including long-established consultants, who will find this book informative, relevant and helpful in their work. I would certainly have liked to have had such a resource available when I was training!

Too often, trainees are offered 'sheep dipping' – that is, a few brief days of management training at the end of their specialist training programme. This does little to equip them for the many and complex challenges ahead. Much of the information in this book is not easily sourced by trainees, nor is it generally covered in formal teaching. The handbook is very readable. It provides an excellent balance between the eminently practical and pragmatic and the more detailed aspects of NHS structure, funding and commissioning. It will have a prominent place in my bookcase, not least to ensure that the trainees are not better informed than I.

Mary Armitage
Clinical Vice President
Royal College of Physicians
August 2006

Preface

We often meet doctors who express the wish that they had received training earlier in their careers in a wider range of non-clinical aspects of their work. Others, who are committed to continuing professional development, seek learning material that will help them to handle the wider issues they confront on a day-to-day basis, and for which initial medical education failed to prepare them. Many trainers find it difficult to access a single source that provides them with material for the non-clinical training of their juniors. This book was written to address these and other needs revealed by our research. Since its publication we have been delighted with the positive feedback received from specialist registrars and other grades of doctors, including many consultants.

Before the book was first published it was piloted extensively, working with a wide range of doctors. Many comments were received which helped us to develop the final version. We have continued to receive positive feedback on the second edition, and this has encouraged us to go ahead with a third.

Since the second edition, changes in the structure, funding and governance of the NHS have continued at a pace. We have incorporated these into this third edition, although inevitably there will be ongoing refinements to, for example, Modernising Medical Careers, as it is carried through to full implementation. Sections relating to the NHS context have also been updated.

We hope you will find the book helpful in your current medical role, and as a means of supporting your continuing professional development.

John Gatrell
Tony White
August 2006

About the authors

John Gatrell works as an independent consultant on the development and delivery of a wide range of training programmes for medical and other healthcare professionals and managers. He has previously held posts in higher education including associate dean of a business school and course director in a faculty of applied sciences. He has a law degree and is a Fellow of the Chartered Institute of Personnel and Development. He has published and presented research papers on a range of topics related to leadership and organisation development. He has worked at trust board level on developing and implementing strategic change programmes, as well as addressing a wide range of other trust management issues.

Tony White is a retired consultant otolaryngologist appointed in Bath where he was clinical director for seven years. He has a PhD from Bath University with a thesis on *The Role of Doctors in Management* subsequently joining Bournemouth University as professor of medical management. He has written six books on medical management, and contributed and edited several other textbooks as well as writing numerous papers. He has lectured widely and organised many workshops on doctors' management development issues. He has been a member of a number of national advisory committees to develop doctors' non-clinical skills, and acted as regular tutor on training courses in various regions.

John and Tony undertook a three-year research project into the non-clinical development needs of doctors. This resulted in publication of the NHS Training Directorate report: *Medical Student to Medical Director*, and also formed a basis for this book.

Acknowledgements

We remain especially grateful to Dr Hugh Platt, whose vision initiated and inspired this work.

Our thanks are also due to those readers who took the trouble to contact us with suggestions for this third edition.

We wish to thank those who provided wisdom and guidance from various medical royal colleges, postgraduate deaneries, the Medical Defence Union, health authorities and hospital and primary care trusts. We freely acknowledge that some ideas may have come from seeds sown during discussions with these people. We apologise if any reference is not attributed or is incorrectly acknowledged; any such errors are ours alone.

Particular thanks are due to Liz Jones, Matron at the Bath Clinic for her help in finding and checking material, Dr Matt Thomas, Consultant, Poole Hospital, for his advice on quality and risk management and Octavia Morgan, Research Consultant, for her research support.

Not least, we are grateful to our wives, Susie and Anne, whose continued support, tolerance and encouragement has made the whole project possible.

Introduction

This book has three main aims:

- to support the development of a range of mainly non-clinical skills related to professional development

- to provide a basis for making the most of a range of learning opportunities that occur during training

- to serve as a source of useful information to doctors in the NHS.

Sometimes it is difficult to ask for advice about non-clinical aspects of our work – it is often assumed that we should acquire this awareness through a kind of osmosis, by picking it up along the way. This book tries to provide answers to questions that you feel you ought to know, but do not like to ask. The book also provides assistance with the development of new skills and capabilities that we know are relevant to professional careers. You may wish to dip into it to help you with a particular problem, or work through whole sections in order to learn more about specific aspects of your work.

Some kinds of learning can be achieved through reading textbooks, some through one-to-one instruction, and others are better undertaken in group training sessions. All require opportunity, an element of underpinning knowledge and a commitment to learn. This book is designed to cover the knowledge element that is the basis for developing professional skill and judgement. It should fit in with your work and be relevant to everyday needs. It supplements other training such as short courses which become available from time to time.

The book emerged from an extensive study of the non-clinical learning needs of doctors at all stages in their careers, and has been further informed by a series of development programmes for doctors. The General Medical Council's *Good Medical Practice Guidelines* remind us that a high level of clinical competence is only one aspect of professional medical practice. Personal insight, effective team working, good leadership, teaching others and skill in dealing with patients need to be supported by clear understanding of the complex structures and systems in the modern NHS.

Following the introduction of Modernising Medical Careers, standardised multisource feedback techniques have been introduced to improve the assessment of interpersonal skills exhibited by doctors in training. This is just one example of the increased breadth of assessment that modern medical trainees must be able to accommodate. Their world has increased in complexity through technological advances on the one hand and political intervention on the other. As future consultants they may be expected to play a much greater role in the organisations in which they work, yet have less power and influence than most of their predecessors. We have tried to cover a wide range of needs in this book. We hope you find it useful and enjoy the experience of using it as a learning resource.

Needs and experience change over time, and it would be helpful if you let us know things that need to be included, things that could be omitted, and things that need changing or moving from one section to another. This process of continuous development and review will ensure that it stays relevant for future readers.

Learning objectives

Key learning objectives of the handbook are listed below. You might find it helpful to start by familiarising yourself with its contents as a whole. If you believe you are already competent in an area, study the action points in that section. This should help you to decide if you need to do more. You may feel that some sections are irrelevant at this stage in your career. Put them to one side, but make a note to return to them later. The book will also act as a reference document into which you can dip as the need arises.

On completion of the book you should be better able to:

- identify your preferred learning style and make better use of learning opportunities
- organise your time so that you can cope with work and enjoy available leisure time
- delegate tasks to others in a way that helps to develop them and permits you to make better use of your own abilities
- make effective presentations to small and large groups
- work effectively in a team
- lead others in the achievement of team goals
- understand and deal with conflict
- deal with stress in yourself and others
- contribute usefully and effectively to meetings
- instruct and train others in skills and knowledge aspects of clinical tasks
- appraise others in the context of training and revalidation
- present clear and concise formal reports and other written communications
- undertake research and prepare articles for publication
- present yourself effectively in the selection process
- deal with patients and close family members in breaking bad news
- request a post mortem
- appear at a coroner's inquest
- support, advise and help to develop colleagues
- identify the key aspects of quality service delivery
- recognise trust and related national systems for risk management
- differentiate between audit and research and apply audit principles to a range of settings
- reflect on your personal values in the context of your career and work as a doctor
- understand something of the current structure of the NHS.

CHAPTER 1

Exploring your approach to working and learning

The aim of this chapter is to enable you to reflect on your approach to your work, to explore your preferred learning style, and to help you to manage your time effectively.

What type of doctor are you?

Doctors usually work in a number of trusts as they proceed through training. This gives them an opportunity to get to know a little of the differing sets of values and attitudes that tend to be a feature of a particular organisation. As they become employees of each organisation, they may consider how well their own values 'chime' with those of their colleagues in each place. This may cause them to reflect on their own values, both as doctor and employee. Older generations of doctors sometimes regard doctors in training as being less able and committed than they themselves were at a similar stage in their careers, and are inclined to believe that deteriorating attitudes to work will have a negative effect on patients.

Without perfect recall we (and they) are unable to prove or disprove this perspective. A high level of self-insight is undoubtedly an important asset for those developing their professional competence and standing. This questionnaire enables you to reflect on the values you bring to the organisation in which you work. It may also help you to understand more about other doctors with whom you work. You may find it interesting to carry out a quick self-diagnostic questionnaire to assess your own values in the context of your work as a doctor. It will also be interesting for you to repeat it after you are appointed as a consultant, and reflect on changes that have occurred.

This questionnaire is derived from *Doctors and Dilemmas* by Hugo Mascie-Taylor, Mike Pedler and Tony Winkless (1996), and is used with permission.

Read each statement and place a tick in the box corresponding to the one option of the four presented that most applies to you.

Question	A	B	C	D
In the development of my work people would describe me as …				
… striving on behalf of the whole.			☐	
… uninvolved.	☐			
… a good corporate citizen.		☐		
… a fighter for my own service.				☐
When I am a consultant I …				
… should not be seen to have to lead very often.	☐			
… should lead from the front (and not expect to be questioned a great deal).		☐		
… lead by creating a vision for the hospital/department and motivating others.			☐	
… have an important role within my team.				☐
My colleagues would tend to say of me that …				
… I am the sort of person who is likely to initiate and deal well with change.			☐	
… I can be relied upon to look after my patients, and play my part in the team.				☐
… I am perhaps a bit of a character and occasionally selfish and pushy.		☐		
… they tend not to talk or know much about me.	☐			
As a consultant it will be important for me to …				
… look after my patients, and be supportive of the hospital.				☐
… look after my patients and develop my service and specialty.		☐		
… look after my patients and avoid wasting time doing other things.	☐			
… look after my patients and contribute ideas for the development of the hospital.			☐	
I believe it is important for research to be carried out in the hospital …				
… so long as it does not interfere with patient care or divert one away from outside interests.	☐			
… so that doctors can treat patients more effectively.				☐
… so as to improve patient services which the hospital offers and to enhance its reputation.			☐	
… so that the reputation of individual doctors and their specialty is enhanced.		☐		
As a future consultant I …				
… should be a leader of my team where appropriate.				☐
… should not be concerned to any great extent with leading others.	☐			
… should become a leader of my specialty.		☐		
… should be a leader in the hospital.			☐	
In my non-clinical working relationships with others in hospital I …				
… single mindedly pursue the self-interest of my specialty.		☐		
… do not have many relationships with others.	☐			
… attempt to work with others to the best of my ability.				☐
… attempt to show others that there is a brighter future.			☐	
In dealing with patients I …				
… resist any restriction which a shortage of resources might bring about.		☐		
… just get on with dealing with an individual patient.	☐			
… make sure the hospital as a whole responds as well as possible to the needs of patients.			☐	
… recognise that there are issues beyond the individual patient.				☐

When I attend a management course, my interest would be in ...
... how to make a team work more effectively, contributing to others and
  the hospital. ☐
... leadership and strategic management. ☐
... understanding the system so that I can get what I want. ☐
... very little of what was on offer. ☐

I believe the curriculum for medical students should comprehensively cover ...
... more medical topics and less of the 'social sciences'. ☐
... methods of effective team working. ☐
... strategic management of the NHS. ☐
... managing the doctor/patient relationship. ☐

In terms of my leadership style I ...
... like to join with people and participate. ☐
... tell people what they need to know. ☐
... consult, then seek to influence. ☐
... have never really thought about it much. ☐

Modern management practices in the NHS ...
... must be resisted at all times by the profession. ☐
... have a useful place. ☐
... are only vaguely understood by me. ☐
... offer the key to the future. ☐

My view of managers in the NHS is that they ...
... are partners in the management of a complex organisation. ☐
... are irrelevant to my practice. ☐
... are an unnecessary imposition. ☐
... have a part to play and contribution to make. ☐

In my view, service commissioners ...
... should find the funds to enable my specialty to expand. ☐
... should be seen as partners in the strategic development of our hospital. ☐
... should ensure balance in developments even if it affects my specialty negatively. ☐
... seem very remote and beyond my sphere of influence. ☐

As a consultant, financial considerations should ...
... be none of my concern. ☐
... be of importance. ☐
... be vigorously resisted if they get in the way of my service. ☐
... have a part to play. ☐

**As a consultant if I were invited by the chief executive to a meeting to discuss
significant cost reductions which might affect my clinical practice I would ...**
... either not attend the meeting or attend and say nothing. ☐
... attend recognising that to resolve the issue requires a team-working approach. ☐
... attend in order to make positive suggestions for taking the hospital forward. ☐
... attend in order to minimise the effect on my specialty. ☐

In discussions with my colleagues about the resource implications of practice I ...
... accept that resource limitations are part of the ethical debate. ☐
... take the view that practice guidelines should not be influenced by resource
  implications. ☐
... persuade other clinicians of the need to seek solutions to such dilemmas. ☐
... tend not to venture a view. ☐

As a future consultant I would like my professional work to be recognised for ...
... strongly influencing the direction of the hospital.   ☐
... providing a good service.   ☐
... solely my clinical work.   ☐
... being influential in the profession.   ☐

I feel that primary care as a service commissioner ...
... has shifted power from hospital doctors in an inappropriate way.   ☐
... emphasises the need for consultants in secondary care to work together.   ☐
... is irrelevant to my practice.   ☐
... has created hospitals which require strategic leadership.   ☐

If it were suggested that the hospital in which I was working should merge with another, in the interests of patient care I would ...
... only support the merger if I thought that my own specialty would benefit.   ☐
... contact my opposite numbers in the other unit to help to forge an effective new alliance.   ☐
... support the merger in the light of the common good.   ☐
... recognise that I would have little influence on the outcome.   ☐

My view of attending conferences is that they ...
... can be useful for networking effectively with other influential doctors and managers.   ☐
... are essential for meeting and influencing other important doctors in my specialty.   ☐
... are not normally part of my life or practice.   ☐
... are something I do in order to keep up to date.   ☐

The leadership of clinical services ...
... rests with the doctor as far as my patients are concerned.   ☐
... is a medical role with some important managerial implications.   ☐
... should be shared on the basis of professional expertise.   ☐
... is the doctor's right.   ☐

A primary care-led NHS ...
... makes me work with other colleagues to meet GPs' needs.   ☐
... is doomed to failure since it removes power from those who really understand.   ☐
... is a piece of jargon which I don't really understand.   ☐
... represents a strategic opportunity for the hospital which should be embraced.   ☐

Consultant job plans are ...
... helpful for consultants to work together.   ☐
... an unnecessary imposition by management on consultant practice.   ☐
... unnecessary given the straightforward nature of consultant work.   ☐
... a useful tool in ensuring that objectives of a hospital are met.   ☐

What I admire most in my colleagues is ...
... their ability to lead.   ☐
... the way they are not distracted from their daily clinical work.   ☐
... their ambition for themselves and their specialty.   ☐
... their being prepared to contribute to the team effort.   ☐

I would like to think that my obituary in the *BMJ* will say ...
... I was first and last an outstanding clinician.   ☐
... I was primarily an outstanding medical manager.   ☐
... I was primarily outstanding in my specialty.   ☐
... I was primarily outstanding in working in a team for the good of the patient.   ☐

Analysis of your questionnaire responses

The ticks for your answers fall under columns headed A, B, C, or D. Add up the totals scores for the whole questionnaire for each column and enter into the boxes

Your highest score suggests one of four possible positions that doctors take with regard to the resolution of common dilemmas which arise in fulfilling their role. Doctors manage at various levels, their personal practice, in teams and groups, departments and units etc. Full details of the use of a Repertory Grid approach to this analysis can be found in Taylor, Pedler and Winkless (1993) who produced four ideal type descriptions or 'identikits' (*see* Figure 1.1).

The caricatures emerge with clarity, but type A turns out to include a variety of subtypes. A cautionary note: people vary in the way they respond to questionnaires by tending to score lowly, highly or opting for the middle option. Also each question is given equal weight, so the salience of questions for you may not be fairly represented. You need to remember these points, particularly if you are making comparisons with other people.

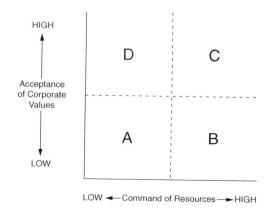

Figure 1.1 Types in relation to resources and corporate values

What type are you?

Type 'D' – the TEAM PLAYER – 'the good corporate citizen'

Focus:

- primarily to the team but with awareness and interest in the whole organisation
- team leader advising rather than leading the organisation.

Abilities and skills:

- takes leadership at team level and is prepared to accept it at corporate level
- plays by rules within corporate goals, a building block of the organisation
- participative, co-operative, loyal, supportive, shares responsibilities, a team worker
- good interpersonal skills, good communicator
- economical with resources
- personable, well respected.

Beliefs and values:

- service orientation
- recognises the added value and complementary skills of management
- democratic process, participation, consultation
- loyalty to medicine and medical values together with valuing the whole organisation.

Implications:

- the backbone of the organisation
- dedicated clinicians – the 'sort you'd like to take your mother to'
- interested in playing their part in the whole
- lack confidence or have insufficient skills to be Type C leaders
- less inclined to take risks than Type C leaders
- prefer to avoid tough decisions
- may choose the quiet life
- may pursue outside interests

- may focus on the medical role
- less likely than Type C leaders to take on formal management roles
- careful with resources
- may be self-sacrificing in meeting demands of others.

Type 'C' – the LEADER – 'who strives on behalf of the whole'

Focus:

- commitment to the organisation
- wide view, broad vision, strategic thinking.

Abilities and skills:

- change agent, politically astute
- high interpersonal skills, influential, good communicator, good listener, assertive and can be tough
- manages resources on behalf of the whole
- develops people and teams
- manages conflict, is constructive and supportive, tolerant of ambiguity and dilemmas.

Beliefs and values:

- quality service and value for money requires doctors and managers to work together
- capability in the whole system is what counts
- pluralistic, different sources of loyalty are legitimate, conflict is inevitable, endemic and needs to be managed
- people (including self) are developing beings and can learn.

Implications:

- the managers may regard you as too good to be true and lacking a 'shadow side'
- although Type Cs are often highly committed and very able leaders, Type Bs and perhaps Type As may see them as having 'gone over to the other side', or as having failed to make it in medicine and now seeking an alternative career

- some Type Cs may be Type Bs in temporary disguise, playing the corporate game in order to secure advantage. Others may indeed be more interested in personal career advancement than with the rather altruistic 'good of the whole'. A strong motivation may be the desire to learn and explore new possibilities, not just of career but of person.
- Type Cs are widely liked and respected for their leadership qualities especially by Type Ds.

Type B – the INDEPENDENT – 'who fights for their own patch'

Focus:

- me and my specialty
- me and my profession.

Abilities and skills:

- confidence, dominance, determined, may be aggressive
- political skills, well connected, knows the 'right people'
- entrepreneurial, energetic and hard working
- uses conflict
- has good ideas, sometimes functional sometimes dysfunctional for organisation.

Beliefs and values:

- self-belief and self-worth
- individuality, individual excellence is what counts
- specialty is all important
- doctors don't need managing but need administration
- rules are to be broken, or are 'my rules'.

Implications:

- little in the way of corporate loyalty or values
- uninterested in corporate management
- see managers (at best) as means of acquiring resources for their patch

- often lack sensitivity to others and may appear aloof, overbearing or arrogant

- arouse strong feelings of admiration, fear or dislike

- express themselves well in advancing their own work or specialty, but are poor at team work, chairing meetings or achieving agreement

- can be extrovert, convivial and amusing

- ability to command resources in the hospital or via external funding while lacking an awareness and concern for the whole makes them often the most difficult people to manage.

Type A – the CONTRACT CLINICIAN – 'uninvolved'

Focus:

- one-to-one patient care and clinical management with no particular interest, awareness or involvement beyond this.

This is a collection of subtypes. Classified as low on both corporate values and command of resources, this type has few abilities, skills, beliefs or values which are relevant from a leadership or managerial perspective.
The four subtypes are:

A1: the new starter

The junior doctor on the way to Type B, C or D. May be naive, idealistic, dedicated with little awareness of how the hospital or health services work and with little energy or attention to spare for learning the role.

A2: the disengager

Winding down and preparing to separate from the organisation through retirement, tiredness or ill-health.

A3: the contract worker

The personal doctor working 'nine to five' who doesn't want to get involved in anything outside one-to-one patient care. May have domestic responsibilities or consuming interests outside

work. Does a job for the hospital within the strict limits of the contract.

A4: the isolate

The loner who may be good, bad or indifferent, but is essentially unrecognised in terms of contribution. May work in remote location or specialty or be isolated for some other reason.

Implications:

- Type As have least impact because they do little to the organisation as a whole beyond their immediate task. This is not a commentary on them as people or as doctors, they may be effective or ineffective at that task. They may be learners or about to retire, they may have a limited contractual relationship with the organisation, or have a deep moral involvement in patient healthcare. They share a certain isolation from the run of events and may be candidates for further personal and professional development.

> **Action**
>
> Note your type now and reflect on what this means for you, your colleagues, the hospital, and your future in healthcare. You may find it instructive to repeat this questionnaire at the end of your first year as a consultant and consider how you have changed and why.

Learning and problem solving – what is your preferred style?

The Calman reforms, which introduced the concept of the specialist registrar, were based on the idea that with more structured training using more appropriate methods, training could be not only shorter but better. *Modernising Medical Careers* follows a similar theme but with a generally more structured approach to performance assessment and feedback. This section seeks to give insight into some concepts behind teaching and learning. An understanding of the thinking behind training methods being used today will help you to get the most from your learning opportunities. We think it would be helpful to introduce you to the work of Kolb, Osland and Rubin (1995).

Career development and the maintenance of professional competence demand that doctors maintain learning habits throughout their working lives. Most of us associate learning with the process we followed at school and university, when tutors provided us with knowledge, often through lectures to large groups of students, and concepts which we dutifully wrote down and memorised and fed back in the essays and project work and examination questions completed as a means of assessing our learning. End-of-term, end-of-year and final examinations helped to confirm the view that demonstrating learning involved satisfying others – our assessors – that we had grasped the necessary *concepts.*

Necessary for what though? 'Real life', as you will already have realised, in the form of daily work with patients, requires a different approach, where problem-solving requires us to gain *experience*, quite different from the unreal world of classroom learning. The concept of learning as we came to know it during school and university often seems less relevant now.

The concept of problem solving also suggests an active rather than passive process. In other words the responsibility for problem solving rests with you, in contrast to teaching, in which the teacher is responsible (for the learning). The problem solver must experiment, take risks and gain experience, in order to address the problem.

This separation of *educational* learning and *work* learning sometimes leads to difficulties for doctors in the transition from medical school to work-based training. Our preferred approaches to learning are usually based on early, school-based experience, which do not always match later learning needs. In this section we will:

- illustrate this concept
- identify your preferred learning style
- show how various learning styles are relevant to different situations

- provide a model for learning which will help you to take full advantage of learning opportunities as they arise
- help you to understand why you find some kinds of learning more acceptable than others.

The inventory on the following page is for describing how you learn – the way you find out about and deal with ideas and situations in your life. Different people learn best in different ways. The different ways of learning described in the survey are equally good. The aim is to describe how you learn, not to evaluate your learning ability. You might find it hard to choose the descriptions that best characterise your learning style. Keep in mind that there are no right or wrong answers – all the choices are equally acceptable.

Learning style inventory

Source: Kolb, Osland and Rubin (1995), used with permission (*see* Related reading, p. 18).

Instructions

There are nine sets of four descriptions listed in this inventory. Mark the words in each set that are most like you, second most like you, third most like you, and least like you. Put a four (4) next to the description that is *most* like you, a three (3) next to the description that is *second* most like you, a two (2) next to the description that is *third* most like you, and a one (1) next to the description that is *least* like you (4 = *most* like you; 1 = *least* like you). Be sure to assign a different rank number to each of the four words in each set; *use whole numbers only.*

Example:

<u>4</u> happy   <u>3</u> fast   <u>1</u> angry   <u>2</u> careful

(Some people find it easiest to decide first which word best describes them (<u>4</u> happy) and then decide the word that is least like them (<u>1</u> angry). Then you can give a 3 to that word in the remaining pair that is most like you (<u>3</u> fast) and a 2 to the word that is left over (<u>2</u> careful) (*see* opposite.

1	_discriminating	_tentative	_involved	_practical
2	_receptive	_relevant	_analytical	_impartial
3	_feeling	_watching	_thinking	_doing
4	_accepting	_risk taker	_evaluative	_aware
5	_intuitive	_productive	_logical	_questioning
6	_abstract	_observing	_concrete	_active
7	_present-oriented	_reflecting	_future-oriented	_pragmatic
8	_experience	_observation	_conceptualisation	_experimentation
9	_intense	_reserved	_rational	_responsible

Scoring instructions

The four columns of words correspond to the four learning style scales: **CE** (concrete experience), **RO** (reflective observation), **AC** (abstract conceptualisation), and **AE** (active experimentation). To compute your scale scores, write your rank numbers in the boxes below only for the designated items. For example, in the third column (**AC**), you would fill in the rank numbers you have assigned to items 2, 3, 4, 5, 8 and 9. Compute your scale scores by adding the rank numbers for each set of boxes.

score items:	score items:	score items:	score items:
2 3 4 5 7 8	1 3 6 7 8 9	2 3 4 5 8 9	1 3 6 7 8 9
Total:	Total:	Total:	Total:
CE =	**RO =**	**AC =**	**AE =**

When the characteristics of learning and problem solving are combined, it is possible to come to a closer understanding of how people use their experience to develop concepts, rules and principles that guide their behaviour in new situations. The process can be conceived as a four-stage cycle as shown in Figure 1.2.

Concrete experience is any experience which has an impact, either physical or emotional, on the person. It is normally as a result of interaction with others that we feel such an impact. This is followed by *observation and reflection* on the experience, taking time to make sense of the context and the experience itself. This should then lead to the formation of *abstract concepts* and generalisations, or explanations which help us to explain the nature and reasons for our reactions to the experience. We may then test out our reasoning by *active experimentation*, or trying out new behaviours and approaches in the fourth stage. This leads on to further experience, and so on. The model shows learning as a continuously recurring cycle. All learning is relearning, and all education is re-education. It may also be assumed that learning is shaped by personal needs and goals, which affect the ways in which we interpret experience. Thus, learning is likely to be erratic and inefficient when personal objectives are not clear.

Interpreting your scores on the learning style inventory

The learning style inventory (LSI) is a simple self-description test based on experiential learning theory. It is designed to measure your strengths and weaknesses as a learner in the four stages of the learning process. Effective learners use four different learning modes: concrete experience (CE), reflective observation (RO) abstract conceptualisation (AC) and active experimentation (AE).

One way to understand the meaning of your scores on the LSI is to compare them with the scores of others. The target diagram in Figure 1.3 gives the norms on the four basic scales (CE, RO, AC, AE) for 1933 (American) adults ranging from 18 to 60 years of age. About two-thirds of the group are men and the group as a whole is well educated (two-thirds have degrees or higher). A wide range of occupations and educational backgrounds are represented. They include teachers, engineers, managers, doctors and lawyers.

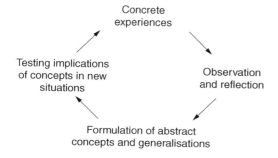

Figure 1.2 Four-stage cycle

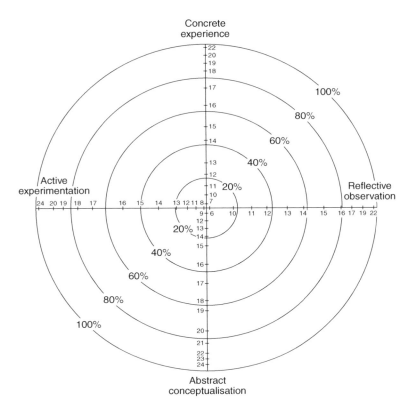

Figure 1.3 Learning style profile norms (© David A Kolb (1976))

The raw scores for each of the four basic scales are marked on the crossed lines of the target. By marking your raw scores on the four scales and connecting them with straight lines you can create a graphic representation of your learning style profile. The concentric circles on the target represent percentile scores for the normative group.

It should be emphasised that the LSI does not accurately define your learning style. It is an indication of how you see yourself as a learner. Your scores indicate which learning modes you emphasise in general. They may change from time to time and situation to situation.

The inventory is designed to give you some indication of which learning modes you tend to emphasise. No mode is better or worse than any other. Even a totally balanced profile is not necessarily best. The key to effective learning is being competent in each mode when it is appropriate.

Orientation towards *concrete experience* suggests being involved in experiences and dealing with immediate human situations in a personal way. It emphasises *feeling* as opposed to *thinking*, and concern with the uniqueness and complexity of present reality as opposed to theories and models, an intuitive, artistic approach as opposed to a systematic, scientific approach to problems. People with concrete experience orientation enjoy and are good at relating to others. They can be good intuitive decision makers, and function well in unstructured situations. They value highly relationships with people, being involved in real situations and keep an open-minded approach to life.

An orientation toward *reflective observation* emphasises comprehending the meaning of ideas and situations by carefully observing and impartially describing them. It emphasises understanding as opposed to practical application. Such people enjoy thinking about the *meaning* of situations and ideas, and are good at discovering their implications. They often look at things from different perspectives and appreciate different points of view. They value patience, impartiality and considered thoughtful judgement, and tend to rely on their own thoughts and feelings to form opinions.

Orientation towards *abstract conceptualisation* focuses on using logic, ideas and concepts. It emphasises thinking as opposed to feeling, and is concerned with building general theories rather than intuitive understanding. Such a person enjoys and is good at systematic planning, manipulation of abstract symbols, and quantitative analysis. They value precision, the rigour and discipline of analysing ideas, and the aesthetic quality of a neat conceptual system.

An orientation toward *active experimentation* focuses on actively influencing people and changing situations. It emphasises practical applications as opposed to reflective understanding, a pragmatic concern with what works as opposed to what is absolute truth. Such people enjoy and are good at getting things accomplished. They are willing to take some risk to achieve their objectives. They also value having an impact and influence on the environment around them, and like to see results.

Action

Greater insight into your preferred learning style should provide you with a basis for exploiting learning opportunities. If possible, discuss your profile with that of colleagues. Compare and contrast them, and consider if it helps to explain your previous performance in learning situations and different subject areas.

Identifying your learning style type

It is useful to describe your learning style by a single data point that combines your scores on the four basic modes. This is accomplished by using the two combination scores, **AC** minus **CE** and **AE** minus **RO**. These scales indicate the degree to which you emphasise *abstract* over *concrete* and *action* over *reflection*, respectively.

The grid shown in Figure 1.4 has the raw scores for these two scales on the crossed lines (**AC – CE** on the vertical and **AE – RO** on the horizontal) and percentile scores based on the normative group on the sides. By marking your raw scores on the two lines and plotting their point of interception, you can find which of the four learning style quadrants you fall into. These four quadrants, labelled *accommodator, diverger, converger* and *assimilator*, represent the four dominant learning styles. If your **AC – CE** score were –4 and your **AE – RO** score were +8, you would fall strongly in the accommodator quadrant. An **AC – CE** score of +4 and an **AE – RO** score of +3 would put you only slightly in the converger quadrant. The closer your data point is to the point where the lines cross, the more balanced is your learning style. If your data point is close to any of the four corners, this indicates that you rely heavily on one particular learning style.

The following is a description of the characteristics of the four basic learning styles based both on research and clinical observation of these patterns of LSI scores.

- The *convergent* learning style relies primarily on the dominant learning abilities of abstract conceptualisation and active experimentation. The greatest strength of this approach lies in problem solving, decision making, and the practical application of ideas. This learning style is called 'converger' because a person with this style seems to do best in such situations as conventional intelligence tests where there is a single correct answer or solution to a question or problem. In this learning style, knowledge is organised in such a way that, through hypothetical–deductive reasoning, it can be focused on specific problems. Liam Hudson's research on individuals with this style of learning shows that convergent persons are controlled in their expression of emotion. They prefer dealing with technical tasks and problems rather than with social and interpersonal issues. Convergers have often specialised in the physical sciences. This learning style is characteristic of many engineers and technical specialists.

- The *divergent* learning style has the opposite strengths of the convergent style, emphasising concrete experience and reflective observation. The greatest strength of this orientation lies in

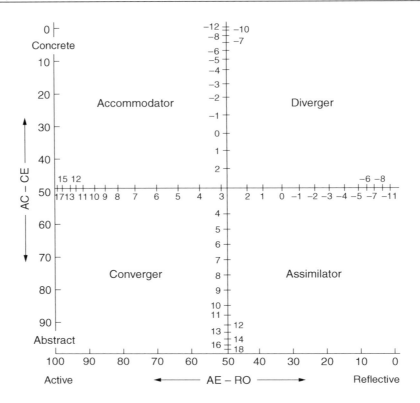

Figure 1.4 Learning style type grid (© David A Kolb (1976))

imaginative ability and awareness of meaning and values. The primary adaptive ability in this style is to view concrete situations from many perspectives and to organise many relationships into a meaningful 'Gestalt'. The emphasis in this orientation is on adaptation by observation rather than by action. This style is called 'diverger' because a person of this type performs better in situations that call for generation of alternative ideas and implications such as a 'brainstorming' idea session. Persons oriented toward divergence are interested in people, and tend to be imaginative and feeling oriented. Divergers have broad cultural interests and tend to specialise in the arts. This style is characteristic of individuals from humanities and liberal arts backgrounds. Counsellors, organisation development specialists, and personnel managers tend to be characterised by this learning style.

- In *assimilation,* the dominant learning abilities are abstract conceptualisation and reflective observation. The greatest strength of this orientation lies in inductive reasoning, in the ability

to create theoretical models, and in assimilating disparate observations into an integrated explanation. As in convergence, this orientation is less focused on people and more concerned with ideas and abstract concepts. Ideas, however, are judged less in this orientation by their practical value. Here it is more important that the theory be logically sound and precise. This learning style is more characteristic of individuals in the basic sciences and mathematics rather than the applied sciences. In organisations, persons with this learning style are found most often in the research and planning departments.

- The *accommodative* learning style has the opposite strengths of assimilation, emphasising concrete experience and active experimentation. The greatest strength of this orientation lies in doing things, in carrying out plans and tasks, and in getting involved in new experiences. The adaptive emphasis of this orientation is on opportunity seeking, risk taking, and action. This style is called 'accommodation' because it is best suited for those situations in which one must adapt oneself to changing immediate circumstances. In situations where the theory or plans do not fit the facts, those with an accommodative style will most likely discard the plan or theory. (With the opposite learning style, assimilation, one would be more likely to disregard or re-examine the facts.) People with an accommodative orientation tend to solve problems in an intuitive trial and error manner, relying on other people for information rather than on their own analytical ability. Individuals with accommodative learning styles are at ease with people, but are sometimes seen as impatient and 'pushy'. This person's educational background is often in technical or practical fields such as business. In organisations, people with this learning style are found in 'action-oriented' jobs, often in marketing or sales.

Making effective use of your time

Time is a remarkable commodity. No matter how we waste time today, tomorrow's entitlement remains untouched. Most junior doctors recognise the problem of time management. You need to organise your time and clinical work around structured sessions, clinics, ward rounds, theatre sessions. You need to organise yourself and your tasks when you are on call, as well as your time on call itself. Your work makes multiple demands on your time, such as writing up discharge summaries, dictating notes from your most recent clinic, preparing a paper to present to the firm at the weekly journal club, and perhaps a promise to read through a paper for a colleague! Then there is your private life outside work and finding time for family, friends – even for yourself! Few have found a simple solution. Most do their best, but some are definitely better at this than others. This is partly based on differing personalities. Some people like their lives to be conducted with a high measure of order and structure. Others prefer to keep their options open and not have plans which might inhibit their flexibility to take opportunities as they arise (Houghton, 2004). Regardless of our natural preferences, work imposes demands which, if not met by careful organisation and planning, can lead to stress and even failure. How well do you use *your* time? Try to answer the following as honestly as you can.

Place a cross (X) in the appropriate column for each item.

Item		Strongly agree	Slightly agree	Slightly disagree	Strongly disagree
1	My work tends to mount up				
2	I tend to put off large or unpleasant jobs				
3	I find it difficult to say 'No' to requests from others				
4	I waste a lot of time in meetings				
5	I have to start and stop jobs frequently				
6	I spend too much time moving from place to place				
7	I have too much paperwork or too many emails to deal with				
8	I spend a great deal of time on the telephone				
9	I always seem to be trying to do too many things at the same time				
10	I never have time to prioritise tasks – I deal with problems as they arise				
11	The only way I can cope is by taking paperwork home with me				
12	I seldom have time to just sit and think				
13	Colleagues would describe me as disorganised				
14	I tend to mislay papers				
15	Other people always seem to come to me for advice				
16	I generally feel out of control of my career and life				

Action

List the items that you marked as strongly agree.

Now take each of these items and consider *why* this is the case. What do *you* do, and what do *others* do, to contribute to your problem? It may be helpful to discuss it with colleagues or friends. Try to identify the work-related and personal consequences of each 'strongly agree' item. Next, prioritise these items in the order in which you would like to resolve them. Take the first item and write down the action you need to take to deal with the problem. Specify the action and support you need from others in achieving this. Do this for each of the other items.

The following guidelines may help you in setting a framework for resolving problems that arise in your use of time.

Goal setting

As a doctor and specialist registrar you need to manage simultaneous tasks, such as dealing with an emergency admission and managing another patient about whom you are concerned and who is located on a different ward. This is before you take account of your private life. The first thing to recognise is that, when thinking about organising your life, it is unhelpful to separate work and 'non-work'.

Take a sheet of paper and write down your 'foreseeable life goals'. These are likely to be attainable within the next two or three years. Think of them as starting from now. They might be personal, family, social, career, financial,

community and spiritual. Work quickly, without limiting your ambitions.

Next, review and refine these goals into statements that imply action. Some may be immediate – 'Spend more time with my family'. Defining and securing your career objectives are likely to figure large. Others may require considerable balancing of resources and long-term planning such as investing to secure early retirement. Some may be unrealistic, and so should be disregarded at this stage.

Prioritise them. This involves taking decisions about yourself. Take into account your own values and circumstances. It can be difficult, but not as difficult as living without purpose. They will all be important, but some will be more important than others. Use them to develop your approach to time management.

Develop a sense of time. How do you really spend your day?

Analyse your working day by keeping a time log for a few days. You can use an ordinary desk diary. Record the activity in which you are engaged at 15 minute intervals throughout the day. This can be frighteningly revealing of the time spent on various activities of which you were not aware.

List the activities and record the time spent on each in a typical week. Ask yourself if this reflects your priorities. Are there activities that take up time but contribute little or nothing? What would happen if you stopped doing them completely? How much of your time do you keep to use at your discretion? Are you spending time on work that could be delegated to others?

Planning and prioritising

Define goals for personal development and professional accomplishment for the coming year. Write them in a way which will permit you to measure your success in achieving them.

Effective planning is impossible without a diary system. There are many options. They include electronic personal organisers, wall charts and desk diaries. Choose the one that suits you.

Set aside time (between 10 and 30 minutes) at the beginning of each day to list your tasks and prioritise them. You may find it helpful to use a simple system of letters or stars to indicate priority, for example:

***   *Must* be done today
**   *Should* be done today
*   *Might* be done today

It is crucial to understand the difference between tasks which are *urgent* and those which are *important*. Urgent but unimportant tasks should be delegated, or done quickly, but given a small amount of your time. Important, non-urgent tasks can be scheduled for later in the day, week or month and given sufficient space in your diary to complete them properly at the first sitting. Some tasks will be a mixture of both. One way of representing this is shown in Figure 1.5.

Work through your list, *completing each task before moving on to the next.* Set a time limit for each task based on its priority. As a doctor and specialist registrar, clearly some of your time may be largely outside your control. But it is not *all* out of your control. You will be surprised to find how much you can control if you choose. Use your daily planning session to make best possible use of the time that you can influence. Do not worry if, at the end of the day, you have not completed all of your tasks. Simply delete those that are no longer necessary, and transfer the rest to your list for the following day. Remember to allocate time to deal adequately with the

demands of quadrant II – this is the way to reduce the number of tasks that find their way into quadrant I.

Working routines

Incoming paperwork should be handled only once. Don't put a pathology or X-ray report down until you have decided what action to take, even if only to ask for advice. Do not put a letter or memo down until you have written or dictated a reply. If you really cannot act immediately, *do something*, even if it is just to decide and diarise *when* you will take action.

Writing clearly, simply and concisely is essential for effective, first-time communication. Consider the purpose of your communication, jot down key points, then arrange them in a logical order. Use short sentences, avoiding jargon and formal language.

- *Emails* can be a time waster or a tremendous time saver. Read and respond to emails only at designated times during the day, for example at the beginning of the day, before lunch, and again before you leave work. If you are a slave to your email system, and particularly if your computer is set up to notify you immediately upon the receipt of any incoming email, turn off the pop-up or noise which notifies you that

	Urgent	Non-urgent
Important	I Activities: Crises Pressing-problems Deadline-driven problems	II Activities: Prevention Relationship building Recognising new opportunities Planning
Non-important	III Activities: Interruptions Some calls, emails, letters Local pressing matters Popular activities	IV Activities: Trivia Some (most?) mail Some phone calls Office gossip

Figure 1.5 Time management matrix

you have received a message. Remember that, used well, email is an excellent way to convey information. It can be more precise than voice-mail, the sender and receiver have a record of the communication, more information can be conveyed than through voice-mail, and the information can be conveyed at a convenient time.

- *Reading* is an important method of personal development for doctors. Develop the following habits when dealing with your paperwork. Scan lengthy documents before deciding that you need to read them all. Perhaps look only at the introduction and summary or conclusions. Highlight key points so that you can refer back to them easily. 'Speed-reading' can be useful for those with many large documents to absorb, but is no substitute for good judgement when deciding *what* to read!

- *Telephones* save time when used appropriately. Try keeping a time log of your telephone use during one week. You may be surprised at the total time taken up. Before using the telephone, make a quick note of what you wish to say. Keep the conversation on track and bring it to a polite end when you have completed your business. Better still, delegate others to make, answer or return telephone calls for you. Mobile phones can be a mixed blessing. Ask yourself 'Does keeping one with me and switched on give me more, or less, control over my life?'.

- *Avoid procrastination.* When faced with large or difficult tasks, most of us are inclined to find diversions in order to avoid starting. These might include tidying our desk, making a cup of coffee or completing other much less important tasks. Your should set starting times for tasks you might be tempted to put off. Forget about finishing the task – concentrate on starting it. Make your deadlines public. Reward yourself for completing unpleasant tasks. Learn to say 'No' to unreasonable or low-priority requests from others. It takes practise to do this assertively, and without offending.

Working with others

- *Meetings* can waste a lot of your time. First, ask yourself if the meeting is necessary, or if

you need to attend. If you have called the meeting, prepare an agenda, set a time limit, and communicate these to others before it starts. Encourage them to prepare for the meeting. Discourage irrelevant discussion. There is a separate section on meetings in this workbook (p. 73).

- *Delegation* can be painful. Giving away tasks you enjoy, or feel you cannot trust others to do, may be the only way to release time for what you need to do to achieve results. There is more on delegation elsewhere in this handbook (p. 38).

- *Saying 'No'* to impossible or unnecessary tasks is often more difficult than it should be. We are brought up to acquiesce to our seniors rather than challenge them, and this creates habits which are nearly impossible to break. Assertive behaviours are dealt with elsewhere in this handbook (p. 30).

Planning working rotas, partial and full shifts

Good continuity of care does not just happen, it has to be planned, implemented and managed if you are to make best use of your time. Here are some key points which might enable you to make best use of your time:

Ensure:

- there is protected time for the handover with an overlap between staff of 15–30 minutes to allow for adequate communication

- information is relayed about all patients, not just the sick ones, placing you in a position to judge easily any changes in a patient's conditions

- you keep a written record of plans. This ensures you cannot forget something important due to pressure of a new emergency. Provide yourself with a daily written update.

Essentially it is about good communications. You can improve your own work simply by taking a little time and trouble, for instance in paying attention to communication at handover.

Setting up this sort of organisation in a department, ensuring there is support, and bringing together the relevant medical and non-medical personnel, is an exercise which will require consultant involvement. Consultants, in turn, will need the support and help of senior nurses and possibly managers. As a junior doctor, your most important role in improving work will be in selling the issue to your peers, particularly to your senior colleagues.

Self-awareness

Insight into yourself and the way you are seen by others can be a difficult thing to acquire. This is made more difficult for people in training to achieve high professional status, because boasting about strengths is not usually seen as acceptable, and admitting weaknesses can feel quite threatening to career development.

The Johari window, named after the first names of its inventors, Joseph Luft and Harry Ingham, is one of the most useful models describing the process of human interaction. It is often used, as here, to demonstrate an approach to developing insight into oneself through interaction with close colleagues. A four-paned 'window', as illustrated in Figure 1.6, divides personal awareness into four different types, as represented by its four quadrants: open arena, hidden, blind spot, and

unknown potential. The lines dividing the four panes can move as an interaction progresses.

The *open arena quadrant* represents things that I know about myself, and that others know about me. The knowledge that the window represents can include not only factual information but also my feelings, motives, behaviours, and perhaps some of my wishes. When I first meet a new person, the size of the opening of this first quadrant is not very large, since there has been little time to exchange information. As the process of getting to know one another continues, the dividers move down or to the right, placing more information into the open window, as described below.

The *blind spot quadrant* represents things that others know about me, but of which I am unaware. Others may know, for example, that I have said something that upset a colleague because he has complained to them, but if no-one tells me, then I remain unaware of the offence I have caused. This information is in my blind quadrant because others can see it, but I cannot. If someone now tells me that I have upset my colleague, then the window shade moves to the right, enlarging the open quadrant's area. Now, I may also have blind spots with respect to many other much more complex things. For example, perhaps in conversation, my eye

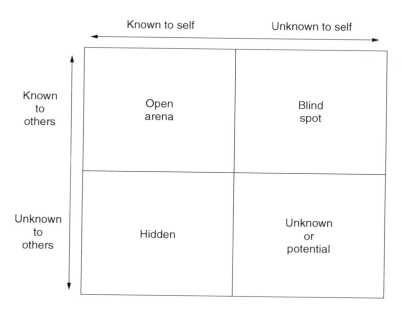

Figure 1.6 The Johari window

contact seems to be lacking. Colleagues may say nothing, in order to avoid embarrassing me by implying that I am being insincere. The problem is, how can I get this information out in the open, since it may be affecting the level of trust that is developing between me and my colleagues? How can I learn more about myself? I may notice a slight discomfort showing in the person I am talking to, and perhaps this may lead to a question. It is difficult for me to identify the problem unless someone else makes me aware of it.

The *hidden quadrant* represents things that I know about myself that others do not know. So for example, if I have not told my colleagues that I enjoy golf, then this information is in my hidden quadrant. As soon as I share my love of the sport, I am effectively pulling the window shade down, moving the information in my hidden quadrant and enlarging the open quadrant's area. Again, there are perhaps vast amounts of information, virtually my whole life's story, that have yet to be revealed to my colleagues. As we get to know and trust each other, I will then feel more comfortable disclosing more intimate details about myself. This process is called: 'self-disclosure'.

The *unknown potential quadrant* represents things that neither I know about myself, nor others know about me. This may include experiences that affect my behaviour and that lie deep in my unconscious and which I may never come to know. Or, I may have the potential to achieve excellence in playing a musical instrument, but because I have never been offered, or have availed myself, of the opportunity, I, with others, remain unaware of this. Sometimes, a novel situation can trigger new awareness and personal growth. I may find myself having to cope with a new, unexpected challenge which I discover I enjoy and can meet with relative ease. The process of moving previously unknown information into the open quadrant, thus enlarging its area, can often be likened to achieving self fulfilment.

Feedback

Giving and receiving feedback requires a high level of skill and confidence which takes time to develop. The Johari window demonstrates that seeking feedback and disclosing information about ourselves in order to elicit feedback from others has the effect of enlarging the open quadrant. Typically, as I share something about myself

(moving information from my hidden quadrant into the open), and if the other party is interested in getting to know me, they will reciprocate, by similarly disclosing information in their hidden quadrant. Thus, an interaction between two parties can be modelled dynamically as two active Johari windows. It helps to choose someone you feel you can trust and whose response will give you some insight into yourself.

As your level of confidence develops, you may actively invite others to comment on your blind spots. You may already seek feedback from students on the quality of a particular lecture, with the desire of improving the presentation. The next stage is to invite comment on your ability to deal with more complex aspects of your role. Self-disclosure – giving the other person something about yourself which helps to build mutual confidence and trust – is an excellent way to start.

Action

Think back over the last fortnight.

- When starting on-call periods, have you always felt adequately briefed about the inpatients under your care?

- When coming on duty in the morning, when and how have you learnt about new patients admitted over the on-call period?

- When going off duty in the evening, have you and your colleagues always fully briefed the on-call team about your patients?

Related reading

- Berens LV (2000) *Understanding Yourself and Others – an introduction to temperament.* Telos, California.
- Buzan T and Buzan B (1996) *The Mind Map Book: how to use radiant thinking to maximize your brain's untapped potential.* Penguin, New York.
- Department of Health (2004) *Modernising Medical Careers – the next steps.* Crown Publications.

- Houghton A (2004) Understanding personality type: how do you like to live your life? Judging and perceiving. *BMJ Career Focus* 329:230–1.
- Hudson L (1967) *Contrary Imaginations*. Penguin Books, Harmondsworth.
- Kolb DA, Osland JS and Rubin IM (1995) *Organizational Behaviour – an experiential approach* (6e). Prentice-Hall, Englewood Cliffs, New Jersey.
- Maitland I (1999) *Managing Your Time*. Chartered Institute of Personnel and Development, London.
- Mascie-Taylor HM, Pedler MJ and Winkless AJ (1993) *Doctors and Dilemmas: a study of 'ideal types' of doctor/managers and an evaluation of how these could support values of clarification for doctors in the health service*. NHSTD, Bristol.

CHAPTER 2

Managing the 'day-to-day'

> The aim of this chapter is to develop your awareness of a range of aspects of dealing with people at work. It provides underpinning knowledge for developing your skills in areas such as leadership and team working. You cannot learn to lead and influence others just by reading a book – but it can help if you have some background information. Much of this section is useful pre-reading for related training workshops.

Leading teams

Doctors usually work as part of a team, and this helps emphasise the importance of leadership. As your professional status and clinical responsibility grow so does your need to lead and direct others. Leadership is about building relationships, setting goals and achieving results through others. Theories and models of leadership are many and varied. There is no simple or correct approach, but many variables which might influence the approach a leader should take to a particular situation. It helps, however, to have insight into some of the established thinking regarding leadership.

Broadly, the development of leadership thinking over the past two centuries has moved through the following stages (Crainer, 1996):

- *great man theories* were based on the belief that leaders are exceptional people who are born with a propensity and capability to lead in any circumstances – this belief has been pretty well demolished by experience and research, although there are still some who may believe in the idea

- *trait theories* are associated with the assumption that successful leaders exhibit a range of qualities or traits that enable them to do the right thing at the right time. It has proven virtually impossible to isolate a consistent set

of traits, despite extensive research into the characteristics of well-known successful leaders such as Ghandi, Churchill, Mandela and Thatcher. One or two do seem to be evident – they are all good communicators, have a vision which followers find attractive and are generally of above-average intelligence (although not super-intelligent). Beyond this there are many inconsistencies which are difficult to resolve

- *power and influence approaches* assume the centralisation of decision making, the exercise of power resulting from this centralisation and passivity in subordinates

- *behaviourist theories* focus on what leaders actually do rather than their innate qualities. Sets of behaviours are categorised and described as different styles

- *situational leadership* sees the leadership process as being determined by the context in which it is carried out. For example, leadership in the field of battle or operating theatre may be different from that in a general practice or high street shop. *Contingency theory* also assumes that the situational variables are the basis for determining best leadership practice

- *transactional theory* emphasises the importance of the relationship between the leader and followers. It is based on a concept of mutual benefit deriving from a form of contract through which the leader delivers rewards and recognition, and the followers provide effort, commitment and loyalty

- *attribution theory* emphasises the power of the followers and their perceptions, who assume their role as followers and thus attribute the leadership role to a particular person

- *transformational theory* is grounded in the concept that leadership is all about change, and the leader achieves change through creating a vision and sharing this with the followers – this requires a complex set of qualities, skills and capabilities that enable the leader to achieve alignment between team members and the goals of the organisation.

Many of these approaches are merged into contemporary models. Some of the more relevant examples are explored in greater detail below.

Do you (have to) possess the right personality traits?

A traditional view of leadership held that a few people were born with special powers and aptitudes which made them natural leaders. These included enthusiasm, self-assurance, initiative, intelligence and so on. Studies of effective leaders have raised doubts about this view, research having failed to identify a consensus on such traits, particularly because there are many notably successful leaders who are deficient in a significant proportion of the defined traits. A few characteristics do seem to be fairly consistent, however. These include a clear vision which followers understand and are attracted to; the ability to communicate effectively, and being of above-average intelligence. While recognising the importance of personal qualities, more attention is now directed to the behaviour and competence of leaders rather than their inherent personal characteristics. Leadership is a complex process which involves a range of skills and qualities which, given aptitude, may be acquired or developed through learning and practice.

Is leadership a matter of style?

Styles of leadership are usually defined as ranging between 'authoritarian' and 'democratic'. The difference between one style and another can sometimes reflect the power relationship between the leader and the led. Authoritarian leaders have power and hold on to it, using it to direct and control the work behaviour of their subordinates. They retain the right to make decisions, to reward and punish. More democratic styles lead to delegation of decision making, or at least to sharing authority and control.

Some writers argue that people are more productive when working in a democratic environment. They reason that supportive styles of leadership help to create job satisfaction, reduce grievance rates and result in less inter-group conflict. Some doubt, however, that such participative styles of leadership are always effective in enhancing group performance. Sometimes circumstances demand a directive style, for example in life or death situations. There may also be circumstances when team members are unfamiliar with the task, or with working together in a team. Here, it may be necessary for a more directive style until the team has matured sufficiently to be able to manage without needing direction from a team leader. Style alone is generally insufficient as a determining factor in success, although it is important.

The following questionnaire helps you to identify your own style. When completing it, try to place your self in a situation in which you might have to lead, even if this is not your normal role.

Task/process leadership questionnaire

Source: Pfeiffer and Jones (1974) – used with permission (*see* Related reading, p. 43).

The objective of the questionnaire is to identify your leadership style through your relative concern for tasks or people, and locate it in terms of three types of leadership: individual, group or shared.

Directions

The following items describe some aspects of leadership behaviour. Respond to each item according to the way you would be most likely act if you were the leader of a team or group. You could think of yourself in a group at work, or in a social, hobby or sports group with a job or task to carry out.

Circle whether you would most likely behave in the described way:

always (**A**), frequently (**F**), occasionally (**O**), seldom (**S**), or never (**N**).

1	I would most likely act as the spokesperson for a group.	A	F	O	S	N
2	I would encourage people to stay late to finish a task.	A	F	O	S	N
3	I would allow team members complete freedom in the way they worked.	A	F	O	S	N
4	I would encourage team members to use standard procedures.	A	F	O	S	N
5	I would allow people to use their judgement in solving problems.	A	F	O	S	N
6	I would stress trying to be ahead of competing groups.	A	F	O	S	N
7	I would speak as representative of the group.	A	F	O	S	N
8	I would nag members for greater effort.	A	F	O	S	N
9	I would try out new ideas.	A	F	O	S	N
10	I would let people do their work the way they think best.	A	F	O	S	N
11	I would work hard to get praise.	A	F	O	S	N
12	I would tolerate delay and uncertainty.	A	F	O	S	N
13	1 would speak for the group if there were outsiders present.	A	F	O	S	N
14	I would keep the work moving at a rapid pace.	A	F	O	S	N
15	I would let people loose on a job and allow them to get on with it.	A	F	O	S	N
16	I would settle any conflicts if they occurred.	A	F	O	S	N
17	I would get swamped with details.	A	F	O	S	N
18	I would represent the group at outside meetings.	A	F	O	S	N
19	I would be reluctant to allow the group any freedom of action.	A	F	O	S	N
20	I would decide what should be done and how it should be done.	A	F	O	S	N
21	I would push for maximum effort.	A	F	O	S	N
22	I would let some people have control which I could have kept.	A	F	O	S	N
23	Things usually turn out as I predict.	A	F	O	S	N
24	I would allow people a high degree of initiative.	A	F	O	S	N
25	I would assign people to particular tasks.	A	F	O	S	N
26	I would be happy to make changes.	A	F	O	S	N
27	I would ask people to work harder.	A	F	O	S	N
28	I would trust the group members to exercise their judgement.	A	F	O	S	N
29	I would arrange how the work was to be done.	A	F	O	S	N

30	I would not explain my reasons.	A	F	O	S	N
31	I would persuade team members of the advantages of my ideas.	A	F	O	S	N
32	I would allow the group to set their own pace.	A	F	O	S	N
33	I would urge my group to better their previous efforts.	A	F	O	S	N
34	I would not consult the group.	A	F	O	S	N
35	I would ask that people used only approved methods.	A	F	O	S	N

P = _____   **T** = _____

Scoring the questionnaire is reasonably straight-forward as long as you the instructions below step by step.

Scoring is as follows:

1. Circle the item number for items 8, 12, 17, 18, 19, 30, 34 and 35.

2. Write the number 1 in front of a *circled item number* if you responded **S** (seldom) or **N** (never) to that item.

3. Also write a number 1 in front of *item numbers not circled* if you responded **A** (always) or **F** (frequently).

4. Circle the number 1s which you have written in front of the following items: 3, 5, 8, 10, 15, 18, 19, 22, 24, 26, 28, 30, 32, 34 and 35.

5. *Count* the *circled number* 1s. This is your score for concern for people. Record the score in the blank following the letter **P** at the end of the questionnaire.

6. *Count the uncircled number* 1s. This is your score for concern for tasks. Record this number in the blank following the letter T.

Now follow the instructions below to plot your **T – P** leadership style profile.

To determine your style of leadership, mark your score on the concern for task dimension (**T**) on the left-hand arrow in Figure 2.1.

Next, move to the right-hand arrow and mark your score on the concern for people dimension (**P**).

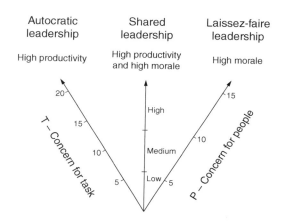

Figure 2.1 Shared leadership results from balancing concern for task and concern for people

Draw a straight line that intersects the **P** and **T** scores. The point at which the line crosses the shared leadership arrow indicates your position on that dimension.

A high score on the **T** dimension and a low **P** score indicates a strong tendency to focus on getting the job done, perhaps at the expense of maintaining good working relations with the team. High **P** and low **T** probably means that team members are at ease with your style, although they might prefer to get more direction at times, even at the expense of having an easy time. The higher your score on the middle (shared) dimension, the more you are likely to be able to adjust your style to suit situations where either a 'telling' style is more appropriate, or to one in which you involve the team in the decision making.

Leadership style is partly about taking into account the situation!

So 'effective' leaders get the task done while maintaining good working relationships with their colleagues and within the team. Appropriate leadership style is about finding a balance between task-oriented and relationship-oriented leadership behaviour:

- *task-oriented behaviour* focuses on directing the actions of others, defining roles, setting goals and giving clear direction

- *relationship-oriented behaviour* concerns the extent to which the leader engages in listening, encouraging and supporting group members, both as individuals and as members of a team.

It is these two dimensions which produce the five leadership styles set out in Figure 2.2.

Choice of leadership style is dependent not only on the situation, but also on the maturity of the group. So to review those styles again we can now say:

- *a telling style* is suited to an immature group which needs high levels of guidance and

structure to get the task done, and is less in need of relationship building. It can also be the only way to lead in a crisis when the outcome might be life-threatening. For example, when leading a team dealing with a cardiac arrest there is little time or opportunity to debate alternative courses of action. This should not mean, however, that the leader in such a situation should not be willing to check from time to time with colleagues in their team and listen carefully to ensure he or she is not missing anything critical

- *a selling style* emphasises both relationship and task behaviours and is suited to groups which are growing in maturity and are in need of support through a team-building process, but need to be regularly reminded of task direction. An example is if you decide you would like to arrange a mess dinner or medical school year reunion, and set out to persuade colleagues of the attractiveness of your idea

- *a consulting style* allows the leader to maintain a degree of control while permitting team members to influence practice and procedures. By listening to suggestions from team members, the leader can often arrive at better decisions

- *a participating style* emphasises two-way communication and support but allows freedom to

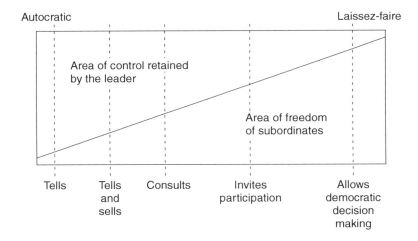

Autocratic   Laissez-faire

Area of control retained by the leader

Area of freedom of subordinates

Tells   Tells   Consults   Invites   Allows
and   participation   democratic
sells   decision
                              making

Figure 2.2 A continuum of leadership styles

the team to make decisions which influence outcomes. This can create a sense of achievement and commitment to the task, but it generally depends on team members being well trained and having a good understanding of team objectives. A decision to undertake a group or departmental audit project, for example, would require co-operation from all group members. Involving everyone in the decision would be most likely to achieve this

- *delegating* can be used only with a mature, well-trained team which is capable of managing its own task and relationships. The leader's role is more 'hands off', but still has accountability for results. This might include enlisting the help of senior house officers (SHOs), nurses or colleagues to manage an influx of work for which you are responsible.

Transformational leadership

We all have a preferred style to which we tend to revert when under pressure, but how can our leadership qualities and skills be developed? Assuming that the views outlined above are valid, then it is *how you deal with people*, rather than *what you are*, that makes the difference. Current thinking on leadership emphasises the role of the leader as one who influences, generates change and develops confidence in followers to take on responsibility for their own work outcomes.

This approach has come to be known as transformational leadership. Such leaders appeal to higher motives in their followers, and focus on positive values when discussing team objectives. They work from a vision of the future, rather than dependence on past history. Transformational leaders commit people to action, convert followers into leaders, and convert leaders into agents of change. It might be helpful here to consider 'heroic' leadership. We tend to have developed our ideas of leadership from our own early life experience. This is likely to include reading novels and watching films or television programmes in which heroic figures lead from the front and always seem to be able to find the right solution to their followers' problems. Transformational leadership does not sit comfortably with leadership as

a 'heroic' process. Heroic leaders assume they should be at the heart of any important activity in which the team is involved. Heroic leaders are relied on by team members to know all the right answers, be aware of all that is going on in their area of responsibility, and be capable of solving problems single-handed. They act as central decision makers and are regarded as being the only people who have the 'big picture'. These assumptions are seldom capable of being fulfilled in the complex world of modern organisations although this does not stop some leaders from trying. Effective *post-heroic* leaders, including transformational leaders, share responsibility, and challenge attempts to depend on them for all difficult decisions. They enable team members to achieve their own successes through coaching, support and personal development.

The psychodynamic approach to leadership developed during the 1960s and brought a humanistic perspective back into the work environment. This approach proposed that leadership style is influenced by family background and psychological make-up. It emphasised that effective leaders and followers are self-reflective and understand their personal preferences and those of the people around them. This recognises that effective leaders and followers have qualities and needs in common. The psychodynamic approach continues to have a wide-reaching influence on contemporary leadership theory and has contributed some of the field's most powerful tools, including the Myers Briggs Type Indicator.

Change is normal in most contemporary organisations. The NHS is no exception. Change can sometimes feel as if it is imposed before there has been time to embed the last initiative. Medical professionals are generally cautious about change unless there is well-established evidence to support it. While this may be a sensible approach for treatments and procedures, it seldom applies to organisational change, which may be driven by economic necessity or by social or political circumstances. There are generally held to be three steps in leading organisational change. The first is recognition of the need for change. Effective leaders transmit this awareness to colleagues and followers, and thus seek to create willingness for change. The second stage is the communication of a new vision which encompasses the long- and short-term needs of the organisation. A critical aspect of leadership is the ability to communicate effectively the benefits of the change to those most affected by it. Avoiding quick-fix solutions is critical to success, and this usually means a period of consultation with colleagues who may be able to refine the process. Finally, the leader institutionalises the change by establishing new cultures and procedures, and restructuring communication arrangements.

The NHS Leadership Qualities Framework was developed from research into effective NHS leaders. It proposes fifteen separate qualities in three clusters that are exhibited by successful leaders. These are:

Personal qualities

- Self-belief
- Self-awareness
- Self-management
- Drive for improvement
- Personal integrity

Setting direction

- Seizing the future
- Intellectual flexibility
- Broad scanning
- Political astuteness
- Drive for results

Delivering the service

- Leading change through people
- Holding to account
- Empowering others
- Effective and strategic influencing
- Collaborative working

This model provides the basis for developing leaders by its use as a 360° feedback tool. You can find more information on each quality and its definitions at the Leadership Qualities Framework website: www.nhsleadershipqualities. nhs.uk.

Getting results through others

Understanding what motivates people to achieve good results

Performance of anyone at work is generally dependent on three variables: their *ability*, which is a combination of aptitude and development; equipment and facilities must be available, so they have the *opportunity*; and they must be *motivated*. In effect, performance is the product of ability and motivation.

Good leaders understand what motivates people and act to get the best from them. They must also harness those energies towards the successful achievement of goals. Motivation (in this context) is concerned with why people choose a particular course of action, and persist in that action in preference to others. The underlying concept of motivation is the existence of *needs* which give rise to *drive* and *action* in order to achieve desired *goals* – thus meeting these needs and creating *satisfaction*.

Human needs were said by Maslow in 1943 to be arranged in a hierarchy, with basic needs dominating higher order needs until the former are reduced. His model is often presented as in Figure 2.3.

Physiological needs include food, water and warmth – the basic requirements of survival. Safety and security needs are met through freedom from threat of physical attack, protection from deprivation, and by predictability and orderliness. Social needs are met by a sense of belonging, friendships and the giving and receiving of love. *Esteem* is focused on the self, and involves the desire for confidence, status, and the respect of others. Self-fulfilment (described by Maslow as self-actualisation) is the realisation of one's full potential. This may vary widely from one individual to another. Some authors have suggested that a sixth need, which follows self-fulfilment, is self-awareness.

Maslow argues that these needs are hierarchical, and that a need which is satisfied is no longer a motivator. Hence, as lower level needs are met, so the driving force of behaviour becomes the higher need. Needs do not have to be fully met. There is a gradual emergence of a higher level need as lower level needs become more satisfied. He also makes it clear that the hierarchy

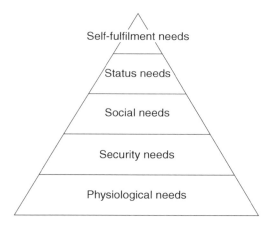

Figure 2.3 Maslow's hierarchy of needs

applies to most, not all, people. It is not necessarily a fixed order. Exceptions will be evident. Some people, driven by a creative and self-actualising urge, will ignore more basic needs. Others, with high ideals or values, may become martyrs and give up everything for the sake of their beliefs. It follows that, in order to provide motivation for changes in behaviour, a leader must direct attention to the next higher level of need.

Maslow's theory is difficult to test empirically. Those attempts which have been made give only tentative support. The theory has been influential, nonetheless, perhaps because of its simplicity and universality.

The work of McClelland in 1976 led to a further content theory of motivation. He and his colleagues identified three main arousal-based, socially developed motive forces. These were: affiliation, power and achievement. These correspond broadly to Maslow's highest-order needs for love and society, esteem, and self-actualisation. Their relative impact on behaviour varies with each individual. It was also possible to identify differences according to occupation. Follow-up research focused on *individuals* with a high need for *achievement*, in whom McClelland identified three common characteristics. You may recognise them in some of your colleagues:

- a preference for personal responsibility
- the setting of achievable goals

- the desire for concrete feedback on performance.

They like to be personally responsible for solving problems and getting results. They also like to attain success through their own efforts, rather than as a member of a team. The recognition of others is not as important as their own sense of accomplishment. A second characteristic is the tendency to set moderate achievement goals and to take calculated risks. If the task is too difficult or too risky, the chances of success would be reduced. If the task is too easy or too safe there would be little sense of achievement from success. Thirdly, feedback on performance should be prompt, clear and unambiguous. It helps to confirm success, and give the sense of satisfaction which comes with achievement.

A second 'family' of motivational theories emphasises the study of process, rather than content. These seek to provide a better understanding of the relationship between variables that influence work behaviour. Process models are generally more able to accommodate individual differences. Among the best known is 'expectancy theory'. It emphasises an individual's perception of the probability that particular outcomes will result from specific courses of action. The model which is best known is based on three variables: *valence, instrumentality* and *expectancy*.

- *Valence* is defined as the attractiveness of, or preference for, a particular outcome to an individual. If a person has a preference for a particular outcome, valence is positive. Where avoidance of a particular outcome is preferred, valence is negative. If the person is indifferent to the outcome, valence is zero. Valence is the *expected satisfaction*, and is distinguished from the value attached to the actual outcome, once achieved.

- *Instrumentality* is best understood if we distinguish between first-level outcomes and second level outcomes. First level outcomes refer to actual performance in the work. For some, this will be an end to be valued for its own sake, as 'a job well done'. For others, the valence of the performance outcomes is determined by the second-level outcomes, which may, for example, be derived from the financial gains resulting from satisfactory completion of the task. Second-level outcomes are need related. Instrumentality is the extent to which first-level outcomes lead to second-level outcomes.

- *Expectancy* is a perception of the probability that the choice of a particular action will lead to the desired outcome. It relates effort expended to the achievement of first-level outcomes. This model, as with others derived from it, is useful in explaining the process by which people weigh and evaluate the attractiveness of different alternatives before committing themselves to specific courses of action. The models do not, however, reflect the actual decision-making steps taken by an individual.

Studies of goal-oriented behaviour provide a further insight into motivation. Goal setting may be viewed as a motivational technique rather than a theory. A number of organisational systems (such as performance appraisal) emphasise the importance of agreeing work goals with employees, whose behaviour is thought to be determined by their goals. People's values give rise to emotions and desires which they strive to satisfy through their responses and actions. Goals direct work behaviour and performance, and lead to certain consequences or feedback. People with specific, measurable goals will perform better than those without. Also, those with difficult, though achievable, goals will perform better than those whose goals may be easily achieved.

In general, theories and models of motivation are unable to provide universal solutions to the challenge of motivating people at work. They do,

however, help us to understand the complexity of the process, and take us away from leadership approaches linked to fear and punishment, once common among traditional managers earlier in the 20th century.

Developing team spirit

There are many kinds of team, some permanent, such as committees, some temporary, such as task forces and working groups. A good example of teamwork is the surgical team, which includes the surgeon and anaesthetist with juniors, nurses, operating department practitioners (ODPs) and others. Each is specialised and knows that each individual's success is dependent on the work of other team members. Bringing together the right number of people to work together does not necessarily make an effective team, this takes time.

Team building and developing team spirit

Initially, there may be confusion over members' roles and leadership. Although there may be a nominal leader, others play leadership roles at times. Gradually members identify their roles but sometimes as individuals working together rather than as a team. Conflicts and interactions occur as personal ideas and agendas are sorted. Gradually the group comes to see itself no longer as a collection of individuals but as a group which has its own identity. There may even be experimentation with new roles. The group usually dies when the task has been completed. Here there may be feelings of sadness or even grief. If the task changes, then some members leave and others join. So the cycle continues, and it is important to be aware of the dynamics of group behaviour.

There are said to be four stages in the development of a team. Obviously, it is seldom this simple if individuals leave and others join. This also disrupts the process of team building. Some teams may never develop into a mature team, for a variety of reasons which may be to do with the mix of personalities within the team, or the transient nature of the work. There is no particular timing to the stages – although they may be accelerated if attention is paid to helping the team through the stages of growth. The four stages are:

- *forming*: this is the early, testing stage, with members being polite, watchful and guarded. Members try to learn about each other and may begin to project their personality through giving formal information about themselves

- *storming*: there may be some confusion in the team, particularly about roles, with controlled conflict and confrontation, some opting out and difficulties experienced in agreeing tasks and goals

- *norming*: the team starts to get organised and develop its skills, establish roles and procedures, giving feedback and confronting issues which are perceived to affect performance

- *performing*: eventually the team may mature to be resourceful, flexible, effective and supportive.

Some writers have added a fifth stage which is sometimes called *adjourning* – that is to say that the team reaches a natural stage in its life when the demands made on it change to such an extent that it no longer needs to function as a team, and so ends its life. Others describe this as the *mourning* stage – the implication here is that the team members become attached to the team to such an extent that personal grief affects team members at the natural end of the team's life.

The characteristics of a fully mature team are listed below:

- team goals are clear and agreed

- information flows freely between members

- relationships between members are supportive, trusting and respectful

- conflict is regarded as natural and helpful, but it is on issues, not persons

- the atmosphere is participative, open, non-threatening and non-competitive

- decisions are by consensus, although the team concedes to individual members the authority to make decisions when it would be most helpful to do so.

Remember it does not follow that, because a group of people works together for sufficient time, it will inevitably develop into a mature team. Nor is there is a single approach to team building which is likely to work for all teams. One view is that the right mixture of personalities to make an effective team needs to be brought together in the first place. This, of course, is not usually possible, since hospital teams are usually decided by the availability of staff at the time the team is formed.

Team maturity has implications for leaders. A recently formed team will require a higher level of direction in order to function. The leader's energies will be mostly taken up with making sure that individuals are clear about their roles, functions and goals. As the team develops and begins to be more focused on goal achievement, issues that arise around relationships will become evident and the team leader will find themselves more engaged in supporting individuals and helping members to develop mutual understanding.

This relates to the storming stage, when the role of the leader is critical to ensuring the team continues to develop. Once the team members are sufficiently clear about team roles and their individual functions, the leader will normally focus on building strong relationships within the team. Once this is established, the mature team can be given increased responsibility for determining its own approaches and dealing with its conflicts (which are inevitable and normally healthy) in an effective manner without too much intervention from the leader.

Research into teams by Meredith Belbin (2003; *see* Related reading, p. 43) indicates that there are a number of separate team roles which, if working together, have a positive impact on team performance. These are often cited in team development programmes. Belbin suggests the following roles are needed:

- *plant*: concerned with putting forward ideas and strategies for achieving the objectives adopted by the group. Performance of this role requires creativity, imagination and innovation

- *resource investigator*: explores the environment outside the group, by identifying ideas, information and resources. Performance of this role involves developing contacts and co-ordination and negotiation with other groups and individuals

- *co-ordinator*: organises, co-ordinates and controls the activities of the group. This involves the clarification of group objectives and problems, assigning tasks and responsibilities, and encouraging group members to get involved in achieving objectives and goals

- *shaper*: challenges, argues and disagrees. Usually an achievement-motivated extrovert who has a low frustration threshold. He/she is a non-chairman leader

- *monitor evaluator*: involved in analysing ideas and proposals being considered by the team to evaluate their feasibility and value for achieving the group's objectives. It is important for the monitor evaluator to point out in a constructive manner the weaknesses of proposals being considered

- *team worker*: creates and maintains team spirit. This involves improving communication by providing personal support and warmth to group members, and by overcoming tension and conflict

- *implementer*: is concerned with the practical translation and application of concepts and plans developed by the group. This entails a down-to-earth outlook, coupled with perseverance in the face of difficulties

- *completer finisher*: ensures that the group's efforts achieve appropriate standards, and that mistakes of both commission and omission are avoided. It also involves searching for detailed mistakes and maintaining a sense of urgency within the group

- *specialist*: is a key provider of the skills on which the team's particular output or service is based. They command the support of the team because of their knowledge, plus their dedication and pride in professional standards related to their particular skills and depth of experience.

More than one of these roles may be performed by a single person, and it can assist team development if individuals can become aware of their preferred roles and work on these for the benefit of the team. Perhaps the most helpful thing to remember is that teams do not naturally fall into maturity – they need help, either from informed insiders or from someone who understands the mechanics of team building and can facilitate the process. If you feel the need for more practical advice you therefore need to read all the other parts of this section which are all relevant to successful team building.

Dealing with opposition – acting assertively

Assertion is not the same as aggression. Assertiveness has been defined as a quality demonstrated by individuals who know what they feel and what they want, take definite and clear action to express their views, refuse to be side-tracked, and ensure others know where they stand. They do not try to serve their own interests at the expense of others. They are prepared to accommodate the interests of the other person while not conceding more than they believe reasonable. Being assertive should usually result in both parties being satisfied with the outcome of the interaction.

- An *aggressive* person seeks dominance, and aggressiveness involves attempts to intimidate others and violate their rights.

- An *assertive* person exercises a right to express a viewpoint and have it fully heard, while respecting the rights of others.

A characteristic of clinical work is the fragmentation and fluctuation in work rate. An essential skill needed by doctors in the protection of their work routines is the ability to prevent others from unnecessary, disruptive interference. This is a common cause of frustration, and impairs performance, particularly for those who hold supervisory responsibilities, no matter how small. Working in teams means you need to be able to manage your work with others. Maintaining good working relationships while avoiding exploitation of goodwill can be difficult. Achieving and maintaining a satisfactory level of independence while still contributing fully to co-operative tasks requires a high level of social and group-working skills. Among these is the ability to act assertively when required – to decline taking on further demands when already fully loaded.

There are many reasons why you may find it hard to say 'No' even to unreasonable demands which are made of you. The more obvious

Managing the 'day-to-day' **31**

reasons are around the difficulty of deciding what tasks should, or should not, be a part of your role. Equally, you may be unable to define what is a reasonable work load. Job descriptions can help, but they are seldom sufficiently detailed to remove all uncertainty and, in any case, constant changes in detail mean they are seldom kept up to date.

It is difficult to deal with colleagues so that good relationships are always maintained, without constantly succumbing to their demands. Unhealthy conflict can arise if we appear to be negative in our responses. It is suggested that, in addition to 'fight or flight' responses to conflict, we have been conditioned to respond passively, by parents who taught us to 'turn the other cheek'. Harris in 1970 describes the impact of early life experiences on our later behaviours. In developing the concept of *transactional analysis*, he outlines the nature of 'life scripts'. These are responses which we learn early in life and which help to shape our view of ourselves, and hence our behaviour when responding to others. Harris suggests that our behaviour is shaped by our use of life data which are derived from early experience of key relationships. Hence, interactions with others are shaped by our tendency to respond from the 'parent', 'adult' or 'child' within us. Since the interaction is two-sided, the response we give is frequently drawn out by the type of initial message we receive. Parental instructions, which are likely to be judgmental and directive, tend to bring out the child in us, and vice versa. Overriding the tendency to behave in this predetermined manner is difficult. It requires the learning of new ways of reacting to requests and demands on our time.

The first and most basic requirement we have in developing the ability to act assertively is to recognise the 'assertive rights' of human beings. Here are a few of these:

- to judge your own behaviour, thoughts, and emotions, and to take responsibility for their initiation and consequences upon yourself

- to offer no reasons or excuses to justify your behaviour

- to make mistakes – and be responsible for them

- be treated with respect as an intelligent, capable and equal human being

- to express your feelings.

Assertive behaviour is not aggressive, nor is it passive. It does not infringe the assertive rights of others. It allows each party to depart with their own self-respect intact. Ideally, it should leave each party feeling 'OK'. It is usually concerned with helping individuals to acquire what is rightfully theirs, to say 'No' to what they do not want, or to enable them to handle criticism.

Most people recognise their own need to behave assertively when they reflect on their inability to refuse requests for assistance from colleagues, friends or family members which they realise place unreasonable demands on their time or other resources. The early life conditioning referred to above is the most common reason for this weakness. Having convinced ourselves that we have a right to say 'No', the next task is to learn how to say it assertively.

There are two sides to saying 'No'. The first is to recognise how simple it is to find the word. It helps to practise saying it without apologising excessively or making complicated excuses. The dominant reason for experiencing difficulty in refusing an invitation or request is the feeling of guilt that results. The rights referred to above will, if remembered, help to assuage the guilt. So, also, will the continued use of the skill, so that it feels normal. A refusal to a request is not a rejection of the person making the request. Once this fact has been learned, the process will become much easier to use. The other side is to develop the skill of saying it using a tone which is at once friendly but firm. The way in which we look and express ourselves has a greater impact on the communication than the words we use.

Sometimes, the person with whom we are dealing is persistent in their demands. This increases the challenge, but need not create a problem. The key to success is calm repetition. This is sometimes referred to as the 'broken record'. It enables you to feel comfortable in avoiding manipulative verbal side-traps, argumentative baiting and irrelevant logic. Simply keep repeating your requirement or refusal in a calm and assertive manner until the other person accepts it.

Handling manipulative criticism can cause difficulty. Assertive responses encompass a range of options. The first is to calmly acknowledge to the critic that there may be some truth in the criticism, yet leave yourself with the right to determine what you will do about it. A stage beyond this is to strongly agree with hostile or constructive criticism as it is given, accepting your faults without resorting to denial. This has the effect of reducing your critic's anger or hostility without making you feel anxious or defensive. There is still no need to apologise if you do not wish to do so.

If it does not weaken your position, or threaten your self-respect, it is acceptable to seek a workable compromise with the other person. This involves recognising that a 'win–win' situation can be achieved by agreeing to concede something of your own position, while retaining your right to protect your own needs.

The objective of assertive behaviour is not to win all your conflicts at the expense of someone else. It is, rather, to maintain your own position and protect your own rights as a person, while dealing effectively with the demands of others around you. It should always be your aim to respect the equivalent rights of others. It is this which differentiates assertive from aggressive behaviour.

Skills of assertion can be identified and learned, increasing the ability to make a positive impact on others; a key factor for those in leadership roles.

So let us consider some guidelines for exercising assertion in the face of the opposition!

- Build your argument step by step thus ensuring people have the opportunity to understand your position.

- Say what you need from others, because people need to know how they fit into larger plans.

- Communicate in language that others understand; this ensures that you convey messages in ways which make sense to the listeners.

- Avoid confused emotions; if you are angry, hurt, or emotionally upset, then others are more likely to respond to your feelings rather than your message. This can confuse the issues.

- Make it simple; people often lose the strength of their argument by excessive complexity or by dealing with several issues at once.

- Work towards resolving questions and concerns of others, which may involve continuing to put your message across until you are satisfied that a resolution can be achieved.

- Do not put yourself down; if something is important to you let others know where you stand.

- Watch out for 'flak'; others may try to divert you from your message. You may feel under pressure. Acknowledge their views, but always return to your position.

- Error does not weaken; we all make mistakes, and error should not make you feel inadequate. A sense of inadequacy will undermine your position.

People who face conflict assertively are said to:

- be open about their objectives

- establish what the other person's objectives are

- search for common ground

- state their case clearly

- understand the other person's case

- produce ideas to solve the differences

- build on and add to the other person's ideas

- summarise to check understanding and agreement.

Action

Reflect on your own situation in putting forward sensitive issues to others or being asked to undertake extra jobs. For example: changes in rotas, changes in routine work, dealing with extra cases, patients added to outpatient lists, having to cover for others at short notice etc.

How do you rate according to the above guidelines?

Resolving conflict in work groups

Our research confirmed the importance doctors attach to the effective working of the teams to which they belong. An occasional consequence of the pressure to which medical practitioners are subjected is the generation of tension and conflict in the team. This section helps to identify your approach to the handling of conflict.

Conflict handling style

What is your preferred style when faced with conflict?

Conflict style inventory

Derived from Pfeiffer and Goodstein (1982; *see* Related reading, p. 44)

Instructions

Choose a single frame of reference for answering all 15 items (e.g. work-related conflicts, family conflicts or social conflicts) and keep that frame of reference in mind when answering all items.

Allocate 10 points among the four alternative answers given for each of the 15 items below. For example: '**When the people I organise become involved in a personal conflict, I would usually … **'

intervene to settle the dispute.	call a meeting to talk over the problem.	offer to help if I can.	ignore the problem.
3	6	1	0

Be sure that your answers add up to 10.

1 When someone I care about is actively hostile toward me, i.e. threatening, shouting, abusive, etc, I tend to …

respond in a hostile manner.	try to persuade the person to give up his/her actively hostile behaviour.	stay and listen as long as possible.	walk away.

2 When someone who is relatively unimportant to me is actively hostile toward me, i.e. shouting, threatening, abusive, etc I tend to …

respond in a hostile manner.	try to persuade the person to give up his/her actively hostile behaviour.	stay and listen as long as possible.	walk away.

3 When I observe people in conflicts in which anger, threats, hostility and strong opinions are present, I tend to …

become involved and take a position.	attempt to mediate.	observe to see what happens.	leave as quickly as possible.

4 When I perceive another person as meeting his/her needs at my expense, I am apt to …

work to do anything I can to change that person.	rely on persuasion and 'facts' when attempting to have that person change.	work hard at changing how I relate to that person.	accept the situation as it is.

5 When involved in an interpersonal dispute, my general pattern is to …

draw the other person into seeing the problem as I do.	examine the issues between us as logically as possible.	look hard for a workable compromise.	let time take its course and let the problem work itself out.

6 The quality that I value the most in dealing with conflict would be …

emotional strength and security.	intelligence.	love and openness.	patience.

7 Following a serious altercation with someone I care for deeply, I …

strongly desire to go back and settle things my way.	want to go back and work it out – whatever give and take is necessary.	worry about it a lot but not plan to initiate.	let it lie and not plan to initiate further contact.

8 When I see a serious conflict developing between two people I care about, I tend to …

express my disappointment that this had to happen.	attempt to persuade them to resolve their differences.	watch to see what develops.	leave the scene.

9 When I see a serious conflict developing between two people who are relatively unimportant to me, I tend to …

express my disappointment that this had to happen.	attempt to persuade them to resolve their differences.	watch to see what develops.	leave the scene.

10 The feedback that I receive from most people about how I behave when faced with conflict and opposition indicates that I …

try hard to get my own way.	try to work out differences co-operatively.	am easygoing and take a soft or conciliatory position.	usually avoid the conflict.

11 When communicating with someone with whom I am having a serious conflict, I …

try to overpower the other person with my speech.	talk a little bit more than I listen (feeding back words and feelings).	am an active listener (agreeing and apologising).	am a passive listener.

12 When involved in an unpleasant conflict, I ...

use humour with the other party.	make an occasional quip or joke about the situation or the relationship.	relate humour only to myself.	suppress all attempts at humour.

13 When someone does something that irritates me (e.g. smokes in a non-smoking area or crowds in line in front of me), my tendency in communicating with the offending person is to ...

use strong direct language and tell the person to stop.	try to persuade the person to stop.	talk gently and tell the person what my feelings are.	say and do nothing.

14 When someone does something that irritates me (e.g. smokes in a non-smoking area or crowds in line in front of me), my tendency in communicating with the offending person is to ...

stand close and make physical contact.	use my hands and body to illustrate my points.	stand close to the person without touching him or her.	stand back and keep my hands to myself.

15 When someone does something that irritates me (e.g. smokes in a non-smoking area or queue-jumps in front of me), my tendency in communicating with the offending person is to ...

insist that the person looks me in the eye.	look the person directly in the eye and maintain eye contact.	maintain intermittent eye contact.	avoid looking directly at the person.

Scoring and interpretation

When you have completed all 15 items, add your scores vertically, resulting in four column totals. Put these on the blanks below.

TOTALS =

Column 1 _____ Column 2 _____ Column 3 _____ Column 4 _____

Column 1: aggressive/confrontive

High scores indicate a tendency to 'taking the bull by the horns' and a strong need to control situations and/or people. Those who use this style are often directive and judgmental.

Column 2: assertive/persuasive

High scores indicate a tendency to stand up for oneself without being pushy, a proactive approach to conflict, and a willingness to collaborate. People who use this style depend heavily on their verbal skills.

Column 3: observant/introspective

High scores indicate a tendency to observe others and examine oneself analytically in response to conflict situations, as well as a need to adopt counselling and listening models of behaviour. Those who use this style are likely to be co-operative, even conciliatory.

Column 4: avoiding/reactive

High scores indicate a tendency toward passivity or withdrawal in conflict situations, and a need to avoid confrontation. Those who use this style are usually accepting and patient, often suppressing their strong feelings.

Now total your scores for **Columns 1 and 2** and **Columns 3 and 4**:

Column 1 + Column 2 = **Score A**
Column 3 + Column 4 = **Score B**

If Score A is significantly higher than Score B (25 points or more), it may indicate a tendency toward aggressive/assertive conflict management. A significantly higher B score signals a more conciliatory approach.

Conflict is certain to occur from time to time when people work closely together, especially if their work sometimes involves making difficult decisions together. Understanding how you normally react to conflict is the first stage in developing strategies for dealing with it in a way that suits your personality, while achieving the best results in your work. Colleagues respond differently according to a wide variety of factors, some of which might involve their current life pressures, others are more to do with their continuing view of themselves and others. Getting to know the things that are affecting other individuals can be as important as knowing yourself.

Handling conflict can, and often does, give rise to anger on either or both sides. We all feel anger sometimes and see it in others. But how can we personally handle our and other's anger?

Dealing with your own anger

We are all different, and the propensity to respond angrily varies greatly from one person to another. Anger is a natural reaction, but it can be destructive if not controlled. Generally, the earlier you tackle the cause, the better. It is, obviously, better to wait until you have cooled down, and if you have been drinking alcohol wait until the effect has worn off. You can release some of your physical tension by exercise, even it is only hitting a cushion. Then coolly analyse the situation and decide what you are going to say to address the situation.

You can be positive and direct, but don't make it personal. Express your feelings – tell the other person how you felt, but avoid saying the person made you angry. Acknowledge some responsibility perhaps for not saying something earlier, but avoid putting yourself down, or invitations to retaliatory criticism, and don't bring up past grievances. Don't stereotype, moralise or bring in third parties. Remember to:

- criticise the behaviour not the person

- be specific and realistic in any request

- avoid humour

- use assertive language.

Dealing with anger from someone else

Sometimes you will find yourself having to handle an angry colleague, patient or patient's relative. Try to remember how you have felt when you were angry, and remember that it was not easy to be rational. The following points will help:

- try to be on a level with the other person, if you are looking down on them they may feel more threatened

- keep your own voice as level as possible – try to communicate calm through the way you speak to the person

- allow them plenty of personal space, so do not get too close, that also may make them feel threatened

- acknowledge the other's feelings by an empathic statement. The other person will then understand that you understand, they no longer have to prove their anger

- indicate that you are listening by reflective listening, repeating back a summary of what is being said

- avoid challenging an angry person

- if you are in a closed space or room check that you are well positioned for leaving quickly, or at least ensure that a large piece of furniture separates you from the complainant!

Use simple assertiveness techniques (*see* p. 30 on assertiveness) such as the 'broken record' to express yourself calmly and persistently, as an angry person often leaps from topic to topic.

These points are also covered on p. 102 on handling patient complaints.

Delegation

You may well feel that you have little need to consider the use of delegation skills. Have you considered how you best use the opportunities to work with other doctors in training, medical students, nurses, technicians, phlebotomists, physiotherapists, pharmacists, auxiliaries, receptionists, secretaries, medical record clerks, audit assistants and others?

Delegation is not just about getting others to do the unpleasant, dirty, tedious or boring jobs that you do not want to do. It is also about sharing out the interesting things. You have a responsibility to help others, including your junior colleagues, to develop themselves and increase their experience. That will not happen unless you take positive steps to make it happen. You may not think this too important now, but the more senior you become, the more you will need to delegate. You cannot do everything yourself. When you become a consultant you will have a great need to be skilful at delegation.

Good time management involves making the most effective use of all staff resources, including your own. Tasks which can be carried out satisfactorily by others listed in the examples above should not necessarily be routinely undertaken by you. The complex nature of healthcare demands specialist knowledge and skills. Rapid change brought on by technological development has increased the complexity of the work of doctors. It is impossible for an individual to carry all the knowledge and skills necessary to ensure effective performance of the unit. Delegation is not just about telling others to perform particular tasks. It provides a mechanism for controlled sharing of workload.

Delegation is achieving results by enabling and motivating others, usually more junior to you, to carry out tasks for which you are ultimately accountable, to an accepted, agreed level of competence. The concept of delegation is simple. The practice is rather different and involves high levels of skill and understanding. Delegation is usually interpreted to mean passing down authority and responsibility to others at a more junior level. It is also possible to 'delegate laterally' to other specialist registrars and colleagues, for example when a surgical specialist registrar hands over the responsibility for preparing a case for theatre, or when a medical specialist registrar hands over responsibility for a severe haematemesis to a surgeon. Even upward delegation may take place when, for example, an SHO is called to an emergency elsewhere in the hospital, the specialist registrar may agree to continue with the ward round or the theatre case that they were carrying out together.

Authority and responsibility

Authority and responsibility go together. Authority is the power and the right to take appropriate action in a given situation. Responsibility is an individual's 'answerability' for the successful accomplishment of a task. It would be unreasonable to delegate responsibility for an activity without giving the person authority to act. For example, if the ward phoned theatre to ask an anaesthetic specialist registrar for analgesia of a previous case which had not been written up, and he sent the anaesthetic SHO to write up the prescription, it would be unreasonable to expect the SHO to have to bring back the treatment sheet to be written up by the specialist registrar himself.

Similarly, if a person is given authority, they should be held responsible for outcomes. If the SHO writes up the wrong dose or the wrong drug, the SHO is responsible for that error. This does not mean that a doctor can delegate *ultimate* responsibility. If the SHO had been a pre-registration house officer (PRHO) and it was their first day, it might be considered unreasonable to delegate that task to them. Or maybe the surgical specialist registrar is operating and the list is running late and it has been suggested that the last case, being done under local anaesthesia, be done in a now empty theatre by another member of the team. The SHO is delegated the task by the specialist registrar, but it would be unreasonable to expect the SHO to have to constantly check every step with the specialist registrar before doing anything. Equally, if that person is given authority, they should be held responsible for outcomes. If the SHO does the wrong operation, the SHO is responsible for that error. If, on the other hand, the SHO had no experience of the procedure, it would be considered unreasonable to delegate the task to them. You should be able to think of other examples within your own specialty.

The role is to delegate effectively and give support, encouragement and reasonable protection to staff. A doctor remains accountable for all the activities, whether medical or managerial, within his or her control.

Performance evaluation

Evaluation of performance and recognition of achievement are additional factors in the process of delegation. Effective control should mean that you will need to check on the satisfactory completion of the delegated task, and feedback given to the successful SHO.

Difficulties arise largely as a result of the emotional link we have with our own work. We worry that another person might not do it as well as we would or, worse, they might show us up by being much better at it! It is often easier to do it than explain to someone else how to do it. Sometimes we feel uncomfortable about asking

others because they are too busy, or the task is unpleasant. There is the need to show trust in our juniors, so that they can develop. A tension sometimes arises because of the relationship which inevitably exists in the 'trust/control relationship'. The amount of control we retain reduces with any increase in trust we demonstrate in the person to whom we delegate.

Motivation

We have already discussed what motivates people when we discussed leadership, but it might be useful just to repeat the key factors, as understanding how to motivate people is fundamental to your success in delegation. The performance of any individual in the conduct of their work is likely to be dependent on three variables:

- the *ability* to complete the task satisfactorily: a combination of aptitude and training

- the equipment and facilities for the job must be available; they must have the *opportunity*

- they must be *motivated* to complete the task.

Much has been written in management literature on the subject of motivation. Most general management textbooks have at least one chapter on the subject.

We have also discussed how good leaders are able to understand what motivates their staff and act accordingly in order to get the best from them.

Guidelines for successful delegation

Doctors work in teams which are made up of individuals who possess complex ranges of skills and are often sensitive regarding their status in the team. Successful delegation requires careful thought and the exercise of skill in dealing with individuals, if good results are to be achieved.

Action

Identify a task that you perform and that you could ask a colleague or junior to do instead of you. It should be a task that you consider to be important, but not something that it would be unsafe to allow others to undertake.

• Identify a person to whom you could delegate the task. Choose the right person, taking into account ability, personality and potential.

• Consult with the individual before finally deciding the extent of the delegated task.

• Delegate the *whole* task, not parts which do not carry significant responsibility.

• Clarify the purpose, limits and outcomes or expected results of the task.

• Instruct them on the best methods and give clear guidance on what they should do if they need help.

• Be prepared to delegate enjoyable tasks as well as those which no-one wants. You will motivate people that way.

• Trust the person to get on with the task and allow them to decide when they need help, subject to agreed monitoring arrangements.

• Review their performance after a reasonable time has passed.

• Review your own performance. Note any improvement in the way in which you are able to carry out your core responsibilities.

The politics of influencing outcomes

Organisational relationships in hospitals are complex and involve most doctors in membership of a wide range of subgroups. Formal structures sometimes exist as diagrams showing divisions, directorates and so on, but these only partly describe the reality of groups or coalitions to which doctors (and others) relate or belong.

There are two broad categories of group – formal and informal. Sometimes informal groups, although not recognised in the formal structure of the hospital, have a very powerful influence on events.

One of the most valuable interpersonal skills is the ability to influence others. It can be used across hierarchical boundaries as well as in traditional managerial roles. Influence rests on the ability to use various forms of power. There are usually said to be five sources of power. Their suitability to exerting influence is affected by access to them, and current circumstances. They are related to:

• *position* in the organisation: authority is vested in a post. This enables people in more senior positions to influence subordinates

• *expertise* held by the post holder: others will usually defer to the person who (they perceive) has expert knowledge

• control over *resources*: sometimes people have power well beyond their status in an organisation because they control access to resources that others need. Information might be regarded as a resource, and control over information is sometimes used by relatively junior employees to exert influence of others

• personal charm or *charisma*: there are a few people we meet who can influence others without appearing to have special powers other than their natural ability to lead. Some suggest these are simply people with unusually high levels of interpersonal skill

• *coercion*: often exerted through an implied threat that induces fear in those who can be influenced by the possible outcome. Not usually regarded as an attractive option, it is sometimes used to achieve change in the face of resistance from those affected by the change.

Another source of power is said to be *who you know* – this is a type of power gained by association, or through access to information and influence not available to others. It can be useful, but also carries a degree of risk if this is a major source of your influence as it is is largely outside your control.

Insight into the sources of power and those who control them can be a useful tool. Power and influence can sometimes be acquired by aligning with those who hold power. At other times it might be wise to avoid them.

Action

Write your name in the centre of an A4 sheet. Now write in the names and/or job titles of all those with whom you interact in your work and work-related activities. Include social contacts, particularly those who may have more influence in your organisation than you.

Group these into formal contacts by drawing lines between connected names. Some names or titles are likely to be part of your *informal* network. Circle these and then list them separately. Consider whether any of these are particularly influential in the context of the organisation. How could they help you to achieve your personal goals? How do you relate to them at present? Could you do more to employ their strengths on your own behalf?

What sources of power do you currently exploit?

Which others could you exploit?

Which do you encourage those working with or for you to develop?

Handling stress

Most professionals become familiar with the concept of work overload at some stage in their careers. For many the effects can be recognised in the deterioration of their capacity for taking on new challenges and maintenance of normal lifestyle and family relationships. A less obvious side-effect is the impact uneven work patterns can have on their health. Stress is often blamed as the instrument which directs the ill-effects. It has been described as a trigger for a multitude of physical and mental disorders, including heart disease and cancer. Most authors prefer to see

stress as describing a spectrum of states of mind, which includes stress as a positive, as well as negative, concept. Thus, it may be described as a demand made on the adaptive capacities of the mind and body. It is only when demand becomes more than the mind and body can handle that its effects become undesirable. Before this stage, it can act as a spur to greater achievement and satisfaction at work.

In order to understand the stress in our lives, we need to assess the external demands that are made on us (and that we make on ourselves), and our own capacity for handling that stress. People vary widely in their personal capacity for dealing with work overload. What appears as a major problem to one person may be an exciting challenge to another.

Personality

Personalities and their approach to work-related stress have been assessed according to type. Complete the following questionnaire. Answer each question 'yes' or 'no'.

1 Do you characteristically do several things at once (e.g. telephoning, reading your post and jotting notes on a pad)?

2 Do you feel guilty when relaxing, as if there is always something else you should be doing?

3 Are you quickly bored when other people are talking? Do you find yourself wanting to interrupt, or get them to hurry up?

4 Do you try to steer conversation towards your own interests, instead of wanting to hear of those of others?

5 Are you usually anxious to finish each of your tasks so that you can get on to the next?

6 Are you unobservant when it comes to anything that is not immediately connected with what you are actually doing?

7 Do you prefer to have rather than to be (to experience your possessions rather than to experience yourself)?

8 Do you do most things (eating, talking, walking) at high speed?

9 Do you find people like yourself challenging and people who dawdle infuriating?

10 Are you physically tense and assertive?

11 Are you more interested in winning than in simply taking part and enjoying yourself?

12 Do you find it hard to laugh at yourself?

13 Do you find it hard to delegate?

14 Do you find it almost impossible to attend meetings without speaking up?

15 Do you prefer activity holidays to dreamy, relaxing ones?

16 Do you push those for whom you are responsible (children, subordinates, partner) to try to achieve your own standards without showing much interest in what they really want out of life?

It has been suggested that personality types can be divided into those who are driven by ambition and the need to achieve (Type A), and those more laid-back people for whom life is a series of experiences which may be outside their control, but can be nonetheless enjoyable (Type B). People with extreme Type A personalities will have answered 'yes' to all 16 questions above. If you have responded positively to 12 or more of the questions, then you are likely to have significant Type A tendencies. Type A people like deadlines and pressures, are impatient to move on to new challenges, and can be intolerant of the failure of others to measure up to their own standards of commitment. Unfortunately, this approach to life can lead to type As drawing more upon themselves than they can reasonably cope with, and finding they have fewer coping mechanisms as the pressure rises to breaking point. If you scored 8 or less you are probably a Type B. The Type B personality is relaxed, uncompetitive, and inclined to reflection and self-analysis.

Lifestyle

Maintenance of a balanced lifestyle, in which sport, leisure and family pursuits are given equal place with work, is seen as an essential pre-requisite for holding on to healthy stress levels. This will help to ensure that the volume and nature of the workload does not outpace the individual's capacity for managing the work. This is usually easier said than done in modern working environments, where pressure to absorb increasing demand is often linked to organisational survival. Techniques of time management, as described in Chapter 1, can be used to begin the process of redressing the balance between work and leisure activities.

Another complementary approach is to increase the capacity of individuals for coping with high levels of stress. Changing lifestyle is not easy, but can be managed, especially if the consequences of failure to do so are taken into account. People with Type A personalities will be able to recognise the kinds of things that can be done to reduce the risk of stress. Paradoxically, they can be most effective in implementing change programmes to improve themselves. Finding and developing non-work interests which provide an antidote to overwork can make a good start to the process. Competitive sports, such as golf or sailing, can help to improve physical fitness and to separate you from work pressure for significant periods of time. Learning to delegate, which is discussed earlier in this section, is also vitally important for people with Type A personalities.

Relaxation

Some writers on stress management advocate the use of relaxation and meditation techniques. These range from undertaking simple physical exercises to the acquisition of understanding of Eastern philosophies and habits of mind. They do not work for everyone. It has been argued that regular meditation, even for only a few minutes each day, builds ability to concentrate and handle emotions, and aids physical relaxation. Some people find it difficult to acquire the mental discipline associated with such an approach, although simple physical relaxation techniques are within the scope of most. A wide range of books on stress management and relaxation techniques is available. Many replicate the same basic approach.

An example of advice on meditative technique is shown below. Try it, in case this is what is right for you. Certain personalities will feel unhappy with this type of approach and it requires practice to become competent, so you should persevere before deciding it does not work for you. Perhaps try it only for five minutes the first few times, rising to ten or more after a week or so.

- Choose a suitable room or place where you are guaranteed peace and quiet, free from interruption. Sit in a comfortable upright chair. Keep your body upright throughout. It may help to imagine that your head is held up by a connection with the ceiling above you. Allow your muscles to relax as much as possible while still keeping an upright posture. Close your eyes.

- Remaining as calm as possible, start to focus on your breathing. You will find it helps to concentrate on either your nostrils or your abdomen, but not on both. Count one for each breath as you finish breathing out. Count up to ten, then down again until you reach one. Keep repeating this process.

- As thoughts arise, allow them to drift without paying attention to them. Do not try to drive them away. Concentrate on your breathing. Allow other thoughts to come and go without hindrance.

- After the meditation session is over, rise slowly from your chair. Try to maintain the poised awareness you experienced while meditating. Apply the same approach to thinking about the sights and sounds around you as you go about your everyday activities.

This approach will not remove the sources of stress. In serious situations radical life change may be necessary, such as a change of career direction. Meditation and other techniques are, arguably, a way of managing stress, rather than allowing it to manage us.

Learning to handle stress

Changing the way we think about our lives is difficult. It has been suggested that the following characteristics are found in those who handle stress most effectively:

- they shelve problems until they are capable of dealing with them. They do not dwell on issues with which they cannot cope

- they deliberately relax after coping with highly demanding and stressful tasks, usually by undertaking contrasting activities

- they take a wider view of situations and do not become bogged down in detail

- they control the build up and pace of stressful situations by planning and intervening to prevent themselves from becoming swamped

- they are prepared to confront difficulties or unpleasant issues

- they know their own capacity and do not permit themselves to become overwhelmed by events

- they can cope with being unpopular

- they do not commit themselves to very tight deadlines which are unlikely to be met

- they actively limit their involvement in work in order to maintain a balanced lifestyle.

The above section on stress management is intended to provide an insight into the issues. It does not deal with the responsibility that those supervising the work of others have in ensuring safe and realistic work programmes for them.

Related reading

- Barr L and Barr N (1989) *The Leading Equation: leadership, management and the Myers Briggs.* Earth Press, Austin, Texas.
- Beels C, Hopson B and Scally M (1992) *Assertiveness: a positive process.* Lifeskills Communications Ltd, London.
- Belbin M (2003) *Management Teams: why they succeed and fail.* Butterworth Heinemann, London.
- Crainer S (1996) *Leaders on Leadership.* Institute of Management Foundation, Corby.
- Fontana D (1989) *Managing Stress.* British Psychological Society/Routledge, London.
- Harris TA (1970) *I'm OK, You're OK.* Pan, London.
- Hirsh SK and Kummerow JM (2000) *Introduction to Type in Organisations.* OPP, Oxford.
- Lindenfield G (1993) *Managing Anger.* Thorsons, London.
- Maslow A (1954) *Motivation and Personality.* Harper Row, New York.
- McClelland DC, Atkinson JW, Clark RA and Lowell EL (1976) *The Achievement Motive* (2e). Irvington, New York.
- Mullins LJ (2005) *Management and Organisational Behaviour.* FT Prentice Hall (Pearson Education), Harlow.

- Pedler M, Burgoyne J and Boydell T (2004) *A Manager's Guide to Leadership*. McGraw Hill Professional, Maidenhead.
- Pfeiffer JW and Goodstein LD (eds) (1982) *The 1982 Annual for Facilitators, Trainers, and Consultants*. University Associates, San Diego, CA.
- Pfeiffer JW and Jones JE (eds) (1974) *A Handbook of Structured Experiences for Human Relations Training*, Vol. 1 (Revised) University Associates, San Diego, CA.
- Quick TL (1992) *Successful Team Building*. Amacom, New York.
- Sadler P (2003) *Leadership*. Kogan Page, London.
- Smith MJ (1975) *When I Say No I Feel Guilty*. Bantam, London.
- www.nhsleadershipqualities.nhs.uk

CHAPTER 3

Effective written communication

The aim of this chapter is to provide you with a foundation on which to develop your written communication skills.

The chapter also covers the role of information in the NHS and the use of information technology in clinical medicine and training.

Effective writing

Communication seems easy enough when we talk to people face to face. Yet mysteriously, those who can charm an audience at a party, when armed with a word processor, use convoluted constructions and obscure words that baffle a reader before the second full stop. Effective writing is the creative use of words in an easily readable form which sends a message from one person to another, accurately and completely. According to Tim Albert (1996), visiting fellow in medical writing at Southampton Medical School, on whose work this information is based, one of the most misleading and pretentious phrases used by scientists is 'in the literature'. The kind of writing dealt with here has nothing to do with pure literature, which is generally written by enthusiasts for themselves, and only rarely considered good enough to be published and shared with others. The kind of writing discussed here is more functional and concerned mainly with putting messages across, not just out. Medical schools encourage young men and women to reject 'real' English in favour of the particular language of medicine. This is acceptable when communicating with other doctors. When communicating with other people it becomes meaningless gibberish. Further traps await. Medicine, like all other professions, is highly competitive. Writing is in black and white. Those who have to commit themselves take great care not to offend their peers and, if possible, try to impress upon them the author's grasp of the subject. This is often an effective way of ensuring that the message fails to get through. The all-important principle is to write with your readers' interests in mind at all times. This principle allows for all other rules to be broken. For instance, if the reader will understand better when you split an infinitive, then you should split one. If the reader has limited knowledge you should simplify. If the reader needs to come away with a vague or softened message, then you should wheel out your euphemisms. Apart from our single principle, there are no absolute, hard-and-fast rules. A written article might need to be revised many times, so do not be discouraged if it takes rather longer than you at first thought. At least the word processor has made this easier.

The process of writing

Forward planning is helpful. Avoid huge undertakings like 'writing a paper' or 'doing a report'. In general writing is a laborious business. Break this down into small units, such as 'five possible topics for an article' or the 'headings' for the report. You do not need to be seated at a desk to do this. As Klauser (1987) points out in her excellent book on the process of writing, 'ruminating time' is an essential part of the writing process. The thought you invest at the beginning pays dividends. The structure and style of a report differs depending on whether it is written for a lay reader or doctor. Writing too much is not a sign that the writer is well informed, but rather that he or she has failed to make basic decisions on what is really important for the audience. And remember your deadline. It should be realistic, allowing ample time for revisions and changes. The best start, as Klauser suggests, is 'mind-mapping'. This involves writing down on a clean sheet of paper the elements of the theme. Then start jotting down questions and thoughts that you will need to deal with, taking them out like the branches of a tree. This technique is explained by Buzan (1989) (*see* Chapter 1, Related reading, p. 18).

Most writers suggest that you write a first draft of the whole piece in one go. Once you have finished this, put it away for a few days (or at least overnight). When you return to it, relatively fresh, you can start the real work. Leave it for as long as possible, and then start revising.

Active or passive?

There is a common argument that professional people should not use the first person. The passive has three disadvantages. It requires more words, it becomes less vigorous, and the writer often fails to state who actually performed the action. We are indebted to Tim Albert for the following example:

Passive:

'The questionnaires were administered and the results were subsequently analysed. It was discovered after analysis that action was indicated.'

Active: the passive statement above could mean either of the following alternatives:

'Trained interviewers administered the questionnaires and processed the results. I analysed the figures and concluded that the Director of Public Health had a problem.'

'A work experience student administered the questionnaire and her boyfriend used his computer to process the results. They looked at some of the comments and decided to send them to the *News of the World*.'

The passive does have a place. It is useful when the object of an action is more important than the subject, or when causality has yet to be established. And it is also useful when a writer, quite deliberately or for political reasons, wishes to make things unclear. Writing in the active, on the other hand, is one of the most effective ways of improving dense prose. As Gowers (1986), one of the leading authorities on effective style, remarks dryly: 'Overuse of the passive may render a sentence impenetrable'.

General reports

There are frequently 'local' rules which should be followed. These are determined by custom and practice within an organisation or profession. The following are general guidelines which can be adapted to the expectations of the population within which your report will be circulated. Define the brief carefully and pay attention to the real audience. Avoid technical words and jargon. Study other reports. Pay particular attention to the structure. You will usually have headings and subheadings. Within each of these sections the usual guidelines apply. Use the conclusion to put across the message you wish to stay in the reader's mind. In addition, give a summary, so that busy readers can at least have a quick overview. Initially we will deal with the general framework or layout for writing a report. This might be a report of an incident or event, an audit report or a medico-legal report. There is no right and wrong way, different people have different views and ideas, but some general principles emerge.

A typical general report

- *Title page*: includes the title and date of the report and the author's name.

- *Contents page*: lists all the main sections and subsections of the report and the pages on which they appear.

- *Acknowledgements*: it is common practice to name and thank sources of help and advice.

- *Aims and objectives/terms of reference*: defines as precisely as possible the purpose for which the report has been prepared and the limits placed on it. Each of these possible section headings has a different meaning: aims are broad statements of intent; objectives are usually stated as 'measurable' outcomes; terms of reference describe precisely the limits placed on the report as well as its aims or objectives.

- *Abstract or summary*: sometimes placed as the front page of the document, this serves to inform the reader of the essence of the whole report in a few words.

- *Summary of conclusions/recommendations*: either or both may be presented at the front end of the report. This is dependent on local practice and the nature of the report objectives. They can be presented in tabular or bulleted form and should be as brief and simple as possible.

- *Introduction*: describes (briefly) the background to the report, the scope and the limitations of the report. The reader should be clear about why the report has been written and, therefore, why it should be worth reading.

- *Methods and/or methodology*: often used to describe the same thing, these two words have different meanings. Methods describe the way data were collected. The reasons for selecting one method rather than another should be explained. Methodology requires more fundamental consideration and explanation. Put simply, it is the way the data are used to obtain results and conclusions. It describes an approach to research. Remember you do not take children to the zoology to see the animals.

- *Results or findings*: outcomes and information presented in some sort of logical sequence, dealing perhaps with one area at a time by dividing into three or four further sections. You may include some discussion or opinion in this section but distinguish between fact and opinion. We have already alluded to the impersonal or personal style of writing. In the past, report writing was very much an impersonal or third-person approach. Indeed

many journals will still not consider any other format. There is now a clear move to greater acceptance of the personal approach to writing thoughts and opinions, certainly as you must be willing to stand by what you write. The placing of tables, diagrams and graphs is a matter of personal choice. This can be a good place to include them if they help to clarify the message within the body of the report. If there is too much information, but you believe the reader should be given an opportunity to see it, then put it into an appendix. Always remember the guiding principle – write with the readers' interests in mind at all times.

- *Conclusions*: should emerge from the results and therefore may be simply cross-referenced to previous sections so that the reader can easily follow the author's arguments. Conclusions should also only be within the scope of the terms of reference. Avoid introducing something new into the conclusions, which has not been explained previously.

- *Recommendations*: should flow naturally from the report and its conclusions and again cross-referencing enables both author and reader to follow the flow of logic. It is worth considering the political implications of your recommendations which would require action by others. Perhaps time spent preparing the ground before the report is published would be time well spent.

- *Bibliography*: sometimes included at this stage, or as an appendix, if the report needs one.

- *References*: may be placed here as an alternative to within the text.

- *Appendices*: start each appendix on a separate page. This section includes graphs, diagrams, charts, statistics, schedules, calculations, plans and source data. Define terms and explain terminology that may be unfamiliar to the target audience.

Memos and letters

The most appropriate structure is known as the 'inverted triangle'. Put the important part – the pay-off for the reader – in the first sentence. The first few words should not be boring, as in: 'I am in receipt of your letter' or 'The car-parking working party of the senior management group ...'. Some people expect a welcoming routine, such as: 'Thank you for your letter' or 'It was good to meet you the other day'. This reinforces our main principle: the interests of the reader are paramount.

Medical records

It might be useful here to say a few words about medical records, their use, what is included and some important qualities they should have. In *Good Medical Practice* (2001), the General Medical Council (GMC) specifies that doctors should:

> keep clear, accurate, legible and contemporaneous patient records which report the relevant clinical findings, the decisions made, the information given to patients and any drugs or other treatment prescribed.

It also says that you should 'keep colleagues well informed when sharing the care of patients'. This requires good medical records.

Currently there is no single model for documenting and communicating information that forms a patient's health record, although some standards have been provided by healthcare regulatory bodies. In 2005 the NHS Information Standards Board and the three largest regulatory bodies, the GMC, the Nursing and Midwifery Council (NMC) and the Health Professions Council (HPC), undertook a review of existing standards. This resulted in a set of health record and communication practice standards for team-based care that brought together the standards that were already in existence and common to all three bodies.

The review found that the standards common to all three regulatory bodies fell into four main categories:

- confidentiality and disclosure

- communication and information

- process principles

- personal and professional knowledge and skills.

They stated that the standards common to all three regulatory bodies were not intended to be best practice but minimum standards to be attained. They are not intended either to replace the standards of the regulatory bodies or any guidance provided by professional organisations. They went on to state that patient safety lies at the heart of clinical governance, and the NHS published a set of core standards setting out the level of quality all organisations providing NHS care in England should meet. The standards they identified in the review relate to the management of records should be implemented in all NHS organisations. For further information you could go to www.isb.nhs.uk and you will find a section on 'Health record and communication practice standards for team based care'.

Some basic considerations

The patient to whom the records refer should be identified clearly, with their name and date of birth and NHS or hospital number on each page (or an addressograph label with that information). If your writing is not very legible then type your notes or have them typed. Sign and print all entries with your name, date (including the year), time by the 24-hour clock, and your status. The entries should be based on the facts you have recorded, and written notes made as soon as possible after an event.

If information has been given to you by anyone but the patient, e.g. relative, staff member, police, ambulance crew, observer, etc, record that person's name and position. It should also go without saying that the records should not be altered or amended later, indeed the records should be such that any attempt to do so should be obvious. So do not leave large gaps between entries or feel tempted to leave space at the bottom of a page to enable you to make a start on a new sheet.

Records should preferably be written in black ink as black photocopies well and, unlike pencil, cannot be altered or rubbed out. It is also claimed that ballpoint pens are less capable of being of being erased than old fashioned ink in a fountain pen. The ball point also transfers well on carbon copy style forms. Felt tip pens should be avoided as they tend to bleed through the paper.

Legibility of records

Legibility is a significant problem, as research has shown that about 9% of entries are not fully legible, some half of healthcare workers' handwriting is 'poor to fair', and that males over 37 years old were found to have the least legible handwriting. However there is good news in that bad handwriting is not a characteristic of being a doctor. In fact, tested under the same conditions, doctors are no worse than other health professionals. The difference may lie in the fact that doctors are often under great pressure to write quickly. Furthermore, the consequences of poor legibility are potentially more serious than in many other professions.

Luckily most general practitioner (GP) surgeries have electronic data entry, thus avoiding problems with handwriting, but this is not usually available to hospital doctors. However, computer records are only as good as the person inputting the data; spelling errors can and do occur, and good keyboard skills are necessary to prevent consultations taking longer.

Ownership of medical records

Questions are occasionally raised as to who owns the records, and a raft of legislation covers access to medical records. In summary however the record is owned by the person(s) entering the data, their employing hospital trust or primary care trust (PCT). Fortunately for you, however, in the NHS, applications for access to records are dealt with by the trust. However, your employing trust may be happy for you to deal informally with an approach for access, providing you are comfortable showing a patient their records, the patient is 'competent', it is unlikely to cause serious harm to the patient (e.g. with psychiatric records), and none of the entries in the record relate to another person who has not given their consent.

Access to medical records

It is also worth knowing that relatives have no automatic rights of access to a patient's medical records, although there may be exceptions with parents/guardians of minors. But be aware that complex family structures may mean that the adult accompanying a child to hospital does not have parental rights. In Scotland, patients can appoint a proxy decision maker, who may have access to a patient's records. In all cases of doubt,

it is best to speak to a senior colleague or your defence organisation.

It can be very difficult when there are anxious relatives who want to know about a loved one. You must consider your duty of confidentiality to the patient, so you could suggest relatives speak to the patient themselves for information, or you could ask the patient how much information they would be happy for relatives to know. Clearly if the patient cannot be consulted because, perhaps, they are unconscious, then exercise common sense as it would be insensitive not to consider worried relatives. Occasionally it might be actively harmful to discuss matters with the patient themselves, and thus it would be in the patient's best interests for you to speak to a relative.

Although there is a duty of confidentiality with regard to medical information on patients it can be disclosed without consent in the following circumstances:

- suspected child abuse

- the patient has a notifiable disease

- the patient is thought to be an active threat to public safety.

It is advised that you contact your senior partner and your defence union if you are considering disclosing information.

Medical records as legal documents

From a legal point of view most written medical records are considered 'hearsay', and are not deemed admissible in criminal court. They are considered 'business records' if they are contemporaneous, written by the person connected with the events and such records are kept routinely.

Thus medical records may be admissible. However, most legal disputes concern questions of fact where the patient's recollection differs significantly from that of the doctor. Experience suggests that courts have a tendency to believe the memory of a patient, for whom it was a once-in-a-lifetime experience; they will have relived the event countless times and they will be well geared up for the trial, whereas the doctor, who may perform many similar procedures daily, may not recall the individual patient and may find it difficult to corroborate events from many years earlier. The doctor's defence relies heavily on the quality of the medical record made at the time.

Therefore, it is important, when discussing operations before patients sign the consent form, to not only highlight potential complications but to try to record any conversation verbatim in the notes at the time.

What should medical records contain?

The medical records should ideally include the problem list, the history, the examination, the diagnosis if known, the information given to the patient, details of consent for any interventions required, treatment plans, follow-up arrangements and progress. This allows care to be seamlessly continued out of normal working hours. It is difficult and wasteful to have to repeat a full clerking every day, but there should be a detailed entry made regularly to update the patient's progress. This is particularly essential before a weekend or bank holiday, when the on-call team is unlikely to know the patient.

It is important that a doctor fills in the medical records as the patient is seen, even perhaps as the consultant is talking. Not all inpatients need daily notes but there should be an entry in the record at least once every 24 hours if they are classified as in 'acute care'. For inpatients in 'rehabilitative care', the minimum recommended standard for review and an entry in the notes is twice per week.

It may not be possible to write in depth when you have 40 patients to see on a post-take ward round. But the following might be regarded as a basic minimum for any entry:

- date and time
- name of senior clinician present
- current problem or diagnosis
- significant changes in clinical status or events since last review
- any significant communication (e.g. patient requests, seen by allied health professional, consent sought or explanations given by medical team, nursing concerns)
- results of any examination made and relevant findings
- significant new test results

- changes in medications or treatment
- planned new investigations
- significant changes to care or management
- a signature and printed name and rank of the author, bleep number if applicable.

If there has been a recent full summary, and nothing significant has occurred since the last review, and no changes are planned, it can be acceptable to write very little.

The patient's perspective is important and should be recorded in the notes as the patient's personal views. Although the patient's opinion can be written verbatim, limit yours to facts.

We have already stated that patient records should never be altered, but suppose you accidentally write things about patient B in patient A's notes and then realise what you have done! Action should be taken immediately the error is realised, but not by anyone attempting to erase, obliterate or attempting to edit notes previously written. Preferably corrections should be by the person who made the original entry. The corrections (and indeed any retrospective entries, and additions) should be clearly marked as such and signed, labelled with the date and time of writing. So draw a single line through the incorrect entry, write 'written in error', add the date and time, and sign and write your name.

Structure of medical records

Most trusts have their own system and some still follow the principle of having separate notes for each specialty. However, the generally accepted policy currently is that documents within the record should reflect the continuum of patient care, and, therefore, be chronologically set out and not separated into different specialties unless legally required (e.g. HIV information). Records can quickly become confusing and misleading unless a strict order of filing is adhered to, and every piece is clearly labelled with at least the patient's name and hospital number.

Most hospitals' record folders have defined places for letters, inpatient entries, outpatient clinic entries, and investigations. If this is not followed information can get lost.

This principle of labelling and filing should apply not only to handwritten notes but also to computerised records, correspondence, laboratory reports, images (photographs, videos and X-rays), printouts from monitors (including electrocardio-grams (ECGs)) and other charts.

What about discharge summaries?

Published literature suggests that standards are highly variable. In one study 17% of discharge summaries had no diagnosis, 19% no procedure stated, and 21% no follow-up. Another published paper suggested that a well-written discharge letter is invaluable to the GP, and 90% of GPs feel that a problem list is helpful and that it improves the continuity of care

Retention of medical records

Finally what about the time medical records should be retained? Governmental guidelines give the following as minimum retention periods for different categories of patient. As it is some-what complicated, the following summary has been taken from a doctors.net module on medical records as it sets it out in a convenient way. This list was stated to be available as a module to download.

- *Children and young people*: until the patient's 25th birthday, or 26th if they were 17 at the conclusion of treatment; or 8 years after death if death occurred before their 18th birthday (hospital records), 10 years after death if death occurred before their 18th birthday (GP records).

- *Donor records*: 11 years post-transplantation.

- *Maternity (including all obstetric and mid-wifery notes even if stillbirth or the child later dies)*: 25 years.

- *Mentally disordered persons (as defined by Mental Health Act 1983)*: 20 years after no further treatment considered necessary, or eight years after the patient's death if they were still receiving treatment (hospital records), 10 years after the patient's death if they were still receiving treatment (GP records).

- *Oncology*: eight years after conclusion of treatment.

- *Patients in clinical trials*: 15 years after con-clusion of treatment.

- *General hospital records*: 8 years after conclu-sion of treatment.

- *General GP records*: 10 years after conclusion of treatment, the patient's death, or they have permanently left the country.

- *GP records of patients serving in HM armed forces*: not to be destroyed.

- *GP records of patients serving a prison sentence*: not to be destroyed.

Summary

Medical records are:

- a permanent record of the patient's medical history treatment and progress.

- tools facilitating communication between hospital doctors, GPs and other staff

- a legal document

- a tool used by hospital quality assur-ance and audit

- sometimes used for retrospective clin-ical research.

Medical records should include:

- handwritten notes

- correspondence

- computerised records

- laboratory reports

- images (including photographs, videos and X-rays)

- printouts from monitors (including ECGs)

- other electrical or electronic charts (e.g. audiograms and tympanograms).

Medical records must be:

- clear

- legible

- identifiable

- objective

- contemporaneous

- first-hand

- original and unaltered.

Medical records and the Data Protection Act 1998

Doctors are sometimes puzzled or concerned about case notes, perhaps relating to private patients, stored at home or in private rooms. The advice of the Office of Data Protection has stated that anyone who keeps healthcare records, whether they relate to NHS or private patients must comply with the Data Protection Act, and if any part of the record is held on or has been processed on a computer the doctor is required to register as a 'data controller'. If entirely hand-written then the doctor can choose whether to register or not; the fee is currently £35.

There is also the question of dealing with safety of electronically stored data. The relevant section of the Act states that 'appropriate technical and organisational measures shall be taken against unauthorised and unlawful processing of personal data and against accidental loss of, or damage to, personal data'. No manual or electronic system can be 100% secure, but you need to be able to justify what steps you have taken to prevent both theft and unauthorised access. While paper records are unlikely to be the target of random theft, computer equipment, especially portable equipment, is very vulnerable. As far as unauthorised access is concerned, there will be the question of passwords although this does not prevent the hard drive from being accessed from another computer, or encryption software. For networked computers there will in addition be the need for firewalls to prevent hackers from gaining access.

Next to consider is the loss of date from hard-ware or software failure, so back-ups will be necessary together with related security. Then there is the problem associated with equipment developing faults and requiring maintenance or repairs. Repairs need to be carried out by a reputable company with a written contract that states that the repairer will not attempt to access data.

Finally there is the question of what to do with old computers. Hard drives are notoriously difficult to erase; even reformatting a hard drive does not make previously held data unrecoverable. There are security products to securely wipe hard drives, and companies that specialise in guaranteeing to wipe hard drives.

Copies of the legislation and guides to electronic data are available at a number of sites that can all be accessed via www.the-mdu.com and typing in 'electronic data' in the search box.

Medico-legal reports

Medico-legal reporting mostly involves reports on people who have been injured by an accident, either road traffic, sometimes industrial or 'slip and trip' accidents in the community. Most reports are provided by GPs or consultants in a particular field of expertise to assess the injuries. These reports try to provide a time-specific prognosis on how long the injuries sustained will take to resolve. GPs in the UK carry out this type of work a lot. Many of the reports involve day-to-day problems such as would be experienced in every-day general practice. Some require a specialist opinion and are carried out by consultants, although some reports may be accepted from senior grade doctors with postgraduate qualifications and experience in a particular field of expertise.

At some point in your career, particularly if you work in a specialty dealing with trauma cases, solicitors may request you provide a medical report. You normally have no obligation to write this and may wish to hand it on to a colleague, perhaps someone more senior. As you progress in seniority and acquire more experience you will probably want to write these yourself, particularly as they carry a fee. The size of that fee will depend on the complexity of the case and the time and work involved, but the British Medical Association (BMA) publishes guidelines on such fees and you can always discuss and compare your experience with colleagues locally. Most reputable agencies pay invoices within three to six months after receipt of the report, but solicitors may not pay until the case is settled, and that may occasionally take years. So you might want to make your willingness to accept the task conditional on a payment on completion of the report. Indeed a few consultants insist on payment after completion of the report but before submitting it!

Initially, some reading and induction to the provision of reports by an experienced colleague is very much advised. Some doctors approach agencies seeking to carry out this type of work. There are many agencies, from small to very large. Again, seek the advice of your colleagues as to who are the best organised and most reliable agencies.

Most agencies have a template. They are all very similar and along the lines suggested below. This involves a formalised approach to reporting that is logical and enables the insurers and solicitors who view the reports to assess the value of the claim. It does not take long to develop the knack of report writing to a structure. The structure is a great help when seeing the patient to ensure that you have covered everything required.

The patients are typically seen in a GP practice, private consulting rooms, or even at the individual's home if they have a problem with transport. Remember, if you see them in hospital, the trust may require you to pay a fee for the use of its facilities. Depending on your experience and complexity of the case, an average time to complete the face-to-face consultation is in the region of 30 minutes.

Most solicitors and agencies expect a report to be returned within four to six weeks of instruction being sent to you. You will normally be asked to address a particular issue. This is your 'remit'. Some will require examination of the patient. Issues you may need to address will include:

- condition

- prognosis

- negligence

- causation.

The medical evidence provided by your report must comply with the requirements of Civil Justice Rules (1998). We recommend, therefore, that before preparing and writing any medico-legal report you obtain a copy of the notes and Part 35 of the Civil Procedure Rules (1998) and the Supplementary Practice Directions.

Try to be proactive with the lawyer who requests the report. Ask questions until you are confident you understand clearly what is being requested. You will need the following:

- hospital records

- X-rays and scans

- GP records

- previous reports

- the patient's statement, if appropriate (personal injury cases).

Hospitals usually charge for these, so it is normal practice for the solicitor to supply them, or at least copies. Well-organised law firms will supply them in chronological order and paginated.

Structuring a medico-legal report

Type with double space and wide margins. The style and layout can vary, although it is largely determined by the Civil Procedure Rules (1998). It is also influenced by the writer and partly by the needs of the solicitor or barrister. We strongly advise you to be proactive and discuss what is expected from you and look at other reports as examples. You will be required to state the extent of your contact with the patient, the history, symptoms and other details as relevant. Avoid technical jargon unless you give an explanation. Remember that lawyers are interested in the strengths and weaknesses of the case, particularly the latter. Give the results of examinations and investigations and state your opinion with reasons. Distinguish facts from opinions and recognise your assumptions.

The Civil Procedure Rules (1998) specify that the following requirements must be met. The report must:

- be addressed to the court

- set out the substance of your instructions

- include details of any literature or other material relied upon

- state who carried out any test or experiment used for the report and whether or not the test or experiment was carried out under your supervision

- give qualifications of any person who carried out any test or experiment

- summarise any range of opinions and give reasons for your own opinion

- set out a summary of the conclusions

- state that you understand your duty to the court and that you have complied with that duty

- set out the statement of truth in the form required

- give details of your qualifications.

Most of the following suggested sections include statements of fact but you need to exercise care with those that require opinion.

* *Summary* – a front page with a summary is usually helpful and might include the identity of the patient, the date of the report, date of injury, the cause, the injuries or at least those relevant to your report, treatment and progress, a summary of your examination findings and, finally, the prognosis.

* *Section 1 – Instructions*: describe the source and substance of your instructions and the documents, literature or other material you have seen.

* *Section 2 – Details of the claimant*: this identifies the patient together with age, sex, date of birth, and age at the time of report of any accident or illness. It is helpful to include subheadings for marital status, family and social history, occupational details and leisure activities. Include a section for other factors which do not fit neatly into other sections but which need a mention.

* *Section 3 – Previous medical history*: you should refer particularly to anything relevant to the present symptoms.

* *Section 4 – Present complaints*: list the patient's symptoms as precisely as possible.

* *Section 5 – History of injury*.

* *Section 6 – Treatment*.

* *Section 7 – Progress of treatment*.

* *Section 8 – Present examination*.

* *Section 9 – Investigations*: it is important to identify any test or investigation undertaken, the qualifications of the person who carried it out, and whether it was under your supervision.

* *Section 10 – Opinion*: this is the most important section and will require careful thought. How do you distinguish facts and opinions? Here are some suggested definitions:
  – *facts* are real and objective
  – *feelings* are emotional responses to situations or events
  – *values* are derived from norms in society, the organisation and the family
  – *opinions* are our personal ideas or explanations about issues, events or situations

  – *assumptions* help to make sense of complexity, but should be distinguished from 'facts'.

In civil proceedings, liability and causation have to be demonstrated on a balance of probabilities. In other words, 'more likely than not'. This could mean a 50.1% chance at least. So the key phrase is 'on the balance of probabilities'. This contrasts with criminal cases, in which the level of proof is generally 'beyond reasonable doubt'. The Civil Procedure Rules (1998) now require that you summarise any range of opinions as well as giving reasons for your own opinion.

* *Section 11 – Period of incapacity from work or normal activity*.

* *Section 12 – Period of partial incapacity*.

* *Section 13 – Residual disability*.

* *Section 14 – Disfigurement*.

* *Section 15 – Psychological aspects*.

* *Section 16 – Special needs*.

* *Section 17 – Recommendations for treatment and rehabilitation*.

* *Section 18 – Prognosis and long-term considerations*.

* *Section 19 – Conclusions*: this is distinct from your opinions and should set out a summary of your conclusions, based entirely on the information contained within the report.

* *Section 20 – Compliance with Civil Procedure Rules (1998)*: review your report and confirm that you have complied with and understand your duty to the court.

* *Section 21 – Your qualifications*: state your qualifications, current post and relevant experience.

* *Section 22 – Data Protection Act 1985*: indicate whether you are retaining the records on a computerised system.

Review your report

It is essential that all reports are typed, proofread and signed by you before dispatch. The important features are that the report should be:

* set out in the form required by the court

- clearly and concisely written
- clearly presented
- clearly structured
- easy to read.

Each page should be numbered; a header or footer with the patient's name is also useful, and the sections should be numbered for easy reference. Sign and date the report – it is easy to forget this! Your fee note should be separate from the report and not referred to in the report.

Some doctors who prepare few reports do their own word processing. Others use the services of a medical secretary, who is often familiar with the structure of medical reports. Please read the section on The Data Protection Agency (p. 52) as you might be advised to register.

Important reminders for medico-legal reports

- You must comply with the Civil Procedure Rules (1998).
- Avoid partiality – you are acting as an independent expert. Partiality will compromise your opinion.
- Never gloss over weaknesses; it is better if they are revealed early in a case.
- Do not stray from your area of expertise as you could find yourself challenged later.

Report submission

What happens to your report after submission? It usually goes to the patient who checks that the history is correct. It may then be sent to counsel who will consider it and write comments. There may be a meeting or conference of experts at this stage, depending on the size of the case. Later you may be asked to review what you have written, as legal issues are often not identical to medical issues. There is nothing sinister in this, but you should not write something to which you cannot put your name or that are not prepared to defend.

The Data Protection Agency

If you are in a practice it is probably already registered with the government's Data Protection Agency, so this is not an issue. It is again something to discuss with colleagues, but if you are unsure it might be wise to register.

VAT and medical reports

In a landmark decision on 20 November 2003, the European Court ruled that doctors will have to charge VAT on medical reports that relate to the following:

- issues of liability and quantification of damages for individuals involved in personal injury litigation
- medical negligence claims
- negligence claims whether by examination of the claimant or a review of the notes
- giving an opinion on a person's medical condition for entitlement to pension or disability benefit
- claims by an individual in support of payment of disability pension.

However the ruling determined that VAT exemptions continue to apply to:

- normal medical examinations and procedures
- examinations on behalf of employers or insurance companies
- the taking of blood for tests conducted on behalf of employers or insurance companies
- the provision of certificates of medical fitness, where this service is intended principally to protect the health of the person concerned.

For doctors earning more than £56,000 a year from medical reports, registration will be compulsory. Clearly if you are in this situation you need to consult your accountant. You may decide to set up a separate business for your medical report writing.

As well as being obliged to register for VAT, some amendments to your book-keeping will be necessary. Proper fee note records showing output VAT will have to be maintained, along with proper records of expenditure showing input VAT to be recovered. There are different accounting systems by which VAT is accounted for; this is normally quarterly on an invoice raised/received basis. However, alternatives to consider are the 'cash accounting' and 'annual accounting' schemes.

These records will be examined by Her Majesty's Revenue and Customs (HMRC) regularly, normally shortly after registration and thereafter every three years or so. Any errors in maintaining records or the submission of incorrect VAT returns results in a package of fines and penalties.

For those earning less than £56,000 a year from report writing, registration for VAT is an option. You will need to decide whether the market will bear the additional 17.5% cost of your reports. It may well do so as reports from experts in other areas already carry VAT. Again your accountant can provide useful advice.

Court appearances

Court appearances are very infrequent, and the structure of report writing is designed to eliminate the expense and time involved in a court case. Court is usually a last resort and very uncommon when related to GP reports, but may just possibly occur with more specialised cases although still rarely.

Being an expert witness

Guidance from the Academy of Medical Royal Colleges (AMRC) on expert witnesses is well worth reading and is available at www.aomrc. org.uk. It is recent, up to date and concise. In summary it gives guidance to doctors prepared to serve as expert witnesses, but in addition guidance for the legal profession and the courts to assist them in establishing the appropriateness of doctors who serve as expert witnesses. The guidance also points out that the duty of a medical expert witness is to the court rather than to the party who instructs them. Again reference is made to the principles set out in the GMC's *Good Medical Practice* (2001). To fulfil these principles, the medical expert witness should ensure that their statements, reports and verbal evidence are: straightforward, rather than intentionally misleading or biased; as objective as possible and not omitting material or information which does not support the opinion expressed or conclusions reached; and properly and fully researched.

The quality and reliability of testimony provided by doctors should be complemented by appropriate professional demeanour. Communication skills of medical expert witnesses should include the careful use of wording that might be regarded as pejorative or prejudgmental. The guidance is also a useful reminder that there is an *Intercollegiate Report on 'Sudden Unexpected Death in Infancy: a multi-agency protocol for care and investigation'* (September 2004) that emphasised that it is the responsibility of courts to decide whether a doctor is competent to give evidence as an expert witness and suggests these prompts:

- what is the expert's area of practice?
- is the doctor still in practice?
- what is the doctor's area of expertise?
- to what extent is the witness an expert in the subject to which the doctor testifies?
- when did the doctor last see a case in their own clinical practice?
- is the doctor in good standing with their medical Royal College?
- is the doctor up to date with continuing professional development?
- has the doctor received training in the role of the expert witness in the last five years?
- to what extent is the doctor's view widely held?

Indeed the AMRC notes recommend that these tests should be applied to all medical expert witnesses. There are some caveats with regard to 'the doctor still in practice?'. There could be merit in evidence from a doctor who, though no longer in active practice, can provide testimony relevant to the period during which, say, alleged clinical negligence occurred. In addition with regard to 'doctor being in good standing with their medical Royal College?' it notes that not all doctors have medical Royal College affiliation. Many non-UK-trained doctors are not members or fellows of medical Royal Colleges, and for these individuals, the 'in good standing' test cannot be applied. Furthermore, 'in good standing' could mean nothing more that being up to date with membership subscriptions and actively participating in a continuing professional development scheme.

Thus, the definition of a doctor as an 'expert' in the context of court proceedings is a matter solely for the court. The mere inclusion of a doctor's name on a list of 'experts' may not be sufficient for the specific aspects of a particular case. Conversely, many doctors not listed in registers or databases of experts may, nevertheless, be sufficiently qualified, trained and experienced to serve as expert witnesses. Several organisations maintain databases or registers of experts, with varying degrees of rigour determining eligibility for entry. These include:

- The Society of Expert Witnesses
- The Academy of Experts
- The Expert Witness Institute
- The Law Society
- The UK Register of Expert Witnesses
- The Council for the Regulation of Forensic Practitioners: launched in 2000, a professional regulatory body independent of government, but currently subsidised by the Home Office pending financial self-sufficiency. It maintains a register of 'currently competent forensic practitioners'. The medical specialists currently eligible for registration are 'physicians (police surgeons and paediatricians)', for details *see*: www.crfp.org.uk.

The notes also point out that neither The Academy of Medical Royal Colleges nor its constituent colleges and faculties operate or endorse registers of expert witnesses, nor do they nominate doctors as experts, or vouchsafe those who serve as experts. Finally the Academy recommends that before agreeing to appear as expert witnesses, you should ensure that you understand the responsibilities and duties, best obtained by attending a relevant course or courses approved for continuing professional development (CPD), and that you should ensure that you have an induction into expert witness work, particularly in those specialties frequently called upon to assist the courts.

Getting published

Researching

Specific provision is made for those who wish to undertake a period of research during the specialist registrar training programme (*see* Chapter 10 in NHS Executive *A Guide to Specialist Registrar Training* (1998)). Others are expected to develop an understanding of research methodology and are encouraged to undertake research. Research can be enjoyable, but is time consuming and can be expensive. In some ways it is like detective work, starting with a problem, going through a process of investigation, building up evidence and moving towards conclusions. The sense of achievement in new discovery can be tremendous, but beyond this personal satisfaction it could be argued that all professional practice should be research based and research validated, and all professional doctors have a responsibility to contribute to the process.

Keeping up with the literature

With so many published journals how do you keep up to date with the literature, especially if you are involved in writing or research? Well for a start keeping up to date goes beyond just reading publications and attending meetings. It is just as important to be able to recall articles quickly, to cite references accurately, and to quote from them correctly. To make this easier, you need to do three things:

- acquire the information
- note the important information
- store references so they can be easily retrieved.

Acquiring information

Your choice of reading depends of course on your research and general interests. It will cover journals, books, conference and other reports, especially review articles and journals that review papers published within a specialty each month. Do not forget that scanning the index of journals will give you a good idea of published material. If you need to do a detailed study or review of a subject you should search computerised bibliographic databases such as Medline, about which your librarian will give you advice. *See* also Literature review (p. 59). From such databases you will obtain citations of all your references, and, in many cases, abstracts. How much time you spend reading new material each week depends on the time you have and the amount of reading you need to do.

Noting important information

This can be done manually with record cards, although most people would now use a computer database. You will need to record:

- the title of the paper

- the authors

- the full title of the journal or book

- the volume number, page numbers and year of publication

- a description of the paper and work (case report or general report, leading article, editorial, review or letter, etc; results of controlled trial, original study, etc)

- the institution where the work was carried out

- key words

- an abstract

- the location of the material (e.g. your own collection, in the library, etc).

Much of the above can be done in your particular shorthand or code.

Is the information relevant and valid?

Ask yourself the following questions when evaluating the research of others:

- is it relevant for your project?

- have rigorous, systematic and objective methods been used? The research should offer the highest-quality evidence. For example, were participants in the study randomly selected or randomly assigned to experimental versus control/comparison? Was there a control group?

- are there other possible explanations for the results that are reported in the research study or how those are interpreted by the authors?

- is there sufficient detail for replication? The research should be described in enough detail so that other researchers can replicate the study

- has it been submitted to independent, expert review? There should be evidence that the research was reviewed by research and content experts other than the researchers. A typical form of expert review would be publication in a refereed journal.

Storing information for retrieval

This is the most difficult of the three tasks but the most important. Your ability to recall the important message from the paper without necessarily reading it all over again will depend on how you file the information. A database is only an electronic filing cabinet. A database is an organised collection of data on a given subject. The database will be composed of a single data file or several files – a file being a collection of records on a theme. All the records on a given subject make up a file, and all the files together form the database.

The record is divided into 'data fields', each holding information on one aspect of the reference, such as the names of the authors etc, as above. One advantage of the computer database is the ability to search for records on multiple variables, to create index files and to use the system in conjunction with word processing programs. You can either create your own system using the database supplied with your computer software, or purchase a separate, more sophisticated package specially designed to handle bibliographic data. These are more expensive but some can communicate with bibliographic databases such as Medline and therefore provide means of obtaining a large number of references from the computer terminal installed in the department, or even at home.

Key stages in the writing process

- Developing your idea

- Background reading and literature search

- Conducting the research

- Analysing the results

- Writing

Literature review

One way to review the literature is to work laboriously backwards through the journals, either scanning the contents lists for suitable papers or reading some of the review journals.

A more efficient way was to use *Index Medicus* for searching for references to a key word or topic. The 2000 edition of the *Cumulated Index Medicus* (CIM) was the last. The National Library of Medicine (NLM) decided to cease publication of this well-known and classic resource with volume 41. CIM enabled researchers to search by either author or subject for an entire year's worth of articles in a single volume. However, CIM became less essential in this computerised age, and subscriptions steadily declined.

Internet searchers tend to use either the NLM PubMed@UCLA or Medline search service that offers free and easy access to the *Index Medicus* citations, or any one of a variety of 'for a fee' commercial products that also provide this information.

The internet is now the almost universal way of searching the literature. It is worth noting here that if you are going to be serious about doing online searches and downloading data from your computer at home, you should consider a broadband package. This is very easy to install and use, and so much cheaper than the time you are taking on the phone line, a whole lot quicker and also means that your phone line is not out of use for telephone calls while your computer is using it.

The Doctors.net.uk website is an ideal place to start, although your own medical school, the postgraduate medical centre, local medical school or university will also be easy sources to use. In addition, many universities and medical Royal Colleges have facilities, although in these latter cases you may need to register. Below are a few sites to help you commence your search:

Doctors.net.uk alone will access:

- Medline, an invaluable resource for health science professionals. Many of the references in this book were checked on this source.

- The Cochrane Library, a source for evidence-based medicine (EBM).

- Bandolier, another useful source for EBM.

- *BMJ*'s Clinical Evidence, a useful source for EBM but only providing abstracts of articles.

- NHS Centre for Reviews and Dissemination (CRD), providing access to information on effectiveness of treatments, with delivery and organisation of healthcare.

- The National electronic Library for Health (NeLH), a digital library which is comprised of some 70 resources.

- Anatomy.tv and a range of specialist libraries.

- Teratology, with detailed information about drug and chemical exposures during pregnancy, management of infective and other conditions during pregnancy, and the effect of drugs and chemicals on breastfeeding.

- Toxbase, the primary clinical toxicology database of the National Poisons Information Service contains specific information on around 14,000 pharmaceuticals, chemicals, and other poisons. Travax includes country specific information on vaccination schedules, malaria prevention, risk assessment sheets, special needs, lifestyles, latest updates on disease outbreaks and much more.

- The Joint Planning and Advisory Committee (JPAC), with guidelines covering the whole transfusion chain from the selection of donors, through collection, testing, processing and use of blood products.

- The National Institute for Clinical Excellence (NICE), where you can update yourself on technology appraisals and Clinical Guidelines.

- The Scottish Intercollegiate Guidelines network (SIGN), where you can select guideline topics on the basis of the burden of disease, evidence of variation in practice, and the potential to improve outcome.

There are also some online textbooks (*Fundamentals of Surgical Practice*, *Oxford Textbook of Medicine*, *Oxford Textbook of Psychiatry*, *Oxford Textbook of Geriatric Medicine*, *Oxford Textbook of Nephrology* and *Oxford Textbook of Paediatrics*) and the following journals:

- *Encyclopaedia Britannica*, the oldest and largest general reference in the English language, with more than 70,000 articles and free abstracts for members.

- *PLoS Medicine*, an open-access, peer-reviewed journal published monthly by the Public

Library of Science. PLoS Medicine publishes the most significant advances in all medical disciplines, including epidemiology and public health.

- Merck Manual of Diagnosis and Therapy, full text of the 17th (Centennial) edition.

- *OMNI* (*Organising Medical Networked Information*) a free UK-based gateway to resources in medicine, biomedicine, allied health, and related topics.

- The *British Medical Journal (BMJ)*, with a full-text access to the current edition (and a restricted-access archive of previous editions). Articles from January 1994 give not only abstracts but full texts.

- *The Lancet*, a journal of review, news, and opinion fully accessible through free registration.

- The *Journal of the American Medical Association (JAMA)*: a subscription is required for full-text articles.

- The *New England Journal of Medicine* (*NEJM*), the oldest continuously-published medical journal in the world. A subscription is required for full text articles.

The Online Librarian has a collection of links to help you navigate the net along with finding out more about searching the net, NLH and libraries you may even want to dip into the 'odds and ends' where one or two curiosities jostle alongside links to medical images. There is also a patient information section with examples of leaflets explaining conditions and treatment to patients. This extensive library enables you to print leaflets off for you to give to your patients.

Most of the medical Royal Colleges have libraries with internet search facilities but vary in the amount of text available other than abstracts. Many universities and medical schools have similar facilities, but most require you to register with them and use passwords.

From these you will obtain citations, in many cases abstracts, and in a few cases copies of articles of your references. Your first attempt can often be daunting. If you can obtain the help of a qualified librarian or an experienced colleague then do so. You first need to precisely define your search subject. Are there synonyms? Alternative spellings (particularly if searching American

sources!)? You also need to decide how far back you want the search to go. The further back you search, the more you will find, the less likely you are to get copies online, and so the more time-consuming it becomes. Good research needs a framework or a set of stages, not necessarily chronological, which should be systematically addressed whatever the scale of the project. Choosing the topic and formulating the problem that is feasible within the timescale is just the beginning.

Information technology in research

The increasing use of electronic media in medicine produces problems with confidentiality and data protection with regard to letters, results systems, clinic schedules, digital photography, radiology pictures, virtual consultations via the web, and email.

There are some basic rules consistent with current advice that applies to all these situations:

- computers must be physically secure and away from public access

- monitors must be placed so their screens face away from public view

- all data must be password protected

- staff with access must be aware of their duty of confidentiality

- data can only be transmitted via the internet with suitable encryption

- all printouts should be treated as confidential and refiled in patients' notes or destroyed after use.

This means that data on a laptop are secure only if it is kept in a locked office, does not leave the building, and has a password lock. You cannot take your laptop home with identifiable patient data on it. Information on computers will not be removed completely from the hard disc, even when deleted. Accidental deletions are a recurrent topic on the doctors.net.uk computing forum, and software is readily downloadable to restore lost files. There are programmes that can make the hard drive impossible to read, but destroying the hard drive is the only really sure method.

Junior doctors and data protection

Junior doctors who make personal records of patient data, for example, for training logbook purposes, should be aware of the provisions of the Data Protection Act. If patient data are recorded on, for example, personal computers, and those data can identify a patient, then the data must be held subject to the provisions of the Data Protection Act. This would require the doctor to be registered for this purpose. Furthermore, the transfer of such data between trusts is a breach of the Data Protection Act.

The BMA therefore advises junior doctors not to record the data with the patient's name, though data which can be matched to a patient only through use of a hospital record system or separate second data set are lawful on an unregistered computer. For example, a hospital number can only identify a patient if cross-referred with the hospital records system. It is probably wise to consult your medical Royal College if you feel you are at risk of being in breach of the Act. Manual records have also been within the scope of the Data Protection Act since March 2000.

Developing IT skills

Developing the necessary skills to make best personal use of IT requires an investment more in time than in equipment, and the earlier the investment is made the greater the potential benefit. Ideally you will have a real need to use IT, such as a research project. This is likely to provide the necessary motivation to complete the learning and integrate it into practice. Essential components are a period of structured training, access to technology and a clear goal to attain relevant IT skills as part of the project. A combination of books, perhaps local courses and direct supervision allow you to focus on skills that are most useful to your project. Progression from simpler tasks (e.g. email, word processing and slide presentations) towards the more complex (e.g. spreadsheets, databases and project management) provides positive feedback and avoids frustration. Some trusts encourage staff to study for and obtain the European Computer Driving License (ECDL). This is a distance-learning course designed to provide participants with competence in all of the main packages available on work-based computers.

Starting the written stages

Aims, objectives or hypotheses

Set out what you want to achieve and how. This will influence your choice of methodological approach and design of the study. The purpose of the research can be set out as a statement of aims, or as a research hypothesis, or both. In health research the range of possible methodologies is vast, stretching from classical quantitative or scientific methods through a variety of structured and semi-structured designs and surveys, to qualitative approaches. You also need to identify resource implications, and may need to seek approval from your local ethics committee.

Pilot study for data collection

Having planned the study, including your forms for data recording, questionnaires, attitude scales, equipment needed to detect flaws in design, etc, a pilot study is essential. When happy with this you can then proceed to full data collection.

Preparation for writing

Having carried out all the work, you then need to prepare the data for analysis and present the findings in a structured way. It might be helpful to re-read the section on writing reports (*see* p. 46). It is also helpful to evaluate and reflect on how the research was carried out and whether parts could have been done differently or better. The research process can be thought of as a cycle, where having worked through all stages you may well find yourself back at the beginning, rethinking the topic and formulation of the study. Each stage is interconnected with every other stage. For example, inadequate funding may mean revision of the scope of the project. To obtain an overview of the process, it is helpful to consider each stage independently.

Writing journal articles

Getting yourself published adds greatly to your curriculum vitae. You may also make a contribution to your professional colleagues' understanding. Publishing research results in refereed journals is, obviously, most attractive, but is also difficult. You are unlikely to approach the record of one published medical researcher, Meir Stampfer, of

Harvard University who, according to *Science Watch Journal*, recently achieved 34,872 citations; surely the world's most prolific medical researcher! You may learn and grow your confidence by getting an article or two accepted by a non-refereed journal. If you are unsure of how to start, ask more senior colleagues to share their experience with you. Having selected a journal, it is essential to obtain a copy of authors' instructions from the publisher. Study the style and approach of examples of previously successful articles before submitting your own.

Creating structure

Here are ten steps to guide you from initial idea to final article. The actual layout you use will be guided by reference to 'authors' notes' set out by the journal you are aiming at, and also the house style of that journal.

1　Consider all the implications of your idea and ask yourself 'so what am I trying to say?'

2　What do you want a reader to do, say or think after they have read your article? In other words what are you trying to achieve?

3　Make a plan of the points in your argument to ensure the article flows from point to point.

4　Try to capture your reader's interest in the first paragraph.

5　Try to keep your reader's interest by telling them what you are going to say and what you have said.

6　Do not assume others have your level of knowledge, so explain and put them fully in the picture.

7　Discuss, analyse and give reasons for your ideas and arguments.

8　Illustrate by using headings, charts, tables, graphs and pictures, wherever necessary, to clarify and emphasise your points and so break up the text.

9　Summarise and finish by presenting your key conclusions, recommendations and ideas for other readers, prompting further research and discussion.

10　Show a draft to one or more colleagues or friends for comments and honest criticisms,

then choose the one you want to take notice of because you will inevitably receive contradictory opinions. Maybe also ask advice and help from people who have published before.

Common style issues

- When using acronyms, the most common style is to use capitals for each letter pronounced (e.g. BBC and NHSE), otherwise, if pronounced as a single word acronym, use upper and lower case (e.g. Unesco and Aids).

- Capitals slow the reader down and should be kept to a minimum. Avoid pompous initial capitals as in 'the Doctors', 'the Nurses' but 'the patients'. Words like 'Department', 'Authority' and 'Mission Statement' do not need initial capitals.

- Christian names are not appropriate for multi-racial societies; it is preferable to use 'first' name.

- Exclamation marks should be used extremely sparingly.

- Avoid stereotyping, for example doctors as male and nurses as female.

- 'Include' is a splendid word for writers because it allows for any complaint that the list is incomplete.

- Monologophobia is the fear of using the same word more than once in the same sentence or passage. This fear is overrated and can lead to confusion when, for example, authors use 'study', 'research' and 'investigation' in one paragraph to describe the same activity.

Some important points to remember:

- check your spelling and grammar. Nothing spoils credibility more. This is the responsibility of the author, not the typist

- avoid padding, which only detracts. Clarity and brevity attract the reader's attention

- ensure accuracy

- do not make assumptions unless they are clearly stated

- check that what you say is justified by evidence from within the report. You may not be there when the reader seeks justification

- If a sentence requires a lot of punctuation, break it up into shorter sentences.

- limit yourself to one idea per paragraph

- do ask someone else to read it and make comments.

Review

Here are ten questions you could ask yourself about the article after it is written.

1 Is it interesting to read?

2 Is it clearly written?

3 Is it relevant to previous work?

4 Is it built on and relevant to the existing body of knowledge?

5 Is there clear evidence and objectivity?

6 Is there quality and logical progression in your arguments?

7 What are the theoretical and practical implications?

8 Does it meet editorial objectives?

9 Have I left it for a while and then re-read it?

10 Have I asked a few others what they think of it?

When your work has been submitted, what will referees look for in your paper? They will consider all the questions set out above. They will also try to identify both strengths and weaknesses of the methods, and examine whether the physical measurements, equipment, questionnaires, attitude scales and so on are appropriate to the question posed. Was there a pilot study and data collection to detect any flaws in the design? With the data preparation and analysis, what analysis was required to test the research hypothesis? Are the data at the appropriate level of measurement for the planned statistical tests? Had it received ethics committee approval? Was the methodology appropriate? Could it have been done differently or better?

It is not just the role of those evaluating research to decide whether or not to make changes or innovations based on the findings. As a practising clinician you need to be able to evaluate papers you read in journals which suggest changes in practice. Researchers make an enormous contribution to innovations and changes in practice, but ultimately they only really provide the mechanism for that consideration.

Action

Do not expect the skills to come easily, particularly at first. Persevere, and learn from your many mistakes – you will find that you have at your disposal an extremely useful tool. Once you are satisfied with a plan, remind yourself of your brief, arm yourself with your plan and start writing. The majority of writers on writing suggest that you write the whole piece (or, if it is a long one, a substantial part of it) in one go. This will ensure that the piece is consistent.

Obtain copies of medico-legal reports carried out by more than one experienced person, and study style and layout. Consider the following and decide whether each is fact, feeling, value or opinion:

- waiting lists are still too high

- for the third year, despite our best efforts, waiting lists have increased

- waiting lists increased by 5% this year compared with last year

- waiting lists have increased substantially.

You may also want to consider writing up a case report of an interesting case or unusual presentation you have seen. You will need to do a literature search to ensure that no-one has already written up a whole series.

Or you might consider writing up a useful piece of audit you have been involved in, with a message that deserves wider dissemination.

Next time you read a paper in a journal, consider whether there are any flaws in the work. Was it a valid piece of work, logical, well reasoned, etc?

Presenting a curriculum vitae

The last part of this chapter is devoted to a subject that many find daunting and about which we have had many questions in workshops. Perversely, it is becoming less necessary as more and more deaneries and trusts opt for application forms, although it is a skill worth having for occasions when you might need to present a curriculum vitae (CV). Better-designed application forms will ask for information similar to the way in which you might have presented it in your CV, so it remains a useful exercise to keep one up to date.

To find the job you want, you need to know and understand the market, which varies among specialties. You can do this by attending meetings, talking to people and doing some investigations. Meanwhile, you should be assembling facts for your CV. You need to ask yourself the question 'Is it the right job for me?'. To do so you need the details, job description and person specification. You might also find it useful to talk to others, including your consultants, who know you, the situation generally, the job and the hospital.

Applications for jobs should be clear and concise, typewritten so that they are easy to read, well prepared and presented, accurate and up to date. They may require submission either via an application form or by a CV, or a mixture of both. The choice for which is used seems to vary. An application form has the advantage for the selectors of excluding information not relevant to the application, thereby standardising the process and making it fairer and easier for short-listing. CVs leave more scope for the applicant to show creativity and initiative. The applicant has more control over the selection process by including or excluding information from a CV. Applicants usually prefers CVs. Selectors prefer well-structured standard application forms.

Short-listing panels are generally under time pressure, so help them by being clear and concise and ensuring your CV is typewritten, well prepared, well presented, accurate and up to date. It should include personal details, qualifications, specialty experience, general experience, research and publications. Examination results and honours or distinctions, scholarships, prizes and other awards may be listed. It is usual to give a full list of your degrees and other qualifications with

dates awarded under this heading. Always add achievements outside your career.

One way of ensuring that your CV presentation is helpful to the selectors is to set it out in the order of items on the person specification supplied to all candidates. For example, if the person specification was as the example given in the BMA *Guidelines for Good Practice in the Recruitment and Selection of Doctors*, your CV headings would match and be as follows:

- Personal details
- Qualifications
- Clinical experience
- Clinical skills
- Knowledge
- Organisation and planning
- Teaching
- Research.

You need to look at the essential and desirable qualities in the person specification in each heading to identify the things to write about; these are mostly fairly obvious. Where this is not obvious, for instance in the example quoted, the features of 'organisation and planning' include audit, IT skills, experience in teams and understanding of the NHS and resource constraints. You would need to quote such examples of your experience in these areas.

Marital status, number of children and nationality are not required on a CV. Items such as GMC registration number and whether you have right of abode in the UK could be requested and should therefore be included. Writing your CV is not a process to be hurried. A word processor makes regularly updating your CV very much easier, and unless you do so it is easy to forget publications or other distinctive experience which will enhance your CV.

It is important to comply with instructions for applicants sent out by the hospital. Supply the correct number of copies (however unreasonable this may seem). Many hospitals require an application form to be completed. This can be a standard form for all members of staff and may therefore be inadequate for more senior medical posts, due to lack of space. It is best to complete the form, referring as necessary to the appropriate page of your CV, but again be aware that some hospitals state that this practice is not acceptable, in which case you will have to do the best you can with their form.

Application forms can be downloaded from the internet and it is becoming increasingly common. You can find out more by accessing www. nhsprofessionals.nhs.uk/doctors/. NHS Jobs is the national NHS site for jobs. It is linked with the NHS Careers site for information about careers in the NHS.

Downloaded application forms may be available in a number of ways. As 'MS word.documents' the form can be filled in directly on the computer, and any boxes enlarged to take account of the amount written within them. Or they may be written as 'Adobe.pdf' files, or maybe as files that can only be printed directly from the computer. Some of the former can be made to accept text with appropriate software so that you can complete the form on the computer. With the latter forms, software such as Paperport will scan the hard copy of the document and enable you to type directly onto the form. This can transform a handwritten form into a much neater and smarter application form. Check the instructions to ensure that you are not required to complete it by hand.

There is debate whether previous appointments should be put in chronological or reverse chronological order. Whatever you decide, include a brief summary of your experience. You may also want to classify these under general and specialty experience. Remember that you may need to emphasise certain parts in the light of the requirements of the job for which you are applying.

When recording your publications, accuracy is important. Interviewers occasionally check one or more publications, more for its quality than its existence, and will understandably be unimpressed if they cannot find it. As your publications become more plentiful you may wish to classify them as original papers, abstracts, editorials, chapters in books, books, reviews or letters, etc, and perhaps also note your contribution where there is more than one author. Add posters and presentations at scientific meetings, but only if you delivered the address. Poster displays are often published in abstract form and would thus normally appear under the list of publications, but it is not unreasonable to indicate both under the one heading.

Learned societies and committee membership may include other non-clinical or medical societies if you feel you can justify their inclusion, and committee chairmanship or a period as secretary would indicate managerial experience.

Other interests, whether cultural, sporting or recreational, should be mentioned, especially if they feature distinguishing excellence. Team sports give the impression of team membership, and a captaincy may suggest team leadership. Similarly, committee membership of a university or hospital club suggests organisational and administrative ability.

A short covering letter should accompany your application, mentioning the post for which you are applying and stating that you are enclosing copies of your CV and the names of referees. Referees are vital to your application and their choice is therefore important. The choice is still likely to be yours, although there is a trend towards requiring your current educational supervisor or supervising consultant to act as one of your referees. The choice requires considerable thought. They obviously need to think highly enough of you to support your application. Referees will sometimes show you the reference they have written for you, and this can be very helpful. Ask your referees' permission before submitting your application and supply them with copies of the job description and person specification, plus a copy of your CV. Also supply them with the likely date of the interview, so that if they are away at least their secretary will be able to notify the appointing hospital. It reflects badly on a candidate if the named referee has not sent a reference, and it may be assumed that the fault lies with the candidate not having allowed sufficient time.

Related reading

- Academy of Medical Royal Colleges (2005) *Guidance for Medical Expert Witnesses.* Academy of Medical Royal Colleges, London. www.aomrc.org.uk (accessed 26 April 2006).
- Albert T (1996) Effective writing. In: White A (ed.) *Textbook of Management for Doctors.* Churchill Livingstone, London. Useful tips on style and grammar.
- British Orthopaedic Association (2001) *Code of Practice for Medicolegal Reports in Personal Injury Cases.* London: British Orthopaedic Association.
- Albert T (2000) *Winning the Publications Game: how to get published without neglecting*

your patients (2e). Radcliffe Medical Press, Oxford.

- Allison GT (1971) *Essence of Decision. Explaining the Cuban Missile Crisis.* Little, Brown and Company, Boston. A fascinating insight into meetings at the very highest level and well worth reading in its own right.
- Berwick DM and Winickoff DE (1996) The truth about doctors' handwriting: a prospective study. *BMJ* 313:1657–8.
- Boyle CM, Young RE and Stevenson JG (1974) Letter: General practitioners' opinions of a new hospital-discharge letter. *The Lancet* 2(7878): 466–7.
- BMA (2000) *Guidelines for Good Practice in the Recruitment and Selection of Doctors.* BMA, London.
- Department of Health (1994) *Research and Development in the New NHS.* Department of Health, London.
- Gatrell J and White T (2000) *Medical Appraisal, Selection and Revalidation.* Royal Society of Medicine, London.
- Greenhalgh T (1997) A useful series of 11 articles in the *BMJ* beginning with 315:80.
- Gulleford J (1994) Preparing medical experts for the courtroom. No need to learn by trial and error. *BMJ* 309:752–3.
- General Medical Council (2001) *Good Medical Practice.* GMC, London.
- Gowers E (1986) *The Complete Plain Words* (3e). Revised by S Greenbaum and J Whitcut. HMSO, London.
- Harris D, Peyton R and Walker M (1996). Teaching in different situations. In: Royal College of Surgeons *Training the Trainers: learning and teaching.* Royal College of Surgeons, London.
- Hoyte P (1998) Writing medicolegal reports: what every doctor should know. *Hospital Medicine* 1:50–4.
- Working party of the Royal Colleges of Pathologists and of Paediatric and Child Health (2004) *Intercollegiate Report on Sudden Unexpected Death in Infancy: a multi-agency protocol for care and investigation* (September 2004). Access full text in 'Publications' at www.rcpath.org (accessed 25 April 2006).
- Klauser HA (1987) *Writing on Both Sides of the Brain.* Harper Collins, San Francisco, CA.
- Mann R and Williams J (2003) Related Articles (2003) Standards in medical record keeping. *Clinical Medicine* 3(4):329–32.
- NHS Executive (1998) *A Guide to Specialist Registrar Training.* NHS Executive, London.
- Roberts REI (1994) The trials of an expert witness. *Journal of the Royal Society of Medicine.* 87:628–31.
- www.nhsprofessionals.nhs.uk/doctors/

CHAPTER 4

Interpersonal communication

This chapter provides a range of tools and techniques for making the most of your effectiveness in face-to-face communications in a wide range of settings, from being interviewed for a job to making a presentation.

Introduction

We communicate with each other in order to seek, give and receive information; to inform, instruct, persuade, negotiate, motivate and encourage; to understand the opinions of others and so on. Interpersonal communication can be easy, happy and positive; it can be difficult, uncomfortable and challenging, or somewhere in between.

Various commentators agree that the impact on the listener in face-to-face communication is made up of 7% words, 38% voice tone and emphasis, and 55% body language. This is sometimes referred to as song, music and dance (see Figure 4.1).

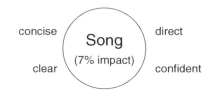

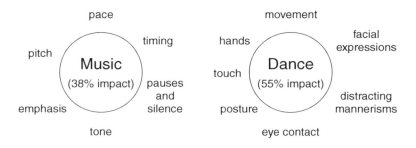

Figure 4.1 Verbal and non-verbal impact

Consider the anaesthetist who is reassuring a patient during the few minutes before they are taken into theatre. The effect of the doctor's hand on the patient's forearm as they hear the words has a far greater positive impact on their feelings than the words themselves.

This is not to suggest that the words that you use in, say, making a case for more resources are not important – they may catch you out if you do not do your research. It is the longer-term impact on the 'concrete experience' of the listener that is enhanced by the other, non-verbal signals they receive.

Core interviewing skills

A great deal of most doctors' time is spent in one-to-one meetings, many of which might be described as an interview. They may not always be labelled as such, but each time we need to find out about a patient, the opinions of a colleague, recruit, appraise or discipline a colleague, break bad news or deal with a complaint, we are using interviewing skills.

Perhaps the most important skill related to interviewing is that of questioning. A clear understanding of the use of different types of question is essential. You should remember, however, that getting the words right is only one part of the process. Your manner, tone of voice, facial expression and posture all go together with the words to influence the interviewee's willingness to 'open up'.

Selection interviewing

As with most things in life, interviews are usually much more effective if the panel has put in enough preparation time before the interview starts. Thought should be given to how a panel will work together, what the priorities are for the interviewers, what style of questioning will be used, how the seating should be arranged to put the candidate at ease, and so on. Panel members should have familiarised themselves with the paperwork and have a good idea about what approach they wish to take to questioning the candidates. The role of the chairperson is critical, particularly during the preparation stages which are aimed at getting the panel to work as a team, and then after the interview when the panel is concerned with making the right decision.

Types of questions and their uses

The following approach to using questions to elicit useful information is framed in the context of selection interviewing. The basic approach is transferable to most other interview situations. It helps if you think of interviews as conversations with a purpose. The most effective interviews will generally feel fairly relaxed, if challenging for the interviewee. The aim should be to help them to feel relaxed and prepared to open up about things that perhaps they had not intended.

Experiential or situational questions

Traditional approaches to medical interviews tended to allow candidates to supply set piece answers to well-signalled questions such as 'What do you understand to be the purpose of clinical governance?', or hypothetical questions which only tell the questioner that the interviewee may have a theoretical understanding of the topic, which has probably already been assessed in an examination: 'What would you do if you were faced with … ?'.

Questions that focus on the interviewee's past experience, their 'real life' events, are generally the most revealing. This requires skill to 'draw out' the interviewee. Such questions might start with 'Tell me about your work in …', or: 'Tell us about a situation in which you had to deal with …'. The answer is then probed in order to gain insight into the person's past behaviour patterns, motives, values, attitudes and personality. An approach whish uses *open* questions, followed by *probing* and *reflective* questions, is most likely to succeed in allowing you to understand the person.

Open questions

Open-ended questions oblige the interviewee to respond with a full answer – they do not permit a 'Yes' or 'No' response. They are likely to start with 'Why … ' or 'How …' or 'Tell me about …'. The aim is to get the interviewee to talk to you in their own words so that you can pick up hints which will allow you to probe more deeply.

Closed questions

These are useful when checking facts. They are generally phrased to attract a 'Yes' or 'No' response. You may need to be absolutely sure you have the information you need: 'Did you pass the examination?' or 'Was your paper published?' Closed questions can be unhelpful in some cases. In history taking, they may lead patients to give answers that match the doctor's assumptions rather than the patient's real symptoms.

Probing questions

Use probing questions to explore in greater detail actions, experiences and associated opinions and feelings which have been hinted at in the answers to earlier open questions. The candidate will not normally mind gentle interruptions with short questions, for example 'How did the patient respond to that treatment?' 'How did you feel when they did that?', or 'What did you do then?'.

Interruptions are usually acceptable if they are in the form of a probing or reflective question and the interviewer continues to show interest in the interviewee. This approach involves careful listening and some practice if it is to work well.

At the end of a response to an open question it can be effective to pause and allow the interviewee to give more detail or to expand on the last point made. A small gesture may be used, or you may merely add a comment such as: 'And … ?' Or 'Go on'.

Silence can also be a very effective way of getting the candidate to open up in areas they had not intended to tell you about. We sometimes feel uncomfortable if a long silence occurs during a conversation. This can lead us to fill it, usually with an ill-thought out and usually unhelpful contribution. Silence can have a positive effect in the interview. It can be used to put gentle pressure on the interviewee. This requires a discipline not always found in less experienced interviewers, who must stop themselves from talking while the seconds pass.

Reflective questions

These are for checking understanding, and also serve to elicit further explanation. They involve selecting a word, or a few words, from the interviewee's most recent response and feeding them back as a question: 'You felt unsure?' or: 'You took responsibility for the patient?'.

These questions work well in counselling situations, but can also be powerful in getting

interviewees in selection or appraisal interviews to go into greater depth regarding their motives and feelings.

Leading questions

Interviewers sometimes try to help the candidate to understand the question by first setting the context for it. The effect is to give the interviewee the answer in the question. These are seldom, if ever, helpful to the interviewer. For example, the interviewer might say: 'We attach a great deal of importance to good teamwork. How do you find you get on in teams?'.

It is far better to use the situational approach described above. Ask for the candidate's experience of particular types of work events (for example, situations they have found stressful), and then try to probe to uncover any successes or problems that have arisen, in particular those that relate to working closely with colleagues.

Presentation skills

Effective communication of ideas is fundamental to the development of professional knowledge. Postgraduate professional development is partly dependent on doctors sharing research and knowledge with colleagues in regular meetings. Your ability to make effective presentations can also have a significant effect on your career opportunities, since self-presentation is a key factor in attracting attention to your potential.

For the purpose of this section, presentations are taken to mean any situation in which you are required to communicate information, ideas, propositions or a report to an audience of any size. These might include presenting an audit report to a department, reviewing a paper, or contributing to a presentation with others. Making an effective presentation means knowing how to present your ideas, your research and yourself confidently and to the best advantage. Of course, you want to be able to do this without spending too long agonising over it. This section will help you make the most of your opportunities in making a good impression as a presenter in both formal and informal situations. It will do this by taking you through the processes involved in preparing a good presentation. That is, first selecting relevant material, then organising that material, and finally delivering it to the best effect.

The first important thing to realise about presentation situations is that, although our basic medium of communication is words, they account for only a small part of the total message. It is generally accepted that less than 10% of what you communicate will be concerned with your words, and some 90% will be concerned with the way you use your voice and with body language, such as facial expression, posture and gestures. You cannot give a good presentation unless you have done the right kind of careful preparation. As part of your preparation you must have the answers to six fundamental questions:

- *WHY am I speaking?* What is the purpose of the talk? Is it to inform, to teach, to make a proposition or to inspire and motivate? Defining your objective, preferably in a single sentence, will make preparation simpler and focus the talk.

- *To WHOM am I speaking?* The size, mix, level of understanding and attitudes of the audience must be taken into account during preparation. Levels of complexity and volume of information and ideas will depend on the likelihood that members of the audience can absorb them in the time available.

- *WHERE am I speaking?* Always visit the venue before your presentation unless it is impossible for you to do so. Check the equipment is working, decide where you will stand and whether your voice will carry without a microphone. Remember that the presence of an audience will deaden the impact and volume of your voice. Make sure the seating layout suits the kind of presentation you have in mind.

- *WHEN am I speaking?* If your presentation is to be made at the end of the working day, you will need to take into account the energy level of members of the audience. The duration of the talk should affect its structure and level of detail. Avoid trying to pack in too much for the audience to absorb in the time available. Audiences will get restless if you run over your allotted time, so keep to your plan. It helps to note the time by which you must finish and to place a watch in front of you at the beginning of your presentation.

- *WHAT am I going to say?* The content will be determined by the objective. Keep returning to your objective statement in order to avoid losing direction. The material is normally organised in one of the following ways:
  - a generalisation followed by detailed explanation/illustration
  - using a time, spatial or geographical sequence, or a sequence based on ascending or descending order of importance of each element
  - contrasting one set of facts/ideas with another
  - dividing a unit up into its component parts and saying a little about each.

Ask yourself which method will help you to present your material most effectively; when you've done that, you are ready to write the first draft. Most good presentations are divided into an introduction, which sets the scene and prepares the audience for what is to come: a main body comprised of three or four main points; and a conclusion, which summarises and emphasises the theme.

- Write your opening and closing sentences in full and learn them 'off by heart'.
- Capture the audience and tell them everything they need to know about the presentation in the opening.
- Make the conclusion really conclusive.

Remember that your presentation will be spoken. When you write your draft, write it in spoken English, not written English. This will help you to sound more natural, even when you are actually reading whole phrases or sentences from your cue cards (as most speakers do from time to time).

To help you achieve a clear, natural style, remember these tips:
- use simple, familiar words that come to you naturally
- only use technical jargon that your audience will understand
- use short sentences.

- *HOW am I going to say it?* Most speakers use notes or prompt cards, but speak from brief notes to avoid reading word for word. The use of voice and gesture as well as audiovisual aids requires careful thought, practice and self-awareness. For speaking notes:
  - use small cards rather than sheets of paper if possible. They are easier to hold and look more professional
  - write key sentences and key words on the cards

– fasten the cards together, or at least number them in sequence.

Effective delivery

This is achieved by paying attention to articulation, pace, intonation and emphasis. Good articulation can be achieved by practising enunciation in front of a mirror. Many speakers are 'lazy' in the way they form their sounds, not moving their lips and tongue enough. Keep your head up. Don't speak with your chin down in your collar.

- Pace should be varied to maintain interest. Nervous speakers always speak too quickly. Avoid racing! Pauses can be used for effect, but they also allow the listeners to absorb the points you are making and react to them.

- Intonation is the rhythm and inflection in the voice. Most people use only two or three tones of the musical scale when they speak. The Welsh and the Western Highlanders, on the other hand, use about an octave and a half. Get colour into your voice.

- Emphasis, often coupled with repetition, is a most useful speaking device. If your voice lacks colour, practise emphasising key words and phrases from your cue cards. Remember that you can also emphasise points by using appropriate (but not distracting) gestures.

In general:

- speak as naturally and conversationally as possible

- stand in a comfortable position with your feet slightly apart

- smile and be friendly

- maintain good eye contact with the whole audience

- check whether you have any distracting mannerisms and work to get rid of them. These may include excessive use of certain phrases or sounds such as 'you know', 'Um', 'Er' or 'You see'. Habits such as jingling keys or coins in a pocket, or pacing up and down like a caged tiger, can also be a barrier to effective communication with the audience.

Visual aids

Good use of visual aids will improve your presentation by helping your audience to remember what you have said more easily than if you use words alone. Visual aids used badly or carelessly can be very distracting and even irritating, and are often worse than none at all. Powerpoint is normally regarded as the most professional way to present, but avoid overdoing it. Too many slides and too much use of special effects can be distracting and even irritating for an audience.

- Check that equipment is in the right place and working properly before you begin.

- Be sure that everything is large enough to be seen by everyone in the room.

- Don't read from visuals – you insult the audience's intelligence.

- Face the audience, not the screen. If you have one, place your laptop so that you can glance at it from time to time.

- Each picture should have only one main message. Complex slides confuse and bore.

- Minimise the words on each visual. A maximum of 20 is a good rule of thumb.

- Words should be printed, and at least 20-point font size should be used.

- Always be prepared with back-up material, to cope if the machinery breaks down.

Handouts are sometimes used to support a presentation. It can sometimes be unhelpful to circulate them at the start of your presentation as they may become a distraction. On the other hand, many people like to have a copy of the presentation so that they can add notes to it as you speak. You should adapt your approach to suit the audience.

Taking questions

Decide whether you will take questions during or after your presentation and tell your audience your decision clearly in the introduction to your presentation. Listen carefully to the question and check that you've understood it. Repetition of the question also helps everyone in the room to

Action

Bearing in mind the above notes, describe in the space below what you see as your strengths and weaknesses as a presenter. If possible seek pointers from a colleague or friend who has seen you make presentations.

Strengths:

Weaknesses:

Now reflect on these, considering which of your weaknesses could be due to lack of experience or learning, and which are unchangeable. Seek to describe them in ways that help you to decide what improvements you need to make in your approach.

Now identify the types of situation in which you expect to make presentations over the next year or so:

At your next presentation, ask a couple of members of the audience (preferably friends who you can rely on to give you helpful feedback) to make notes about the way you make your presentation and tell you what they thought of it afterwards. You and they may find the checklist in Box 4.1 useful as a guide. Do not mention your perceived weaknesses to them beforehand, but quiz them about these aspects of your presentation when you get your feedback.

Good luck!

Box 4.1: Presentation feedback sheet

Content
Introduction

- Was the purpose clear?
- Was a link made with the audience?
- Did the speaker make an impact within the first two minutes?

Main body

- Was the talk pitched at a level to suit the audience?
- Were there clear stages?
- Did it follow a logical sequence?

Conclusions

- Was there a summary of key points?
- (If relevant) was there an indication of action to be taken, and by whom?

Voice

- Volume too loud/soft?
- Tone varied to maintain interest?
- Pace too fast/slow?

Timing

- Start and finish on time?

Stance

- Relaxed posture, facing audience?

Mannerisms

- Free from distraction, such as pacing, verbal habits?

Visual aids

- Relevant/simple and clear/technically proficient?

know exactly what is being answered. Do not expect questions to come as soon as you stop talking. You are expecting the audience to go into a different mode, so be prepared to wait or 'plant' a question in the audience to get things going. Keep your answers short as you may bore the rest of the audience.

Contributing to meetings

Meetings are a feature of professional life. They are a common event for clinicians representing colleagues, nurse managers and business managers. They are also expensive. They can waste time, for example when there is no clear objective to the meeting, or a lack of effective leadership and control, or there are too many or the wrong participants. Time is often wasted on debate about 'Why?' rather than 'How?'. In addition, a lack of clarity on outcomes produces unclear final decisions or even no decisions. Meetings which do not achieve results not only waste time, but can even lead to more meetings.

Types of meeting

There are many different kinds of meeting, including small group, support, events, clinical, staff, departmental, open or public, committees, workshops, learning sessions, conferences and so on. Every well-run meeting, whether formal or informal, is based on three prerequisites:

* clear aims

* careful planning

* effective teamwork.

Aims

Clear aims will be related to the purpose of the meeting. A departmental meeting may be for talking, listening and sharing problems. A committee normally aims to make and agree decisions, whereas a learning session is about sharing ideas through teaching and learning.

Always go to meetings knowing what you want to achieve. Advance preparation is vital, and that

applies to all participants. How often have you been at a presentation of a new idea and when participants have been asked to comment, nearly everyone has suggestions for improvements? No one had been given the opportunity to study the proposal in advance, everyone was seeing it for the first time. Discussions are lengthy and suggestions numerous. Other time wasters include fighting losing or lost battles by discussing items decided elsewhere or that are not within the group's power to decide.

Some reasons for meetings

Meetings can be called for all sorts of reasons other than reaching a decision, and these can be classified as follows:

* creating and developing ideas, for example brainstorming sessions

* sharing out work and responsibility – usually valuable for small groups only

* delegation of work or authority within a group

* sharing responsibility for a difficult problem

* providing or receiving information – there may be better ways

* persuasion – best done before the meeting

* networking, which become 'talking shops'

* an alternative to preparing a short written report

* committees in the habit of meeting without a real purpose, even with lengthy agendas

* socialising – acceptable at the beginning of a meeting, but do keep it short

* perhaps as a substitute for work.

Decision making at meetings

Decision making on tasks or issues may be a valid reason for calling a meeting, but you need to ask yourself if it is:

* consulting before a decision is made

- gathering information for a decision to be made elsewhere

- gaining agreement on a decision

- seeking a decision that requires the agreement of more than one group

- enhancing commitment to a decision

- making a decision.

Why go to a meeting?

Any meeting you attend is your meeting too. Do you know why you're going? At every meeting you should have a personal objective(s).

Planning for a meeting

Make sure you are fully prepared, otherwise you are failing to be an effective member. It may be the opportunity to put across a message. A seed sown today might be important for later. You can often turn someone else's question into a bridge for your own message. A question directed at you, in any situation, will always give you an opportunity to say what you want. Always answer the question and then make your point. If you are asked a question and you don't know the answer it is perfectly acceptable to say: 'I don't know but I'll find out and let you know' and then go on to your statement, via a suitable link. You can also use the same technique in response to a statement, by agreeing with that statement, before linking to your own statement. Here the speaker becomes the leader and controls the meeting while speaking. This is observable at medical committees.

Seating arrangements

Semicircles are good for problem-solving meetings and provide a good balance of control and sensitivity for the leader. Long tables are control mechanisms and inhibit brainstorming sessions. It is impossible to see others down the same side of the table, and discussions between participants is limited. The more the eye contact and the more people it is made with, the more control you have.

To some extent where you sit will depend on your purpose. If you want to be uninvolved pick a position that permits that. If you are seeking to win a point or plan seizing control, pick a controlling position. At a long table this will be at either end. At a three-sided arrangement this will be either side of the chair or at either end. At a long table, an ally at the other end of the table will give you maximum support in handling a difficult meeting.

Next time you are at a meeting observe where people sit and see how it influences their roles. If you are going to be a competitor to the chair, sit as far away as possible. The ideal position is opposite, so that you can talk directly to the chair and include others as well.

General meeting techniques

Interruptions

Knowing when to interrupt to gain control is a useful tool. Asking a question is a useful way of interrupting and changing the direction of the meeting. Always maintain a moderate tone and remember that the greatest impact you have will be through your non-verbal communication.

- 'Have you considered … ?'

- 'Could I add … ?' and continue speaking.

- Call the person by name, 'John, don't forget …', and continue speaking.

- Just start speaking and raise your voice above the level of the other person.

Do not wait for permission to be granted before you interrupt, but continue talking. It is often difficult to hang back while someone presents something that you consider inappropriate. But do think twice before making yourself vulnerable by interrupting the speaker, as your own point may not be quite as perfect as you thought.

If you want to prevent yourself being interrupted:

- insist on finishing by saying: 'Please, just let me finish …' and continue

- hold your hand up, palm outwards, and continue.

Criticism

If your suggestion should be the subject of criticism, ask the critic to present an analysis of your proposal with workable alternatives for the next meeting. Emotion can resist logic. When someone is emotionally aroused, your best ploy is to remain silent until their emotion peters out.

Opposition

When you are up against opposition your objective should always be to determine your opponent's objectives. There is nothing wrong with having a different objective. Ask yourself what your opponent wants and why they want it. Better still, ask them. Only when you know your opponent's priorities can you plan your own strategy.

Confrontation

If you are disagreeing with someone, try to provide your opponent with a way out, a way to save face. If you disagree, first state what you agree with, thus supporting their position as modified by your own. Make criticism less personal by claiming you are acting as the 'devil's advocate'.

Contribute early

Research indicates that when a person contributes early in a discussion, they are likely to exert a greater influence throughout the discussion. Asking questions for clarification or to challenge assumptions is a positive way to contribute at an early stage. This will help you to establish where others stand before committing yourself. This also obliges others to respond to you, but be prepared to come back into the discussion to combat opposing arguments.

Being interviewed

Before we address the interview, it might be worth reflecting on the importance of your CV (*see* p. 64) or application as a basis for firstly, being short-listed and secondly, providing a sound basis for the panel to prepare questions.

Action

There is an important difference between a stimulating discussion and a productive meeting. For the next meeting you attend, ask yourself:

- what is the purpose of this meeting?
- what should I achieve by the end?
- how will I distinguish my success from failure?

After the meeting ask yourself:

- was I correct about the task?
- were the other participants clear about the task and objectives?
- did I achieve the meeting's objective as stated in the agenda?
- was the meeting a success or failure?
- if it was a failure, why?
- what could be done to improve the next meeting?
- what was done that should be discontinued?
- what could the chairperson do to improve the meeting?
- could you have done without the meeting?
- if so, how?

You should remember that at least some of the panel will never have met you, so their first impressions will be coloured by the quality of your application paperwork. There is useful guidance on this topic in a couple of articles from *BMJ Careers* which are referenced at the end of this chapter (*see* pp. 77–8).

Prepare everything the day before and allow plenty of time by arriving early and having all possible questions and your answers totally revised and memorised. You need to convince the panel that you will achieve your goals or, in the case of a consultant appointment, make a delightful colleague.

The size of appointment committees tends to grow in relation to the seniority of appointment, although there are guidelines and statutory regulations for the composition of selection committees. In the case of consultant interviews, it is not uncommon for the main interview process to be enhanced by a series of smaller interviews with small groups (say three or four persons) from the multidisciplinary team. These are used to help other future colleagues to have a say in who they will be working with, as well as giving you greater insight into the culture of the organisation. Apart from consultants within a specialty, members of the main selection committee will not all know one another. You can be reassured that even some of the panel members may feel in strange surroundings, and many panel members also confess privately to some nervousness.

As a general rule you should dress to reassure and fit the stereotype of the post for which you have applied. Go into the room positively, smiling and determined to enjoy it. It will not be as bad as a viva examination. Try to:

• be relaxed but business-like

• sit upright

• be friendly, smile with perhaps a degree of authority

• look initially at the chairperson, who should put you at your ease

• show enthusiasm for the job.

Interview questions

Routine questions (usually from the chair) about your journey or finding the place help to 'break the ice' and are usually followed by some more routine questions to clarify any queries with your CV, such as unusual features or gaps. The questions then tend to move on to asking you your reasons for wanting the job or what attracted you to it. This is an opportunity to show that you have researched the hospital. Perhaps you have identified a significant challenge that the institution faces. Take care to avoid appearing critical of the trust or its management; they are unlikely

to warm to someone who hardly knows them and who finds fault. The next questions are likely to explore your future career direction. Be enthusiastic and do not give evasive answers. The questions are usually fairly straightforward, and simply aimed at getting you to talk about yourself. Do so with a mixture of confidence, enthusiasm, honesty and maturity as appropriate to the question (it is as easy as that!). Always address your answer initially to the questioner but look around and try to engage all the panel members with your answer.

Be neither monosyllabic nor loquacious; balance is important. Even if asked closed questions, avoid the temptation to give simple 'Yes' or 'No' answers. Try and expand the answer to allow the interviewer time to recover. You will gain no friends by making him or her feel uncomfortable.

The panel will normally have agreed in advance to split up questions into a number of areas, each covered by one panel member. You might be asked about your vision for the hospital and department, what you think of the hospital, or what you have to offer. Typical questions ask about research you have done or intend to do, your experience of clinical audit, government reports that affect you, and the NHS generally, as well as possible future plans and changes in NHS.

There may be questions that seek to reveal 'what makes you tick'. These are usually about hobbies and outside interests. Avoid suggesting these might interfere with your work! Aptitudes and outside interests are a measure of whether you are a well-rounded personality.

Talking about strengths and weaknesses

The interviewers may try to reveal your virtues and weaknesses, perhaps by asking about your mistakes or weakness directly, or your aptitudes and ambitions. Answers tend to reveal your personal values. Questions about weakness, mistakes, tasks that you could have done better, or opportunities missed gauge your self-awareness, intellectual honesty, maturity and dependability, and may relate indirectly to your team-membership characteristics. There are no right answers to these questions, but it is worth thinking in advance about mistakes you have made, difficult situations you have been in, and times when you have felt out of your depth and hope you coped, and what you learned from these experiences. Pressure questions about previous failed interviews may also give clues about your ability to cope with stress, your maturity and your emotional stability.

Questions about your greatest achievements, challenges or responsibilities are an attempt to obtain a record of your standards, your qualities of management and relationships, as well as your leadership style and ability, and whether you are a process- or people-oriented person. Questions about relationships are trying to assess relationships with colleagues by view of personality: social or self-contained; conforming or independent; extrovert or sensitive; phlegmatic or excitable.

Handling difficult panel members

These are the ones who ask tricky questions that are intended to impress the committee with the questioner's skill. If you are asked that sort of question, stay calm, and if you find you are struggling remember that only better candidates get asked difficult questions to separate them, and that committee members usually have sympathy for candidates being given a difficult time by colleagues.

Handling silence

If there is silence after your answer you are being invited to continue. Do not be embarrassed by silence, even if you need time to think about your answer. Allow yourself time to think before answering, so that your replies are considered and logical. Do not be tempted to leap in and say something ill-considered. You need not be embarrassed to have a question clarified if you are not clear what you are being asked, but do not waste time looking for hidden catches. Remember the interviewers are usually seeking reassurance. Do make sure you are answering the question asked. With multiple questions try to remember the individual questions or clarify before answering.

Conclusion

Try to appear friendly, cheerful and smiling. Body language helps with a businesslike authoritative attitude, professional appearance and energetic approach. At the end of the interview you are generally invited by the chair to ask the panel any questions you might have. While it will not count against you to ask a question, it is acceptable and possibly desirable not to do so.

Panel presentations

This is a developing method of helping to assess candidates for consultant appointments, and is thought to be a reasonable way of assessing the vision of candidates in relation to the future of a unit. Whether the candidate has grasped the problems of the unit in pre-interview visits and has a realistic expectation of what they are coming to will also be apparent. Some candidates like it as a way of being in control of the first part of the interview, whereas others feel uncomfortable making presentations, particularly as it will not usually be a part of their everyday work. It does illustrate the importance of making sure you collect useful information from the clinical director, medical director, chief executive and chairman when paying your pre-application visit.

Related reading

- Allison GT (1971) *Essence of Decision. Explaining the Cuban Missile Crisis.* Little, Brown and Company, Boston.
- Heshan Ariyasena, Tewari N and Livesley PJ (2005) The search for the perfect curriculum vitae. *BMJ Careers* 331:167–9.
- Bradbury A (2000) Successful Presentation Skills. Kogan Page, London.
- Erin S (2004) Writing a Winning CV. *BMJ Careers* 328:225.
- Gatrell J and White T (2000) *Medical Appraisal, Selection and Revalidation.* Royal Society of Medicine, London.
- Gray C (2005) Fair interviewing is harder than it looks. *BMJ Career Focus* 331:68–9.

- Reynolds P and Harrison M (2005) Consultant interviews are different. *BMJ Career Focus* 331:73.
- Scoote M, Elkington A and Thaventhiran J (2004) How to prepare for your first specialist registrar interview. *BMJ Career Focus* 328: 233–5.
- White A and Gatrell J (1996) Being interviewed. In: A White (ed.) *Textbook of Management for Doctors*. Churchill Livingstone, London.
- White A (1996) Managing meetings. In: A White (ed.) *Textbook of Management for Doctors*. Churchill Livingstone, London.

CHAPTER 5

Non-clinical involvement with patients

The aim of this chapter is to guide you through the process of obtaining consent, breaking bad news, handling patient complaints and dealing with administrative aspects of post mortems and coroners' inquests.

Consent

Consent means more than simply getting a signature on a consent form. While there is no English statute setting out the principles of consent, it is a general legal and ethical principle that valid consent must be obtained from the patient before starting any treatment or physical investigation or procedure, or providing any personal care. Case law has established that touching a patient without valid consent could result in action under civil or criminal offence of battery. Should the patient claim lack of knowledge, and he/she suffers harm as a result of treatment, this could be a factor in a claim of negligence against an individual health practitioner.

The patient should, therefore, be given sufficient information to understand the treatment or procedure, and should be fully aware of what can go wrong. Health professionals should also be able to provide evidence that such consent and information has been given. If something is not documented, in a court of law it will generally be assumed that it has not been done. If the basic requirements have not been met and something goes wrong, the door is open for litigation – and the continued growth in litigation is something of which all doctors must be aware.

Case law on consent evolves constantly. Doctors must also be aware that it is their duty,

and in their interests, to keep themselves abreast of legal developments. Advice from a senior doctor or lawyer should be sought if you have any doubt about the validity of an intervention.

Other legislation affecting consent include The Human Rights Act 1998, The Human Tissue Act 1961, The Care Standards Act 2000, The Family Law Reform Act 1969 and The Children Act 1989.

In November 1998 the GMC published a booklet 'Seeking Patients' Consent: the ethical considerations'. Since then there have been a number of legal developments that need to be reflected in the guidance, including legislation relating to adults who lack capacity, and on the retention, use and storage of human tissue. The contents of the booklet are therefore under review during 2006 but the original 1998 booklet can been seen online at www.gmc-uk.org by typing 'seeking patients' consent' in the search facility or clicking on 'guidance for doctors' then 'guidance library' and then 'consent' in the left hand column.

Seeking consent

You must only seek consent from a patient if you are knowledgeable about the intervention that is proposed. For consent to be valid it has to be given voluntarily by a person (the patient or, where relevant, another person who has parental responsibility for a patient under 18 years (see below)) who has the capacity to give consent.

So, if you are seeking consent you must consider the following:

- does the patient have capacity to give consent?
- is the consent given voluntarily?
- has the patient received sufficient information?
- is there a likelihood of additional procedures?
- what are the associated risks?
- are there any alternative treatments?
- is there going to be any tissue removed?
- is there going to be video recording or clinical photography?
- is the patient going to be involved in any research or innovative treatment?

It is, therefore, quite clear that when you are asked by a senior colleague, or other healthcare professional, to seek informed consent, procedures have to be explained in detail to patients, and you have to be aware of your responsibilities in the event of a positive response to the previous questions. In this situation, theoretical knowledge may not be able to replace practical experience. In the case of more major and complex procedures, consent should therefore be obtained by someone more senior, if only because there can be more complications.

Dealing with patients in obtaining consent provides an important learning opportunity. You must remember that patients may be extremely nervous, very anxious or fearful, and they may not be able to understand the implications of what they are being told.

Many problems can be considered at the time at which you list patients for elective surgery. Many consultants do discuss the procedure with the patient at this stage, so it makes sense to obtain consent at the same time, although it is not always clear what patients will need before they come into hospital. There is also the problem of a long wait prior to the admission. It is held as best practice guidance to seek consent again if six months have passed. There is however no statute at present to enforce this, in that it is held that valid consent once given, has infinite duration. It must be remembered that the patient's condition could change, new information may be available, or the benefit of the proposed intervention may have altered.

Patients can also withhold or withdraw consent – further information is given about these circumstances later in this chapter (*see* p. 81).

You should use every opportunity possible to develop your skills in dealing with patients at this stage. Ask to sit in with experienced consultants when they have to obtain consent in difficult circumstances. There are certain circumstances where consent cannot be obtained due to the condition of the patient immediately before the procedure is to be carried out, or if an individual is incapable of giving consent.

Emergencies and the temporary incapacity to give consent

An adult who is usually able to give consent can be rendered temporarily incapable to provide consent due to an emergency situation such as a road traffic accident or sudden illness. Unless there are advance refusals of treatment, then a doctor is permitted by law to make interventions that are necessary and are reasonably required in the patient's best interests. As a general rule, treatment given without consent should be the minimum amount necessary, and any treatment which could be reasonably postponed, be delayed until the patient recovers capacity.

Permanent or long-standing incapacity

Where an adult is permanently incapacitated, or if the incapacity is likely to be long-standing then it is lawful to carry out interventions which are in the best interests of the adult. Case law judgements have stated that the patients' best interests extend beyond their medical interests, but also covers routine procedures such as basic care, and the provision of nutrition and adequate fluids.

Although it has no validity in court, it is best practice to involve the adult's family or friends closest to him/her in the requirements for the patient, and to ask them to sign the standard consent form.

Fluctuating capacity

It is possible that incapacity is transient or can fluctuate. It is therefore good practice to gain consent when the patient is capable, and to remember to also obtain consent in advance for . interventions that may be necessary when the adult is incapacitated.

Consent for medical research

The same legal principles apply to obtaining consent for research as to seeking consent for investigations or treatment. The GMC states that particular care should be taken, as you must remember that there may be no benefit for the individual to participate in research projects. The patients must be given ample time to think about the implications of the research, and they must never be pressurised.

All research projects involving patients will generally have had to receive formal and written approval by the hospital's ethics committee.

The same applies to requesting patients' permission to use their medical images in any way. A patient consent form is available on the *BMJ* website.

Children and young people

The legal position for children and young people under the age of 18 years concerning consent (and refusal of treatment) is different from that of adults.

As a general principle consent for the treatment of children of less than 16 years is obtained from an adult holding parental responsibility for the child.

Young people aged 16–17 years are entitled to consent to their own medical treatment. All the same principles pertaining to consent, and to capability to give consent, apply to these young people as they do to adults. However, this consent may be overridden by an adult with parental responsibility, or a court.

Children under 16 years – the concept of 'Gillick competence'

Following the case of *Gillick* v. *West Norfolk & Wisbech AHA* (1986) the concept of 'Gillick

competence' must be understood by all doctors involved in obtaining consent from children.

Following this case the courts have held that children who have the ability to demonstrate sufficient understanding and have the intelligence to understand fully what is involved in a proposed treatment also have the capacity to consent to that treatment, or indeed to refuse treatment.

Junior doctors finding themselves in complex situations should seek advice from their senior colleagues, and if necessary, from legal advisors. Such circumstances are likely to be fraught with distress and emotion, and must be approached with empathy and caution. The legal situation is highly complex, and the courts have significant powers under certain circumstances.

Advance statements/directives (also commonly referred to as living wills)

The purpose of an advance statement/directive is to enable individuals to let people know of their preferences about future medical treatment that they would like to have, or refuse, especially if they are in a condition which prevents them from making their own views known. People who understand the implications of their choice can state in advance how they wish to be treated if they suffer a loss of mental capacity.

All junior and senior doctors have to come to terms with their own response to the statement: 'every adult has the right to consent to or to refuse treatment' – and that includes resuscitation. Many health professionals, particularly doctors and nurses, have considerable difficulty in *not* giving treatment to patients, and struggle with the personal objectives of helping people versus the need to respect each individual's decisions. This is something that you need to consider before you are face to face with these specific situations.

Common law establishes that a decision to receive or refuse treatment made by an adult who has been fully informed and who can understand the implications has the same legal power whether it is spontaneous or made in advance.

The advance statement of a person under 16 years is not legally binding. However, where capacity has been assessed as present, their wishes should be considered.

In order for all decisions to be legally binding, the individual must have envisaged the situation that has subsequently arisen.

There are generally three types of advance statements:

- one made when an individual is in good health, making a general statement about how they wish to be treated should certain conditions or circumstances arise

- one made at a time when an individual is faced with a serious diagnosis, and has various treatment options

- one made which nominates a person who should be consulted about an individual's treatment.

If you are consulted by someone who wishes to write an advance statement, you must consider whether there are any reasons to doubt the person's capacity to make the decisions in question. Capacity is assumed unless evidence suggests the contrary. Your signature as a witness may well imply that assessment of capacity has taken place. You must also be aware that a patient cannot demand inappropriate treatment or treatment that is currently illegal, such as euthanasia.

An advance statement may be verbal or written, as long as it is witnessed. It does not have to be witnessed by a doctor.

Wills

A will is any properly signed and witnessed document that provides instructions for the disposal of an individual's property after death.

You should never advise a patient as to the content or method of expression within a document intending to be a last will and testament.

If you are asked to act as a witness to a patient's will, you should record this in the patient's health record along with a short note as to the patient's mental capacity at the time. It is advisable that you do not know the patient professionally or personally if you are asked to witness a will.

Do not attempt resuscitation (DNAR) statements and withdrawal of treatment

The information under this heading bears some similarity to that given previously if the DNAR statement is part of an advance statement. However this often is not the case and the purpose of this section is to provide guidance in the event of having to identify those patients who would not benefit from attempted cardiopulmonary resuscitation (CPR) in the event of arrest.

Good communication is important. The involvement of the patient, those people close to the patient and the entire healthcare team is essential in this process of decision making, as is the communication of those decisions to all the relevant healthcare professionals.

It is also important to enable your patients to discuss their wishes with you, and hospitals are now frequently making written statements available in patient information leaflets, or on wards, to encourage them to do so.

When a DNAR decision has not been recorded in the patient's health record, and the precise wishes of the patient/relatives are unknown then CPR should be initiated if cardiac or respiratory arrest occurs. However, this is a general assumption. It is likely to be considered unreasonable to attempt to resuscitate a patient who is in the terminal phase of illness or for whom the burden of treatment clearly outweighs the potential benefit.

A DNAR decision should only be made after appropriate consideration of all respects of the patient's condition including likely clinical outcome, the patient's known wishes, patient's human rights (right to life, right to be free from degrading treatment), and the perspectives of all members of the healthcare team.

Patient confidentiality must also be maintained. The views of the patient's relatives and close friends should be considered, but these do not have to be determinative. Acknowledgement of the patient's spiritual wellbeing and religious beliefs is vital, and the healthcare team must facilitate any actions needed to meet the patient's spiritual needs.

The same principles should also apply when a decision is being made about the withdrawal of treatment.

It is preferable that decisions about resuscitation should be made as soon as the diagnosis and prognosis is known, rather than at a time of crisis. It is appropriate to consider a DNAR or withdrawal of treatment decision in the following circumstances:

- where the patient's condition indicates that effective CPR is unlikely to be successful

- where CPR is not in accordance with a valid advance directive

- where successful CPR is likely to be followed by a length and quality of life that would not be acceptable to the patient.

A DNAR decision alone applies only to resuscitation, so this does not preclude the right of the patient to receive all other treatment and care.

All decisions relating to DNAR and withdrawal of treatment must be recorded in the patient's health record, together with the reasons for the decision and with whom this has been discussed. As with any other aspect of care, decisions must be able to be justified.

All hospitals should have a DNAR alert record system in place, and this should be completed. A DNAR decision should be withdrawn if the patient is discharged from hospital, and reconsidered if readmission occurs. DNAR decisions should also be reviewed regularly, and the timing of those reviews decided upon conception of the first DNAR statement.

In the case of incapacitated adults, people close to the patient often have the perception that they have the final say about whether CPR is attempted or not. This is not the case, in that doctors have the authority to act in their patient's best interests where valid consent is unavailable. If the clinical decision is seriously challenged, then some form of legal view may be necessary.

The use of chaperones

Recent publicity over the practice of some former doctors has raised public concern that chaperones are not being used effectively. This is of most concern in primary care and community settings. Most hospitals have a chaperone policy, and this usually states that all patients are entitled to ask for a chaperone to be present for an examination or procedure, although not all requests will be able to be fulfilled. If no chaperone is available, patients have the right to refuse a procedure unless they are not considered able to make a decision and by not having the procedure they would put their life, or someone else's, at risk. Chaperones are most often requested when a male doctor is performing an 'intimate' examination or procedure on a female patient. Research published in the *BMJ* found that male doctors use chaperones in

around 68% of cases, and female doctors in only 5% of cases.

The NHS Clinical Governance Support Team was asked by the Shipman Working Group to investigate current practice and to review the use of chaperones in primary care and community care settings. They developed a model chaperone framework and provide guidance and examples of good practice and this can be accessed at www.cgsupport.nhs.uk. The framework includes advice on record keeping, and explains the different types of chaperones, the roles of informal and formal chaperones, training and obtaining consent. It also offers a sample chaperone policy that can be used as a template. It does not replace recommendations and guidance from professional organisations such as the GMC (*see* below). The framework also addresses two major obstacles – time constraints on doctors and the availability of someone to act as a chaperone – as well as lone working, all of which may restrict the offer and use. Certainly it is good practice to let patients know that chaperones are available. This can be made clear through leaflets or posters in the waiting area, but should also be mentioned verbally at the beginning of a consultation, allowing the offer and response to be recorded in the patient's notes.

The GMC guidance on *Good Medical Practice* (May 2001) has a supplementary section added in December 2001 (to read go to www.gmc-uk. org/guidance/library/intimate_examinations.asp)

This explains that the GMC regularly receives complaints from patients who feel that doctors have behaved inappropriately during an intimate examination that can be stressful and embarrassing for patients. The GMC advises that when conducting intimate examinations you should:

- explain to the patient why an examination is necessary and give the patient an opportunity to ask questions

- explain what the examination will involve, in a way the patient can understand, so that the patient has a clear idea of what to expect, including any potential pain or discomfort (*see* also the previous section on informed consent or go to paragraph 13 of the GMC booklet: *Seeking Patients' Consent* (www.gmc-uk.org/ guidance/library/consent.asp) which gives further guidance on presenting information to patients)

- obtain the patient's permission before the examination and be prepared to discontinue the examination if the patient asks you to

- record in the notes that permission has been obtained

- keep discussion relevant, and avoid unnecessary personal comments

- offer a chaperone, or invite the patient (in advance if possible) to have a relative or friend present

- if the patient does not want a chaperone, you should record that the offer was made and declined

- if a chaperone is present, you should record that fact and make a note of the chaperone's identity

- if, for justifiable practical reasons, you cannot offer a chaperone, you should explain that to the patient and, if possible, offer to delay the examination to a later date

- you should record the discussion and its outcome

- give the patient privacy to undress and dress, and use drapes to maintain the patient's dignity

- do not assist the patient in removing clothing unless you have clarified with them that your assistance is required.

The advice also adds that for anaesthetised patients, you must also obtain consent prior to anaesthetisation, usually in writing, for any intimate examination. If you are supervising students you should also ensure that valid consent has been obtained before they carry out any intimate examination under anaesthesia.

Medical negligence

Legal actions in negligence arise when a person who owes a duty of care to another person, because of the relationship which exists between them (for example a doctor and patient), breaches that duty and causes loss or suffering to occur as a result of the breach. Hospital trusts are vicariously liable for employees' actions carried out in the course of their employment. Doctors

are therefore not normally sued directly. Medical defence organisations have no role in litigation against NHS hospitals because from 1990 NHS hospitals began indemnifying their employees against patients' allegations of medical negligence. Trusts thus became defendants in legal proceedings, and the NHS accepted financial responsibility for claims. When a patient issues proceedings, the health authority or trust – depending on the date of treatment – is the named defendant.

NHS indemnity provides invaluable support to doctors facing litigation. It is, however, strictly limited in its scope. These limits apply only to civil litigation. It does not indemnify doctors in respect of disciplinary proceedings within the NHS or brought by the GMC. In the former instance, the relevant NHS body is likely to use its own lawyers to prepare a disciplinary case against a doctor. Criminal proceedings are occasionally undertaken against doctors. The NHS provides no indemnity in such cases, but defence bodies, at their discretion, may be prepared to fund such representation. Doctors providing any private treatment, whether in an NHS hospital or elsewhere, will become a named defendant because they have a legal relationship with the patient separate from NHS indemnity.

So while your NHS indemnity covers you for the consequences of alleged negligence in NHS hospital or community work in the UK, you could be at risk from the following:

- claims arising out of Category 2 work including insurance medical reports, medico-legal reports and signing cremation certificates

- disciplinary procedures by your trust or the GMC

- Good Samaritan acts outside the hospital

- lack of access to a 24-hour ethical and medico-legal advice line

- criminal charges as a result of your practice within the NHS.

So it is prudent for doctors to maintain their own indemnity to cover those instances where their employer's indemnity may not help, or the employer may even act against them.

The first medical defence organisation was established in 1885 following outrage in the medical community over the case of a Dr David

Bradley who was wrongly convicted of a charge of assaulting a woman in his surgery. Although the doctor later received a full pardon, he spent eight months in prison.

Traditionally, medical defence organisations have provided medical indemnity to doctors on either an insured or discretionary basis. An insurance policy is a contractual agreement that will always provide financial assistance under the terms of the policy. Discretionary benefits give a doctor the right to ask for financial support, but not necessarily the right to receive it.

Medical defence organisations can help with preventive advice through their advisory, education and risk management services, to reduce the risk of complaints and claims. They can provide the safeguard of defence if you are faced with a claim or complaint. An advisory helpline, in some cases available 24 hours a day, 7 days a week, may have in-house legal teams and provide assistance in Good Samaritan acts worldwide.

In 1990 the government introduced NHS indemnity for doctors employed by health authorities or trusts, but defence organisations continue to provide their members with advice and assistance on medico-legal matters including disciplinary charges and complaints.

Medical defence organisations defend the professional reputations of members when their clinical performance is called into question. They may pay legal costs in the civil courts, professional tribunals and criminal courts on behalf of their members. They may also pay compensation to patients who have been harmed by medical negligence during their treatment.

They support members throughout their general professional lives, not just if they face a complaint or claim. For example:

- assistance might include advice on confidentiality

- a solicitor writes requesting to see a patient's notes, should you disclose the information?

- should you approach the GMC if you are concerned about a colleague's fitness to practise?

- what do you do when a patient refuses to undergo the treatment he needs?

- journalist enquiries – some have a 24-hour press office to help you deal with enquiries from the media.

The potential size of the problem

The size of clinical negligence compensation within the NHS has grown enormously. To give you some idea of the statistics, in 2003–2004, the NHS Litigation Authority (NHSLA) (see below) made payments totalling £432.64 million in respect of its five schemes. These figures relate only to expenditure incurred by the NHSLA itself. An estimate of expenditure by the NHS as a whole in recent years is given in the Chief Medical Officer's report *Making Amends*, published in July 2003 by the Department of Health. An excess is payable on the non-clinical schemes (Liability to Third parties Scheme (LTPS) and Property Expenses Scheme (PES)), and the cost of these excesses is carried by individual NHS organisations, and is not included in the NHSLA's figures. As at 31 March 2004, the NHSLA estimated that it had potential liabilities of £7.88 billion.

The amounts paid out by the NHSLA for legal costs relating to clinical negligence claims closed in 2003–2004 were £110.74 million, and only related to costs paid by the NHSLA This did not include costs met by claimants themselves or by the Legal Services Commission (LSC).

In 2003–2004, the NHSLA received 6,251 claims (including potential claims) under its clinical negligence schemes, and 3,819 claims (including potential claims) in respect of its non-clinical schemes. The authority had 19,706 'live' claims as 31 March 2004, and Clinical Negligence Scheme for Trusts (CNST) claims are now settled in an average of 1.36 years, counting from the date of notification to the NHSLA to the date when compensation is agreed. The greatest number of claims appears to be in respect of surgery, but the greatest value of claims is for obstetrics and gynaecology.

As of March 2004 of the total outcome of claims, approximately 35% were abandoned by the patient, 43% were settled out of court, just over 1.5% were settled in court in favour of claimant, just under 0.5% settled in court in favour of the NHS, and nearly 20% remained outstanding.

The NHS Litigation Authority

This special health authority was set up in 1995 to oversee the CNST, a voluntary pooling scheme to assist trusts in managing their clinical negligence liabilities.

The NHSLA handles negligence claims made against NHS bodies through five schemes. Three of these relate to clinical negligence claims (CNST, Existing Liabilities Scheme (ELS) and the ex-regional health authorities (RHAs) scheme), while two cover non-clinical risks, such as liability for injury to staff and visitors and property damage (LTPS and PES, known collectively as the Risk Polling scheme for Trusts (RPST)).

- The CNST is a voluntary risk-pooling scheme for clinical negligence claims arising out of incidents occurring after 1 April 1995, funded out of members' contributions. Currently all NHS trusts and PCTs in England choose to belong.

- The ELS covers clinical negligence claims arising out of incidents which occurred before April 1995. It is not a contributory scheme: the costs of funding settlements made under ELS are covered centrally by the Department of Health.

- The Ex-RHAs Scheme covers any clinical liabilities incurred by the regional health authorities before their abolition in April 1996, with the NHSLA itself acting as defendant.

- The LTPS covers non-clinical 'third party' liabilities such as public and employers' liability claims. Like the CNST, it is a voluntary scheme funded through members' contributions.

- The PES covers 'first-party' losses by NHS bodies such as property loss or damage. Again it is a voluntary scheme, funded through members' contributions.

Under NHS indemnity, NHS employers are ordinarily responsible for the negligent acts of their employees where these occur in the course of the NHS employment.

The Clinical Negligence Scheme for Trusts (CNST)

Administered by the NHSLA, the CNST provides an indemnity to members and their employees in respect of clinical negligence claims arising from events which occurred on or after 1 April 1995. It is funded by contributions paid by member trusts. The scheme relates to incidents occurring in the context of NHS trust employment

Clinicians' own medical defence organisations (MDOs) continue to provide an indemnity in respect of private practice and independent GP and dental practice. In all cases, major or minor, it will be alleged that clinicians have failed to work to a suitably professional standard (the Bolam/Bolitho test) and that, in consequence, the patient has suffered injury and/or loss.

The NHSLA has a panel of specialist solicitors and allocates practices to trusts. There is a panel of 13 specialist firms of solicitors who are instructed on clinical negligence claims, and a panel of nine firms instructed on non-clinical claims. Once a panel firm has been instructed, it will represent the interests of the authority, the member trust, and the trust's employees. One of the objectives set for the NHSLA by Parliament is 'to minimise the overall costs of clinical negligence to the NHS and thus maximise the resources available for patient care by defending unjustified actions robustly [and] settling justified actions efficiently'. It is for the panel firms, in conjunction with the NHSLA, to work out the chances of a claim succeeding at trial, and the damages likely to be awarded, and then to advise on whether/how the claim should be defended or settled.

The patient is required to prove that the treatment fell below a minimum standard of competence, that he/she has suffered an injury, and it was more likely than not that the injury would have been avoided, or been less severe, with proper treatment. There is a time limit for a claim of three years from the date of injury, but it can be longer in some circumstances, if:

- the patient is a child, then the three-year period only begins on the eighteenth birthday

- the patient has a mental disorder (Mental Health Act 1983) so as to be incapable of managing their affairs, then the three-year period is suspended

- there was an interval before the patient realised or could reasonably have discovered they had suffered a significant injury possibly related to treatment

- a court is persuaded that it is fair to allow a longer period.

The NHSLA calculates two elements to an award. The first recognises 'pain, suffering and loss of amenity' and varies from about £4,000 for an unnecessary laparotomy scar, through about £140,000 for blindness to about £200,000 for quadriplegia. The remainder of any award is wholly related to the financial losses and extra expenses caused.

The role of the doctor(s) is crucial. The NHSLA relies on the doctor's view regarding the relevant factual issues at trial so that they can accurately work out the chances of the claim succeeding. If you are involved in such a case the NHSLA will need to know:

- what you did
- the reasoning behind any decision you made
- what your notes say.

In some claims the NHSLA may need you to think through what you would have done in a hypothetical situation. What you think is acceptable/understandable may not be so for someone outside your field. You need to explain even apparently obvious actions.

Lawyers claim they are very conscious of the time taken to resolve claims, and this may seem odd to clinicians who routinely have to deal with major problems in minutes or hours. The reasons given for the time taken include:

- time for the condition to stabilise before an accurate valuation on prognosis can be made. This can take years where the claim is on behalf of a young child with a brain injury
- time for other calls on the time of medical experts. There are frequently issues which cannot be resolved without both parties having had independent expert advice, and it is not unusual for respected experts to have an 8–12-month waiting list
- it may also take time before a trial date can be allocated.

Finally, very few claims go to trial, currently fewer than 2%. Most claims are either settled by negotiation or mediation for whatever proportion of their full value matches the chances of success of trial.

For further, comprehensive, information visit the website at www.nhsla.com.

Action for Victims of Medical Accidents (AVMA)

AVMA, founded in 1982, provides independent advice and support to patients injured and harmed during the course of medical treatment. It has been estimated that in the region of 320,000 adverse events occur each year in hospitals within England, with 40,000 deaths and 20,000 cases of serious disability (Vincent, 1995). AVMA is a charitable organisation and employs a team of medically trained caseworkers and support staff to help patients with their complaints about medical treatment. AVMA also works closely with selected members of the legal profession and occupies a unique position in the field of medical accidents since it is authorised by the LSC (Legal Services Commission, formerly the Legal Aid Board) to accredit and monitor selected solicitors in the field of clinical negligence. For more information visit the AVMA website at www.avma.org.uk.

Breaking bad news

It is an unfortunate consequence of working in healthcare that you will be called on from time to time to be the bearer of upsetting information. That news can include any information that changes a patient's, or their loved ones', view of the future in a negative way. In this context bad news can come in many forms for doctors. It may refer to:

- terminal illness
- diagnosis of a chronic illness (e.g. diabetes mellitus)
- disability or loss of function (e.g. impotence)
- a treatment plan that is burdensome or painful
- death of a patient.

Hippocrates recommended that doctors be wary of breaking bad news because 'the patient may take a turn for the worse'. In *Medical Ethics* for 1803 Thomas Percival gave a similar warning, as did the American Medical Association (AMA) in its first code of medical ethics in 1847.

In fact, withholding bad news from patients was commonly practised until quite recently. In 1961 a survey of 193 doctors revealed that 169

(88%) routinely withheld cancer diagnoses. Furthermore, they often used euphemisms such as 'growth' to describe cancer. The policy was to tell as little as possible in the most general terms consistent with maintaining co-operation and treatment. The same study revealed that most patients really wanted the truth about their diagnoses. In fact, many recent studies have found that most patients want to know the truth about their illness.

So a paternalistic model of care has been replaced by one that emphasises patient autonomy and full disclosure. Honest disclosure allows patients to make informed decisions. Withholding bad news diminishes patient autonomy. When a patient eventually realises the nature of their illness he or she may no longer trust the doctor. In fact, good practice now indicates that only under rare circumstances is non-disclosure of bad news ethical.

Breaking bad news can be difficult task. How it is done may affect patient comprehension of, and acceptance of, the news, to say nothing of their relationship with their doctors. Some of the barriers to effective communication of bad news have been identified as:

- fear of being blamed by the patient

- not knowing all of the answers sought by the patient or relatives

- inflicting pain on the patient

- doctors' personal fears, even own fear of illness and death

- little or no formal training in how to break bad news

- lack of time to give to the task

- cases with multiple doctors making it unclear who should break the bad news.

Breaking bad news requires expertise, knowledge and skill, but also requires compassion. You should give careful thought to your own perspective on the kinds of issues that will arise for the person receiving the bad news.

The basic principles

Who

The consultant is normally the lead person, but does not necessarily need to be the person who does it. Make sure you are clear about what the person is to be told. Remember the recipient may like to have another person with them. This could be a relative or friend, or someone for support such as a priest or social worker.

Where

Ideally a specially designated area should be used. In any event, it must be private. An office might suffice, but ensure there are no interruptions from people entering, the telephone going or from your bleep. Try to arrange for comfortable seating without the barrier of a desk.

How

In order to give information at the earliest appropriate opportunity, find out what the patient knows about their illness. Make eye contact. Start with:

- 'I've come to discuss your situation'

- 'What have you been told already?'

- 'What have you been told about your condition?'

- 'Do you recall why we did this test?'

- 'Do you know what I have come for?'

- 'What have they told you already?'

Assessing a patient's perceptions and level of understanding also allows you to correct misinformation and tailor the news to the patient's level of comprehension.

Avoid medical jargon. Patients and families will be confused, so don't make it even worse. Be honest, if you do not know something, say so. But let them know if there is someone who does. Check their understanding, and when you have finished, make sure there is someone to accompany them after your meeting.

Use appropriate eye contact, voice tone and body language. Remember the old saying; only 7% of the message is in the words, there is 55% in the 'dance' and 38% in the 'music'. Ensure that you know what the recipient wants to know and that the time is appropriate for them. All people being told are given the same information, with the same options, including an offer of a second opinion. The information should be factual. Give recipients an opportunity to return for further information or clarification.

Ensure that time is allocated not just to breaking the news but to supporting the recipient. In order to ensure that the patient's GP can deal effectively with them, make sure he is informed promptly of what the patient has been told. Your hospital will have a time scale for this, normally within two days. The medical record should be fully updated with notes of your consultation with the patient.

The practicalities

The essentials in preparation are:

- check the case details thoroughly

- make sure you have all information and results to hand

- take the notes with you in case you need to refer to them for details

- remember that another member of staff present is helpful, not only for you, but to help and support the relative(s).

Your appearance is important. Is your white coat really necessary for this? If you must wear it, it should go without saying that you should make sure there are no blood stains, particularly if it is a case of major trauma.

Find a suitable private room, furniture arranged, tissues to hand, and make sure that you will be undisturbed. Make sure you allow enough time. Adoption of an appropriate mood can be difficult if one is pressed for time, stressed or unprepared. First check identities and relationships, it is not the time to get names and relationships wrong. Offer your own identity and status and that of anyone with you.

A brief neutral conversation to establish rapport may be beneficial, but do not delay getting on with the purpose of the meeting. You might explain why you have brought someone with you. The reason for meeting should be explained. It is helpful to find out what they already know or

have been told, it cannot be assumed that they have previously been prepared for the possibility. Empathise, comfort where necessary, allow time for information to sink in, do not argue, and allow relatives their expressions of anger without criticism. Check their understanding, invite questions and try to be practical.

Finally offer to remain with them for a while in case they wish to ask questions perhaps, although they may wish to be alone. When finished summarise and check what the relatives wish to do immediately. They may wish to see the body. Give them the opportunity to attend to their appearance if they have been crying.

Some further thoughts

There are countless articles and books on this subject, and a review of nearly 100 showed that there are few trials of strategies for breaking bad news. Most writing on the subject is opinion, albeit by experienced practitioners. It is said that the most important factors for individual patients when they receive bad news are the doctor's competence, honesty, and attention, the time allowed for questions, a straightforward and understandable diagnosis, and the use of clear language. Families rank privacy, the doctor's attitude, competence, clarity and time for questions as important. Knowing the doctor well and the doctor's use of physical contact (for example, by holding the patient's hand) rank lower.

You might sometimes need to get the patient's permission to share bad news, particularly for patients from some non-Western cultures in which autonomy of the individual may not be paramount, and healthcare decisions are frequently shared with others.

Also, informing patients about possible outcomes before ordering tests or procedures may help prepare patients for potential bad news. You can ask patients if they want only basic information or a detailed disclosure. Remember that although patients need enough information to make informed healthcare decisions, they need to understand. So, for example, the word 'spread' should be used in place of 'metastasised'. Also it is helpful to check frequently that the patient understands perhaps by asking 'Am I making sense?' or 'Can I clarify anything?'. Undue bluntness and misleading optimism should be avoided.

An empathic doctor acknowledges a patient's emotional response to bad news by first identifying the emotion and then responding to it. 'I can see that you are upset by this news' is an empathic statement. Deliberate periods of silence allow patients to process bad news and vent emotions. After receiving bad news, a patient may experience a sense of isolation and uncertainty. Doctors can minimise the patient's anxiety by summarising the areas discussed, checking for comprehension, and formulating a strategy and follow-up plan with the patient. Written materials such as handwritten notes, or prepared materials listing the diagnosis and treatment options, may be helpful.

The use of an empathic communication may improve the experience for you and reduce the patient's anxiety. Helpful phrases include:

- 'I wish I had better news' (as opposed to 'I'm sorry, I have bad news')
- 'I admire your courage'
- 'I will be here for you'
- 'What gives you hope and strength?'

Unhelpful statements include:

- 'It could be worse'
- 'We all die'
- 'I understand how you feel'
- 'Nothing more can be done'

Action

Ask if you can sit in with someone who is experienced and skilled at breaking bad news.

When you feel confident enough try doing it yourself, maybe with a more experienced person sitting in to help if things get difficult.

Afterwards reflect on what went well and what less well, and ask for some feedback from the person who sat in to help.

Only when you feel confident, try doing these interviews on your own.

Children and bereavement

Children who are forewarned of the imminence and inevitability of death have lower anxiety levels as a result than those who are not forewarned. Young children are often said to need the concrete experience of seeing the parent after death. The bereaved adult may find this difficult, and the doctor may be able to offer to accompany the child. Further counselling is normally the responsibility of the primary care team using appropriate counselling services as required. Cruse – the national charity for bereavement care – publishes literature for bereaved children and their carers as well as providing training and counselling services. The Macmillan Children's Bereavement Service provides help for children and young people to talk about bereavement or a life limiting illness.

According to the BBC News and Information website (May 2004), a child is bereaved of a parent every 30 minutes in Britain, one in three loses a sibling during childhood, and 70% of schools are expected to deal with related problems. The National Children's Bureau (NCB) says teachers are often afraid of saying the wrong thing, and has called for issues surrounding death to become part of science and religious studies lessons. The NCB has written a booklet *Childhood Bereavement: developing the curriculum and pastoral support* of advice for schools that recommends ignoring euphemisms, such as 'passed away' and 'sleeping', for fear children will think the deceased parent is going to return. Sometimes children and young people want to talk openly about their loss, but find that it is those around them that avoid the issue.

For those requiring more on this subject we would refer you to the further reading list at the end of this section (p. 106).

Last offices

A last office is the care given to a person who has died. It should demonstrate respect for the dead, should be carried out with privacy and dignity, and must be focused on fulfilling cultural and religious beliefs and traditions. It also has to comply with legal and health and safety requirements.

It is unusual for doctors to be directly involved in the performing of last offices, as it has traditionally been a nursing role. Many nurses view this task with symbolic significance as it is the final demonstration of care given to the patient, and this should be respected by doctors. Last offices also give the family the message that care continues even after death. It is, however, crucial that doctors are aware of legal requirements for the care of the dead, and the correct procedures to be followed.

Some hospitals have taken the last rights procedure away from hospitals, giving the responsibility to the undertakers or the mortuary. This can cause difficulties for staff in following some cultural and religious processes.

Death and religion

Behaviour that is in ignorance of the religious beliefs and needs of a dying patient and relatives may cause great distress and offence. The following are only guidelines, as there are wide variations within all the world's faiths. Problems are likely to occur with patients whose cultures and beliefs differ considerably from those of your own religion. If in doubt, consult the family or use the contacts listed below. In many cultures, grief is expressed more openly than in the West, and wherever possible a side ward should be made available to allow families and friends time with the deceased if they wish. Jewellery and insignia of possible religious significance should not be removed from the body without the permission of the relatives. It is, of course, imperative that the bodies of those belonging to any religious sect are treated with respect and dignity according to any traditions.

Bahai

- The body of the deceased should be treated with respect. Bahai relatives may wish to say prayers for the deceased person.

- Normal last offices may be performed by the nursing staff.

- Bahai adherents may not be cremated, nor may they be buried more than an hour's journey from the place of death.

- A special ring will be placed on the finger of the deceased and must not be removed.

- Bahais have no objection to post mortem examination and may leave their bodies to scientific research or may donate organs if they so wish.

- Further information can be obtained from the National Spiritual Assembly of the Bahais of the UK, telephone number 020 7584 2566.

Buddhism

- There is no prescribed ritual for the handling of the body of a Buddhist person, so customary last offices are appropriate.

- A request for a Buddhist monk or nun to be present may be made.

- There are a number of schools of Buddhism – relatives should be contacted for advice as sects may have strong views on how the body should be treated.

- When the person dies, the monk or nun should be informed (the relatives often do this), and the body should not be moved for one hour after death.

- There are unlikely to be objections to post mortem examination or organ donation – although some Far Eastern Buddhism may object to this.

- The patient's body should be wrapped in an unmarked sheet.

- For further information contact The Buddhist Hospice Trust, PO Box 123, Ashford, Kent TN24 9TF.

Christianity

- There are many denominations and degrees of adherence with the Christian faith. In most cases customary last offices are acceptable.

- Relatives may wish staff to call the hospital chaplain, or minister or priest from their own church to either perform last rites, say prayers, or give Holy Communion. The latter may be held with family members also taking communion.

- Some Roman Catholics may wish to place a rosary in the patient's hands, and/or a crucifix at the patient's head.

- Some Christian Orthodox families may wish to place an icon at either side of the patient's head.

- For further information consult the hospital chaplain or local denominational minister.

- The Free Church and Church of Scotland have different practice, so check with relatives.

- A useful website is www.nhs-chaplaincy-spiritualcare.org.uk.

- Quakers (The Religious Society of Friends) have no clergy, but the presence of another Quaker or the hospital chaplain is usually acceptable.

Hinduism

- If required by relatives, inform the family priest or one from the local temple. Relatives may wish to read from the *Bhagarad Gita* or make a request that staff read extracts during last offices.

- The family may wish to assist in last offices and may request that the patient is dressed in their own clothes. If possible the eldest son should be present. Relatives of the same sex as the patient may wish to wash the body, preferably in water mixed with water from the River Ganges.

- A Hindu may like to have leaves of the sacred Tulsi plant and Ganges water placed in his/her mouth by relatives before death. It is therefore very important to inform relatives that death is imminent.

- If no relatives are there, staff of the same sex as the patient should wear gloves and apron, straighten the body, close the eyes and support the jaw before wrapping it in a sheet. The body should not be washed. Jewellery or sacred threads must not be removed.

- The patient's family may request that the patient be placed on the floor, and they may wish to burn incense.

- The patient is usually cremated as soon as possible after death.

- Post mortems are viewed as disrespectful to the deceased person, so are only carried out when strictly necessary.

- For further information contact the nearest Hindu temple (see telephone directory) or contact the National Council of Hindu Temples UK, telephone number 01923 350093.

Jainism

- Relatives may wish to contact their priest to recite prayers with the patient and family.

- The family may wish to be present or to help with the last offices.

- The family may ask for the patient to be clothed in a plain white gown (which they may supply), and then wrapped in a plain white sheet.

- Post mortems may be seen as disrespectful, depending on the degree of orthodoxy of the patient.

- Organ donation is acceptable.

- Cremation is arranged whenever possible within 24 hours of death.

- Orthodox Jains may have chosen the path of Selleklana which is death by ritual fasting. This is rarely practised today but may still have an influence on the Jain attitude to death.

- For further information contact The Institute of Jainology, telephone number 020 8997 2300 or the Jain Centre, telephone number 0116 254 3091.

Jehovah's Witnesses

- Routine last offices are appropriate. Relatives may wish to be present, and may read from the Bible or pray.

- The family will inform staff should there be any special requirements, which may vary depending on the patient's country of origin.

- Post mortem examinations will be refused unless absolutely necessary.

- Organ donations may be acceptable.

- Further information may be obtained from the nearest Kingdom Hall (telephone directory) or the Watch Tower Bible and Tract Society (Medical Desk), telephone number 020 8906 2211.

Judaism

- The family will contact their own Rabbi, or the hospital chaplain will advise.

- Prayers may be recited by those present.

- Traditionally the body is left for eight minutes before being moved. A feather may be placed over the lips and nose to detect signs of breath.

- Staff members are permitted to perform procedures for preserving dignity and honour. The body must be handled as little as possible, and staff must wear gloves. The body must not be washed. Staff may straighten the body, leaving the arms parallel and close to the body with the hands open.

- Bodies must remain in the clothes in which they died. The body will be washed by the Holy Assembly which performs a ritual purification.

- Watchers stay with the body until burial (normally within 24 hours). In this period a quiet non-denominational room is appreciated when the body can be placed with its feet towards the door.

- If death occurs on the Sabbath (sunset Friday to sunset Saturday) then watchers will remain with the body until the Sabbath is over, as funerals cannot take place during this time.

- In some areas, the Registrar's Office will arrange to be open on Sundays and Bank Holidays to allow for registration of death.

- Post mortems are only permitted if required by law.

- Organ donation is sometimes permitted.

- Burial is preferred, but non-orthodox Jews may choose to be cremated.

- Further information may be obtained from The Burial Society of the United Synagogue, telephone number 020 8343 8989 or the Office of the Chief Rabbi (Orthodox), telephone number 020 8343 6301.

Mormonism (Church of Jesus Christ of the Latter Day Saints)

- No special requirements.

- Relatives may wish to be at last offices.

- Relatives will advise if the patient wears a one- or two-piece sacred undergarment, if so, they will dress the patient as necessary.

- For further information contact the local church or the Head Office, telephone number 0121 712 1145.

Islam (Muslim)

- Where possible the bed should be turned so that the body is facing Mecca feet first. If the bed cannot be moved, the patient should be turned onto their right side so their face is towards Mecca.

- Muslims may object to the body being touched by someone of a different faith or opposite sex. If there is no family present, staff must wear gloves to close the eyes, straighten the body, support the jaw and turn the head to the right shoulder.

- The body must not be washed or nails cut.

- The body should be covered in a plain white sheet.

- Cremation is forbidden.

- Burial takes place within 24 hours wherever possible.

- The body is normally taken home or to a Mosque where it is washed by another Muslim of the same sex.

- Post mortems are only permitted if required by law.

- Organ donation is not always encouraged, although a Fatwa (religious verdict) has been issued by UK Muslim Law Council which allows Muslims to donate.

- Further information is available from the Islamic Cultural Centre, telephone number 020 7724 3363.

Rastafarianism

- Usual last offices are permitted although the patient's family may like to be present to say prayers.

- Post mortems are refused unless absolutely necessary.

- Permission for organ donation is unlikely.

- For further information contact The Rastafarian Society, telephone number 020 8808 2185.

Sikhism

- Family members, especially the eldest son, and friends will be present if able.

- Usually families will perform last offices, but staff may straighten the body, close the eyes and support the jaw and wrap it in a clean white sheet.

- The '5ks' must not be removed, these are personal items sacred to a Sikh:
  - kesh: do not cut the hair or beard or remove the turban
  - kanga: do not remove the semi-circular comb which fixes the uncut hair
  - kara: do not remove the bracelet from the wrist
  - kaccha: do not remove the special shorts worn as underwear
  - kirpan: do not remove the sword (usually miniature).

- The family will wash and dress the patient's body.

- Post mortems will be refused unless required by law.

- Sikhs are always cremated.

- Organ donation is permitted but is rare as they do not wish the body to be mutilated.

- For further information contact the nearest Sikh temple or the Sikh Missionary Society UK, telephone number 020 8574 1902.

Zoroastrianism (Parsee)

- Usually normal last offices are permitted. The family may wish to be present or to participate.

- Orthodox Parsees require a priest to be present if possible.

- After washing, the body is dressed in the Sadra (white cotton or muslin) and Kusti which is a girdle woven of 72 strands of lamb's wool symbolising the 72 chapters of the Yasna (liturgy).

- The head may be covered with a white cap or scarf.

- The funeral will take place as soon as possible after death.

- Burial or cremation is acceptable.

- Post mortems are forbidden unless required by law.

- Organ donation is forbidden.

- Further information may be obtained from the Zoroastrian Information Centre, telephone number 020 7328 6018.

Helping or counselling

Nursing staff are helpful in advising bereaved relatives on the procedures for registration of death, cremation certificates, and finding a suitable undertaker. The hospital chaplain may take on these duties and may be able to put relatives in touch with members of their own religion or community when no relatives are easily accessible.

Death, certification, coroners and cremation

This section is not a complete overview of the current system, as this is under review primarily as a result of the Shipman Inquiry. It should also be noted that there are variations in interpretation between individual coroners and crematoria, and indeed trusts are likely to have policies for dealing with the death of a patient. The practice outside England and Wales may show differences although much also applies to Scotland and the Procurator Fiscal.

It might be helpful to highlight one or two common misconceptions. Death certification is not the same as verification of death. Depending on circumstances, a number of individuals other than doctors can confirm a death including a senior nurse or paramedic. A doctor who has attended the deceased during the last illness and who has seen the deceased in the last 14 days is normally required to issue the Medical Certificate of Cause of Death (MCCD). This is often know as certifying death, and in hospital could be done by any member of the medical team, while outside hospital it is usually done by the GP of the deceased. A doctor not in attendance during the last 14 days of illness may also certify, provided they attended the last illness and have seen the body after death or have the coroner's permission.

Requesting a post mortem

There are two possible reasons for requesting a post-mortem. The first arises as a statutory requirement if a coroner's inquest is to be held. The second is when it is felt that significant benefit would be gained from further investigation into the cause of death. Several studies have shown that even when patients have been intensively investigated in hospital, the cause of death is wrong in about 10–15% of cases, with major unexpected conditions in up to 75% of cases. Furthermore doctors have been shown to be poor at predicting those cases likely to exhibit unexpected findings.

Some communication skills, such as the breaking of bad news, are transferable between different areas of clinical practice. Autopsy requests represent a specific requirement for communication skills training that is probably not transferable, and therefore requires specific attention.

Even clinicians with little or no interest in autopsies may still have to inform relatives of the requirement for a medico-legal autopsy, and all clinicians should therefore be capable of providing adequate reassurance regarding the autopsy to bereaved relatives. It is often those clinicians who cannot provide adequate reassurance regarding the fears and reservations expressed by relatives who are reluctant to request autopsies because of the personal discomfort experienced when approaching bereaved relatives for consent.

The process of requesting an autopsy from recently bereaved relatives is stressful for doctors, and any sense of personal discomfort will decrease the motivation of clinicians to request autopsies. This difficult request of relatives often falls to junior staff. A request for a post mortem is of necessity made at a time of grief and distress for relatives, especially as they tend to be associated with a bereavement which is sudden, unexpected or traumatic. There is likely therefore to be denial, perhaps dissociation in addition to the grief. The relatives' mental state may understandably therefore be difficult to deal with, thus you may encounter anger, resentment or rejection.

Many studies have highlighted the problems of obtaining permissions for autopsies, and most clinicians have no formal training in how to obtain permission. Studies have also shown that provision of training in how to request permission for autopsies can contribute to the improvement of autopsy rates. Those clinicians who have received appropriate training have more confidence, and consequently may be more willing to take the time to educate relatives in the nature and the importance of the autopsy. The manner in which permission for autopsy is sought is important, and can in some cases influence the decision of the family.

Although formal training is thought to be appropriate between the beginning of the final undergraduate year and the end of the PRHO year, some further assistance is useful later. Active methods, such as demonstration video sessions, video feedback sessions based on the performance of participants, and role-play techniques, have been found to be more desirable than the more passive training methods such as written guidelines and lectures. Your local trust may well provide such opportunities.

It may be better to break the bad news separately from the gaining of permission for a post mortem. You also need to agree who is going to do it and who you are going to ask for permission.

Key people involved with agreeing post mortems

The doctor

Breaking bad news is difficult enough for any doctor; having to deal with distressed relatives and give bad news is a significant stress for all doctors. Being less experienced and less senior adds to that stress. Adding to that, the difficulty of requesting a post mortem adds further to the stress.

It is easy to think that your main task is to get permission. But that takes no account of your personal attitude to dying, death and post mortem examination, to say nothing of your feelings about what a post mortem may say of the correct diagnosis which may reveal errors in earlier diagnosis and treatment.

Although the responsibility for obtaining consent is often passed to more junior doctors, ultimately it is the responsibility of the consultant. It is important however that the doctor making the request should have sufficient knowledge of the case and procedure to inform the relatives and answer any of their questions adequately. Trusts often have policies on this issue, and may specify the grade of doctor making such a request. Some trusts have bereavement officers responsible for these policies.

Family members

It is also easy to forget in the emotionally charged atmosphere that the family may want answers too, not for any reason of possible litigation but in the natural desire to know why, what happened, how did it happen?

Relatives and family will have personal, religious and cultural attitudes towards death and medical science. They may have a fear about the body being cut up, that their relative may not really be dead. A poorly handled request for a post mortem can be a source of additional stress to relatives. In some cases, although a full post mortem may be ideal, the next of kin may impose limitation, such as head not being opened, or examination being limited to certain organs, maybe the heart or lungs or specific areas such as the abdomen or chest. The next of kin can also specify whether material may be kept for histology, teaching or research.

The pathologist

This is not a two-party process, but a triangle with the person carrying out the post mortem involved too. It can be easy for them to forget about their colleagues who have to discuss issues face to face with relatives. Delays in getting results to medical staff can be frustrating, contribute to tensions and be worrying. For relatives, the delays can be agonising.

The approach

The individual approach of the doctor can be helpful and soften the blow, whereas for others this may exacerbate the emotional trauma for relatives. Relatives seem to gain support when they perceive that the informant is also distressed. A cold, impersonal, 'professional' approach might even cause offence. There are basically three ways of approaching the problem:

- blunt and insensitive: accepting that relatives will be upset whatever is said

- kind and sad: but without any positive support or encouragement or optimism

- understanding and positive: with flexibility, reassurance and empathy.

The right approach is obvious, but you will be aware that there are many complicating factors – most of which we hope we have covered in the preceding sections.

Making the request

In olden times, messengers bringing news of battles lost were often executed. There is still a tendency to blame a messenger for bad news. Doctors are no exception. Patients and doctors often harbour unrealistic expectations about modern medicine. Guidelines for breaking bad news are relevant here (*see* p. 87).

People respond according to their personality, which is often difficult to predict. Stunned silence, disbelief, guilt, anger, acute stress can all occur. Anger and acute stress are especially problematic, but stunned silence and disbelief are also difficult. Anger may be directed at the doctor, the medical profession, medical science, the hospital or at the NHS in general, but meeting this with anger only exacerbates the situation.

Allowing the relative to cry can be important to them. People value doctors who can cope with tears without being embarrassed. The doctor's instinctive reaction is usually to treat tears like haemorrhage – stop them as quickly as possible. Doctors should be able to display emotion, particularly as cool professional detachment can so easily be interpreted as evasive and unsympathetic.

Remember that the most difficult aspects for the clinician are often not those of most concern to the relative, so remember the importance of checking continually on the responses and feelings of a relative and allowing time and opportunities for things to sink in and think about ask questions.

Reporting cases to the coroner

As already indicated, at the time of writing the whole system of 'death, certification, coroner and cremation' is under review. There are also significant variations in interpretation of existing rules between individual coroners and crematoria. All trusts will have their own policies in relation to dealing with the death of a patient, and you are strongly advised to read these.

The coroner's officers must be informed of all reportable deaths. These are usually civilians employed by the local police, or police officers. They seldom have a medical background, and this should be borne in mind when giving medical information, although their experience is usually sufficient for one not to be aware of this. The cases requiring reporting are categorised in instructions to registrars of deaths, but the cases you are likely to be involved with would include the following:

- deaths in hospital
  - within 24 hours of admission
  - during an operation
  - before recovery from anaesthetic
  - within 24 hours of leaving theatre
  - where the conduct of a member of staff is called into question.

In addition there are cases which you might experience in accident and emergency (A&E) and which usually result in an inquest. They are generally non-natural causes of death:

- cause unknown
- has occurred in suspicious circumstances
- due to violence or neglect
- due to an accident whether at home, at work, or any other situation
- occurs in or shortly after prison or police custody
- alcoholic poisoning
- drugs or poisons
- abortion

- stillbirth if there is any reason to believe that the child was born alive
- industrial disease or industrial poisoning
- septicaemia associated with an injury or industrial disease
- possible homicide or manslaughter
- death due to trauma
- suspected suicide
- death not due to natural causes
- the patient has not been seen in their last illness (normally 14 days)
- sudden unexpected death including epilepsy or cot death.

Cases relating to violence or injury are still reportable even later, when death occurs less than a year and a day after the event causing the injury. An injury includes burns, choking, fractures (pathological fractures are usually excluded), foreign bodies, concussion, cuts, drowning, hyperthermia and hypothermia, sunstroke, lightning, electric shock etc.

Unless it is clear that the death is due to a known natural cause, it will normally be necessary for a post mortem examination to be carried out. The permission of the relatives is not needed, but they of course must be informed and notified of the time and place unless this would unduly delay the examination. The relatives and other recognised persons are entitled to be represented at the post mortem examination by a medical practitioner.

Action

Check out the written guidelines your hospital has for reporting cases to the coroner.

An inquest

Following a coroner's post mortem an inquest may be held, the purpose of which will be to establish who died, when they died, where they died and how they died. Your most likely appearance is in the coroner's court at an inquest. Some families may regard the inquest as an extension of the funeral and may find it a very distressing experience. For this reason alone it may be advisable to dress soberly and act appropriately, and avoid using medical jargon or words not easily understood when answering any questions from the family.

When the coroner's office issues the request they are generally helpful and happy to informally liaise with the coroner and give information and assistance to the doctor preparing his report. Should the original records be released to the coroner, it is advisable to make a complete copy.

The coroner

A coroner is an independent judicial officer of the Crown whose duties as assigned under the Statute of the Coroners' Act 1988. The coroner must be either a registered medical practitioner, barrister or solicitor of a least five years' standing, and they investigate the circumstances of certain deaths. Nowadays most are lawyers and indeed changes are anticipated that will make this mandatory. Each year in the UK about 180,000 cases are reported to a coroner, over half by doctors. An inquest is a fact-finding enquiry, to establish who died, where, when and how, and the cause of death.

There will normally be guidelines written for your trust particularly for dealing with cases that may have implications for the reputation of the hospital or the staff, and especially in cases in which there may be media interest, although a coroner is not allowed to apportion blame for a death. At an inquest a coroner may allow questioning by lawyers representing the family of the deceased. Trusts normally provide appropriate managerial, legal and personal support. Common verdicts include accidental death, misadventure, suicide, industrial disease, natural causes, and an open verdict.

The coroner has the power to subpoena a witness and to impose a fine of up £1,000 or imprisonment for contempt of court for non-attendance; however they are usually mindful of a doctor's other commitments and will often accept a written report from a doctor, such as the deceased's GP. If you are planning any leave in the period that may coincide with the inquest, it is strongly advised that you notify the coroner's office as soon as possible so that attempts can be made to avoid a clash. In cases where the medical issues are complex, it is possible that the coroner may ask for the opinion of an independent expert.

It is also worth noting that a coroner can accept so-called hearsay evidence of another person, unlike a criminal court. This usually takes the form of the results of tests, X-rays, or biopsies by another doctor not present in the court.

Giving evidence

Careful preparation and familiarity with the events of the case are important. Witnesses are generally put at ease, and the procedure is more informal than in other courts. Witnesses still take an oath or affirm. Each witness is taken through their statement by the coroner, and questions asked where necessary. Family or their representatives may then ask questions. When family members are unhappy or angry they may have legal representation and their lawyer may also ask you questions. Defence organisations will often be prepared to give you advice if you are worried by the experience of appearing at an inquest.

The normal approach to dealing with legal decisions in English courts is by adversarial debate. Coroner's inquests are different. This is an inquiry, not adversarial, so coroners will not usually tolerate hostile questioning of witnesses. Where there is disagreement between witnesses, the coroner will hear all evidence and the evidence thus presented enables the coroner to reach a verdict.

Solicitors may view an inquest as a preliminary investigation to a claim, but it is not for the coroner to apportion blame or deal with matters of negligence or civil liability. If your professional conduct or competence should be called into question you may seek an adjournment of the inquest from the coroner and contact your defence organisation for further advice. You are not obliged to answer questions that may incriminate you.

If there has been prior criticism of a doctor, or you know that the family plan to be represented by a solicitor then often your defence organisation will instruct a solicitor on your behalf. This situation is rare.

Lawyers often advise witnesses to follow three 'golden rules'. They are:

- dress up
- speak up, then
- shut up!

So, it is sensible to dress for the occasion, to take notes with you to refer to, having rehearsed them so that you can deliver your message with confidence, and, when you have said what you planned to say, sit down as soon as you have given simple answers to any questions. Do not dig a hole for yourself. If you do not know the answer, be honest and say so. Speculation or trying to be helpful is a pitfall to avoid at all costs. If you wish to refer to the records, ask to be allowed to do so.

In a trust it is usual for an individual to be designated the task of co-ordinating the gathering of information and providing this for the coroner. The report should be factual and accurate. You should refresh your memory as to the sequence of events using medical records, which are an essential part of the investigation. Avoid technical language and detailed explanation of complex procedures. Times of events should be given as precisely as possible. An account of the practitioner's personal involvement should be in sequence. Other staff should be identified so that their comments can be sought where necessary. If the deceased was a trust patient the trust solicitor may attend on behalf of the hospital.

Summing up and conclusions

At the end of the hearing the coroner will sum up the evidence that has been given, and if a jury has been sitting, will direct them on points of law. This would happen if the death:

- occurred in prison
- occurred in police custody
- was due to a notifiable disease
- was due to an accident
- occurred 'in circumstances the continuance or possible recurrence of which is prejudicial to the health or safety of the public or any section of the public'.

The verdict will include the deceased's name, the injury or disease causing the death, the time, the place and circumstances in which the injury occurred, the determined cause of death and the registration particulars.

The coroners' rules allow no verdict to be framed in a way that appears to determine criminal or civil liability. Inevitably, the verdict that gives rise to most concern is lack of care. The court of appeal has recommended that this be replaced by 'to which neglect contributed'. The coroner is not permitted to apportion blame for the death.

The most common verdicts are:

- accidental death
- misadventure
- suicide
- industrial disease
- natural causes
- open verdict
- lawful killing
- unlawful killing
- stillbirth.

The decision of the coroner can be subject to judical review, where the facts and evidence do not justify the verdict.

In Scotland there is no coroner's officer and a fatal accident inquiry is heard by the procurator fiscal who investigates all sudden, suspicious, accidental, unexpected and unexplained deaths. The procurator fiscal should hold the inquiry before the sheriff issues the final report (known as the 'Sheriff's Determination').

Witnesses will be paid their fees and reimbursed all reasonably incurred expenses immediately after the inquest. These fees are set by the Home Secretary and you are advised to contact the clerk of the court after the hearing to claim your fees.

Confidentiality

If a coroner asks for a statement or disclosure of the medical records, then consent from the deceased's representative is not necessary, although you may wish to inform the family. If, however, information about living patients related to the deceased is requested, you will need their consent.

The duty of confidentiality however does not end with a patient's death. After inquest there may be questions from the press. It is acceptable and courteous to convey publicly to the family sympathy at the death and distress. It is not appropriate without consent of the family to volunteer further information. Never talk to the press without professional guidance. With regard to dealing with the media in a crisis remember the following:

- remain calm
- think before you speak, preferably from a prepared statement
- don't get drawn into any conversation
- don't breach patient confidentiality
- don't lose your cool
- be reassured that even the media have to take account of guidelines and the laws of libel
- call your defence society as early as possible and seek help.

For members of the Medical Defence Union (MDU), a 24-hour press office helpline (020 7202 1535 office hours and 0800 716 646 out of hours) is available to assist its members with media enquiries in these circumstances.

You should go to the GMC website for further useful information on the following:

- the duties of a doctor registered with the GMC
- patients' right to confidentiality
- principles
- protecting information
- sharing information with patients
- disclosing information about patients
- circumstances where patients may give implied consent to disclosure
- sharing information in the healthcare team or with others providing care
- disclosing information for clinical audit
- disclosures where express consent must be sought

- disclosure in connection with judicial or other statutory proceedings
- disclosures required by law
- disclosures to the courts or in connection with litigation
- disclosures to statutory regulatory bodies
- disclosures in the public interest
- disclosures to protect the patient or others
- children and other patients who may lack competence to give consent
- disclosures in relation to the treatment sought by children or others who lack capacity to give consent
- disclosures where a patient may be a victim of neglect or abuse
- disclosures after a patient's death.

Cremations

The doctor who certifies death will often be the one to complete the first part (Form B) of the cremation form although this is not a requirement. Before a body can be permanently disposed of by cremation, the second part of the form (Form C) has to be completed by an independent doctor of at least five years' standing. This means five years fully registered in the UK, and does not therefore include pre-registration house jobs.

Ideally the doctors should meet, but in practice a phone call is regarded as acceptable practice. However both doctors must have seen the body after death and the doctor signing Form C must speak to at least one other person such as a third doctor, a nurse or a relative of the deceased or any person who has knowledge of the deceased's last illness and circumstances surrounding the death.

If there is a post mortem, Form C is not required to be completed, provided the post mortem was carried out by a doctor of at least five years' standing and Form B was completed by that doctor after the post mortem, thus with knowledge of the result.

It is also worth noting that a pacemaker can explode on cremation, causing damage to the crematorium equipment, and therefore a doctor signing Form B must state that any pacemaker has been removed; the crematorium referee will check this confirmation before authorising the cremation.

Guidance for doctors asked to complete forms B and C is available from the Home Office and can be downloaded from their website www.dh.gov.uk/cmo for links. The guidance is part of a drive to tighten the authorisation procedures following the Shipman Inquiry.

Action

If you have time then why not go and see an inquest. A call to the coroner's office will tell you when the next cases are scheduled. You may find it helpful to refer to the following for more information:

Books

- Levine M and Pyke J (1999) *Levine on Coroners' Courts*. Sweet and Maxwell, London.

- Burton J and Rutty G (2001) *The Hospital Autopsy* (2e). Hodder Arnold, London.

Online with full text

- Report of the Joint Working Party of the Royal College of Pathologists, the Royal College of Physicians of London and the Royal College of Surgeons of England (1991) *The Autopsy and Audit*. If you go to www.rcpath.org you will need a user name and password, but a Google search of 'The Autopsy and Audit' will take you direct to the report in either html or as a pdf file.

- O'Grady G (2003) Death of the teaching autopsy. *BMJ* 327:802–3. Go to www.bmjjournals.com and search by author or title or a Google search of 'Death of the teaching autopsy' will take you directly to it.

- Underwood J (2003) Commentary: resuscitating the teaching autopsy. *BMJ* 327: 803–4. Go to www.bmjjournals.com and search by author or title or a Google search of 'Resuscitating the teaching autopsy' will take you directly to it.

- McDermott MB (2003) Obtaining consent for autopsy. *BMJ* 327:804–6. Go to www.bmjjournals.com and search by author or title or a Google search of 'Obtaining consent for autopsy' will take you directly to it.

Other online sources

- Royal College of Pathologists www.rcpath.org

- Home Office www.homeoffice.gov.uk

- The Shipman Enquiry, www.the-shipman-inquiry.org.uk

- Department of Health www.dh.gov.uk

- King's College, London has some useful information on Coroners' rules www.kcl.ac.uk

- The Coroners' Society of England and Wales www.coroner.org.uk

- Cremation Society of Great Britain: arrangement of regulations www.srgw.demon.co.uk/CremSoc/

- For links to the Pathology Specialities Forum and Medico-Legal Forum, www.doctors.net.uk

---

Complaints

Complaints fall into three main areas:

- complaints, whether clinical or non-clinical, may be made against you or the hospital by dissatisfied patients and relatives with whom you have direct contact

- complaints about the whole team, medical outcomes, administrative and support service, and the hospital generally. These can be made by patients and relatives or organisations representing patients' interests

- internal employee complaints made against the hospital.

In the next section we will deal mainly with those instances where you are faced with a patient bringing a complaint. The following section outlines the procedures for dealing with more formal complaints. Employment complaints are normally the subject of internal trust procedures and are monitored by the personnel department. If you do become involved in a complaint related to employment, we suggest you contact the local BMA office and seek the advice of the industrial relations officer.

Dealing with an informal patient complaint

Patients initially have three options for complaining or obtaining advice on complaints.

- The Patient Advice and Liaison Service (PALS) staff or complaints manager at the NHS trust hospital or PCT involved in the complaint. They may be able to resolve the problem on the spot or will provide details of how to complain.

- NHS Direct on 0845 4647.

- The Independent Complaints Advocacy Service (ICAS).

Complaints are usually due to one or more of the following:

- actual or perceived failure of a doctor to deliver the expected standard of care

- unrealistic expectation of a patient or their relatives

- failure of communication.

A complaint is not a claim but it could become one. It is important that it should be handled well. Usually this means a prompt explanation to any patient or their relative involved in any event that has given rise to the complaint. Minor criticism should be dealt with by conciliation not confrontation. Deal with the situation sympathetically. An apology can be given, as an apology is not an admission of legal liability.

If you find yourself first in line when a patient or relative complains it is helpful to remember that the complainant is usually angry so:

- try to be on a level with the other person; if you are looking down on them they may feel more threatened

- allow them plenty of personal space and do not get too close; this also may make them feel threatened

- acknowledge their feelings by an empathic statement. The other person now understands that you appreciate their position and they no longer have to prove their anger

- indicate that you are listening by reflective listening, repeating back a summary of what is being said

- avoid questioning an angry person

- if you are in a closed space or room check that you are well positioned for leaving quickly, or at least ensure that a large piece of furniture separates you from the complainant!

Use simple assertiveness techniques (see p. 30 on assertiveness) such as the 'broken record' to express yourself calmly and persistently, as the angry person often leaps from topic to topic.

They may use criticism as a weapon, and again the 'broken record' technique is useful. It can be helpful to use another assertiveness technique called 'fogging'. This is simply a method of taking the wind out of your critics' sails by saying that there may be some truth in what they saying, or agreeing in principle with them.

Safety considerations

In 2005 the Healthcare Commission reported that a quarter of NHS staff reported abuse or harassment by patients in the previous year, with 14% being physically attacked. Despite claims of a 'zero tolerance' approach to violence against staff, the most recent figures from 2002–2003 found that 116,000 incidents of verbal and physical abuse had been reported by NHS staff. The number of successful prosecutions against people who assaulted NHS staff rose sharply in the previous year, according to statistics from the Department of Health that show that in 2004–2005 there were 759 successful prosecutions, compared to 51 in the previous year.

Employers are responsible for ensuring that employees are kept safe at work, and the Health and Safety Act (1974) and ensuing amendments emphasises the need for assessment of risks and adequate training. There is also a responsibility on the employee to take reasonable steps to safeguard their own safety and health at work. The following pointers may be useful:

- there should be security systems in place

- layout of the room should be considered, doors opening outwards, with observation panels and removal of potential missiles

- there should be protocols for seeing patients with another member of staff nearby

- CCTV, panic buttons and personal alarms may be necessary

- staff should be trained in personal safety and breakaway techniques

- it is always important to review a patient's history for previous violence, mental health problems and history of alcohol or drug abuse

- for any home visits there must be a protocol for letting people know where you are and your expected return time.

Personal safety

- Use your work address in the Medical Directory.

- Use an ex-directory home telephone number.

- Be aware of the dangers of ties and scarves when seeing risk patients.

- Be aware of body language signs.

- Avoid prolonged eye contact.

- Position yourself in a room nearest the door, and if necessary leave door open.

- Know about the safety procedures in your unit and the position of panic buttons.

During an interview about a complaint, or even during a consultation be aware of the possible signs of pending violence:

- raised tone of voice

- raised volume of voice

- red face

- clenched fists

- pointing fingers

- invasion of personal space

- verbal threats

- refusal to communicate

- restlessness

- pacing about.

Use your communication skills to take the heat out of the situation once you see signs of impending violence. Once things have progressed beyond a certain point this may be futile, and at this stage you should leave the situation as soon as possible. However before you have made that decision you could try:

- active listening with open questions

- reassurance and acknowledgement of grievances

- good, but not persistent and prolonged eye contact which might be considered threatening

- keeping your distance, but away from corners where you could be trapped

- ask for any weapons to be put down rather than handed over

- use the panic button or call for help

- leave the room and get assistance from security or police.

If an incident occurs, it has further implications for the individuals concerned and other members of staff, so the following will be required:

- fill out an incident report form

- discuss the incident with colleagues

- document it in the patient's notes so that subsequent staff are aware of the history

- consider pressing charges

- in general practice consider removing the patient from your list

- seek counselling if required

- consider the Criminal Injuries Compensation Authority or NHS Injury Benefit Scheme

- consider how you handled the situation and whether you need further training.

When a patient assaults a doctor they forgo a degree of their right to confidentiality, in that while reporting the incident to the police, the doctor can only provide essential details but no clinical details. Under certain circumstances, however, clinical details may be disclosed if the withholding of such information places the patient or others at risk of serious harm or death. If you are attacked you can also discuss these issues with your defence organisation. Also note that the NHS Security Management Service (NHS SMS) has launched a comprehensive strategy to better protect staff and property in the NHS, with a particular emphasis on tackling violence. *See* www.cfsms.nhs.uk/ where you will find more detailed guidance and information on this subject and what the NHS is doing to try and tackle the problem.

Formal complaints procedures

More serious complaints should be reported and handled by formal procedures, as they may lead to a claim for compensation. These should be referred to a person of sufficient seniority for advice, and for them to deal with the situation as required. Most trusts have well-documented procedures for handling complaints, and these should always be followed.

NHS complaints procedure

If a patient is unhappy with their treatment or the service they have received from the NHS they are entitled to make a complaint, have it considered, and receive a response from the NHS organisation or primary care practitioner concerned. The NHS complaints procedure described applies to the NHS in England, except for NHS foundation trusts (*see* below).

Current legislation

The National Health Service (Complaints) Regulations 2004 (the 'Complaints Regulations') came into force on 30 July 2004. All NHS trusts and health authorities have to provide information to all patients about their right to complain, and provide advice about how to use the complaints procedure, and what help is available to complainants.

The LSC encourages people to use this system as an alternative to litigation. It is designed to resolve any problems quickly and efficiently, and to the complainant's satisfaction. There are two parts to the procedure: local resolution and independent review. It is hoped that most complaints can be resolved within the local resolution stage, but some go on to an independent review. There is no right to an independent review, but if a complaint has not been resolved within local resolution, the complainant may request an independent review. The request will be considered by a convener and an independent lay chair, and a decision will be made to either: convene an independent review panel, refuse a panel, or refer the complaint back for further local resolution. The patient also has the right to complain to the health service ombudsman, but there are limits to what he can investigate.

There is normally a time limit to complain – within six months of the event(s) concerned, or within six months of becoming aware that there was something to complain about. Primary care practitioners and complaints managers in NHS organisations have discretion to waive this time limit if there are good reasons for a delay.

There are two elements to the system, local resolution and independent review both of which should be managed by an appropriate person.

Local resolution

This involves the provider of the service trying to resolve the complaint to the patient's satisfaction, in the majority of cases on an informal basis, as quickly as possibly. A PALS has been established in every NHS trust and PCT. The PALS is not part of the complaints procedure itself, but might be able to resolve concerns informally or can tell a patient more about the complaints procedure and independent complaints advocacy services.

Your trust is certain to have written guidelines on its complaints procedure. As a first step, complaints should receive a response immediately or within a specified time scale. The patient will receive an oral response first, supported by a written response. This may include the offer of investigation or conciliation if appropriate. A complainant should receive a response from a primary care practitioner within 10 working days or from a chief executive of the NHS organisation concerned within 20 working days, and be kept informed of progress if this is not going to happen.

The clinical director, department head or complaints officer, follows this up either orally or in writing, within a period of 21 to 28 days. The complainant has the right to receive a full and prompt written reply from the chief executive to a formal complaint. In particularly serious cases or where the complainant remains dissatisfied, the investigation may well need to be detailed and may include obtaining independent advice. Complainants must also be made aware of both the role of the ICAS and any other patients' advocate services available to assist them in pursuing complaints and how they may be contacted.

NHS foundation trusts

NHS foundation trusts have their own systems for the internal handling of complaints which may differ from the 'local resolution' process described so far. The 'independent review' stage carried out by the Healthcare Commission applies to NHS foundation trusts, which are also covered by the health service ombudsman.

Most dissatisfied patients require explanations or apologies for poor service, and assurances that defects will be remedied, rather than financial compensation. Only a relatively small number of complaints proceed to litigation.

Independent review

If the patient is unhappy with the response to their complaint, including a complaint about an NHS foundation trust, they can ask the Healthcare Commission for an 'independent review' of their case. The Healthcare Commission is an independent body established to promote improvements in healthcare. More details are available at www.healthcarecommission.org.uk.

Health service commissioner (ombudsman)

Complainants who remain dissatisfied after the NHS complaints procedure has been completed may ask the health service commissioner (ombudsman) to investigate their case. The ombudsman is completely independent of the NHS and of the government, and can consider complaints about most aspects of NHS services

and treatment. However, he is not obliged to investigate every complaint put to him.

The health service commissioner has the power to investigate written complaints from the public about the provision of services or mal-administration. The commission has the power to examine internal papers and clinical records. Any doctor faced with a request to give a report should take advice.

Further information about the ombudsman can be seen at www.ombudsman.org.uk.

Roles of parties to a complaint

There may be any number of parties involved in a complaint. The following is a summary of those who might be involved and some aspects of their roles.

A patient's advocate

If the complainant is not the patient it is important to be clear just what the nature of the complaint is and the complainant's perspective: is the complainant acting on behalf of the patient and if so, do they have the authority of the patient to do so?

A patient's family or carers

It should be established whether the complainant is acting on behalf of a wider group, or drawing upon a wider knowledge base than is immediately obvious.

A convenor

The convenor is a non-executive director appointed by the board to manage the independent review panel process. Where a complaint relates in whole or in part to action taken in exercising clinical judgement, the convenor must take appropriate clinical advice.

The Independent Complaints Advocacy Service (ICAS)

Set up in September 2003, the Independent Complaints Advocacy Service can help patients to make their complaint or give help with making a complaint. Trained advocates, also known as case-workers, with knowledge of the NHS complaints procedure help clients to understand whether they wish to pursue a complaint and, where needed, provide support to clients to do so. This support may range from helping with initial preparation in ordering their thoughts and thinking about what a good resolution would look like, through to attendance at resolution meetings, and helping with correspondence.

Four voluntary sector organizations deliver ICAS: the Citizens Advice Bureau (CAB), the Carers' Federation, PohWER and the South East Advocacy Projects (SEAP). The four providers took over cases from the old Community Health Councils (CHCs).

For more information look at their websites:

CAB – www.nacab.org.uk/

Carers' Federation – www.carersfederation.co.uk/

PohWER – www. pohwer.net/

SEAP – www.icassoutheast.org.uk/

Or go to www.dh.gov.uk/ and search for 'complaints advocacy'.

Healthcare professionals

A complaint can harm a professional's career, especially if it is poorly handled. To ensure they do not feel excluded from the process the professional normally drafts the response that will go to the complainant. If an apology is required this can be the clinician's own letter with a follow-up by the chief executive, thus ensuring compliance with the regulations.

Professional bodies

Allowances are made in the planning for the involvement of a professional's representative body. The representative body can also provide independent support to a professional.

Trade unions

Trade unions or other staff bodies will be interested in the complaints procedure and likely to play an active part in supporting its members.

The media

The NHS is a popular topic for both local and national media. The episode may come under media scrutiny. Some letters may appear in the press if the complainant is unhappy.

The board

Complaints have to be reported to the board quarterly. The board has to produce an annual report on complaints handling and circulate it widely.

The health service commissioner (ombudsman)

If a complainant is not successful in getting an independent review panel established, or is unhappy with the outcome of the panel then he or she can approach the ombudsman.

Action for Victims of Medical Accidents (AVMA)

AVMA can provide patients or relatives with information about how to proceed with a complaint.

Action

Look at the summary document of your trust's complaints procedure.

Related reading

- AVMA website www.avma.org.uk (accessed 27 April 2006).
- Baile WF, Buckman R, Lenzi R et al. (2000) SPIKES – a six-step protocol for delivering bad news: application to the patient with cancer. *Oncologist* 5:302–11.
- BMA (1995) *Advance Statements about Medical Treatment*. BMA, London.
- BMA Medical Ethics Department www.bma. org.uk (accessed 27 April 2006).
- BMA, Resus Council, Royal College of Nurses (2001) *Decision relating to Cardio Pulmonary Resuscitation*. BMA, Resus Council, Royal College of Nurses, London.
- Buckman R (1992) *How to Break Bad News: a guide for health care professionals*. Johns Hopkins University Press, Baltimore.

- Burton J and Rutty G (2001). *The Hospital Autopsy* (2e). Hodder Arnold, London.
- Chief Medical Officer (2003) *Making Amends*. Department of Health, London.
- Data Protection Act (1998) See www.opsi.gov.uk/ACTS/acts1998/19980029.htm (accessed 27 April 2006) or www.dh.gov.uk and type in search box 'Data Protection Act' concerning its application to the NHS
- Department of Health (1992) NHS Guidelines: *Patients who Die in Hospital* (1992) HSG(92). Department of Health, London.
- Department of Health and Social Security (DHSS) *Informed Consent*. DHSS Circular, HC (90)22. DHSS, London.
- Dyregrow A (1991) *A Grief in Childhood: a handbook for adults*. Jessica Kingsley, London.
- Department of Health (2002) *Reference Guide to Consent for Examination or Treatment*. Department of Health, London.
- Ellis PM and Tattersall MH (1999) How should doctors communicate the diagnosis of cancer to patients? *Annals of Medicine* 31:336–41.
- Evans J (1999) *Clinical Negligence in NHS and the Law. Wellard's NHS Handbook 1999/2000*. JMH Publishing, East Sussex.
- Faulkner A (1998) *When the News is Bad – A Guide for Health Professionals*. Stanley Thornes, Cheltenham.
- Fogarty LA, Curbow BA, Wingard JR et al. (1999) Can 40 seconds of compassion reduce patient anxiety? *Journal of Clinical Oncology* 17:371–9.
- Frances G and Job N (2004) *Childhood Bereavement: developing the curriculum and pastoral support*. National Childrens Bureau, London.
- Gillon R (1985) Telling the truth and medical ethics. *BMJ* 291:1556–7.
- Girgis A and Sanson-Fisher RW (1998) Breaking bad news 1: current best advice for clinicians. *Behavioral Medicine* 24:53–9.
- GMC (1998) *Seeking Patient Consent*. GMC, London. (This is being updated during 2006) see www.gmc-uk.org (accessed 27 April 2006).
- GMC (2001) *Good Medical Practice*. GMC, London.
- GMC (2002) *Withholding and Withdrawing Life Prolonging Treatments: good practice in decision making*. GMC, London.
- Health and Safety at Work Act 1974 See www.hse.gov.uk, www.pcs.org.uk/, www.health andsafety.co.uk or www.opsi.gov.uk (accessed 27 April 2006).
- Heegaard M (1991) *When Someone very Special Dies – children can learn to cope with grief*. Minneapolis. Woodland, Minneapolis.
- Heegaard M (1991). *When Something Terrible Happens – children can learn to cope with grief*. Woodland, Minneapolis.
- Hippocrates (1923) Decorum, XVI. In: Jones WH. Hippocrates with an English Translation. Vol II. William Heinemann, London.
- Human Rights Act 1998, Article 2 'Right to Life', Article 3 'Right to be Free from Inhuman or Degrading Treatment', Article 8 'Right to Respect for Privacy and Family Life', Article 10 'Freedom of Expression', Article 14 'Freedom from Discriminatory Practices'.
- Jurkovich GJ, Pierce B, Pananen L et al. (2000) Giving bad news: the family perspective. *Journal of Trauma* 48:865–70.
- Levine M and Pyke J (1999) *Levine on Coroners' Courts*. Sweet and Maxwell, London.
- McDermott MB (2003) Obtaining Consent for Autopsy. *BMJ* 327:804–6.
- McLauchlan CA (1990) Handling distressed relatives and breaking bad news. *BMJ* 301: 1145–9.
- MDU Publications: *Can I See the Records*; *Confidentiality*; *Consent to Treatment*; *The MDU Guide to the Complaints Procedure*; *Problems in General Practice – Delay in Diagnosis*; *Clinical Negligence*; *Inquests – a Practical Medico-legal Guide*; *GP Registrars – a Practical Medico-legal Guide*. MDU. London
- Mitchell JL (1998) Cross-cultural issues in the disclosure of cancer. *Cancer Practice* 6:153–60.
- Neuberger J (1991) *Caring for Dying People of Different Faiths* (2e). Mosby, London.
- NHS Executive (1990) *A Guide to Consent for Examination*. NHS Executive, London.
- NHS Litigation Authority website www.nhsla.com (accessed 27 April 2006).
- O'Grady G (2003) Death of the teaching autopsy. *BMJ* 327:802–3.
- Parker PA, Baile WF, de Moor C et al. (2001) Breaking bad news about cancer: patients' preferences for communication. Journal of Clinical Oncology 19:2049–56.
- Ptacek JT and Eberhardt TL (1996). Breaking bad news: a review of the literature. *Journal of the American medical Association* 276: 496–502.

- Quill TE, Arnold RM and Platt F (2001) 'I wish things were different': expressing wishes in response to loss, futility, and unrealistic hopes. *Annals of Internal Medicine* 135:551–5.
- Report of Joint Working Party of the Royal College of Pathologists, Royal College of Physicians and Royal College of Surgeons (1991) *The Autopsy and Audit.* If you go to www.rcpath.org you will need a user name and password, but a Google search of 'The Autopsy and Audit' will take you direct to the report in either html or as a pdf file.
- Resuscitation Council www.resus.org.uk (accessed 27 April 2006).
- *The Royal Marsden Hospital Manual of Clinical Nursing Procedures* (6e) (2004) Royal Marsden Hospital, London.
- Underwood J (2003) Commentary: resuscitating the teaching autopsy. *BMJ* 327:803–4.
- VandeKieft GK. (2001) Breaking bad news. *American Family Physician* 64:1975–8.
- Vincent CA and Bark P (1995) Accident investigation: discovering why things go wrong. In: CA Vincent (ed.) *Clinical Risk Management.* BMJ Publications, London. pp. 391–410.
- Walsh RA, Girgis A and Sanson-Fisher RW. (1998) Breaking bad news. 2: what evidence is available to guide clinicians? *Behavioral Medicine* 24:61–72.

CHAPTER 6

Teaching, training, appraisal and assessment

This chapter aims to help you make the most of your structured learning opportunities, to provide you with the 'tools' to support others, and to help them learn from you.

Teaching and training

Continuing medical and professional development is fundamental to career success and to safe and effective delivery of service to patients. The training of specialist registrars was laid down by the Calman Implementation Steering Group and is the subject of a training agreement. The following chapter provides an insight into all aspects of your training responsibilities as a specialist registrar. It also introduces assessment and appraisal aspects of *Modernising Medical Careers*.

Differences between competence and confidence, and between teaching and training

Experience by itself is insufficient to develop competence. There is evidence to suggest that confidence levels (but not skill levels) grow with experience alone (Marteau *et al.* 1990). Feedback on performance and an unflagging commitment to learning are prerequisites for continuing professional development. This feedback comes from other, usually more senior, colleagues. This is often referred to as teaching or training. There is some confusion about the meaning of the terms 'teaching' and 'training'. We will employ definitions for the purposes of this handbook which are outlined as follows, although you will hear

them used in many differing contexts in everyday language.

We tend to think of learning as a formal process, although much real learning is informal. It occurs on a day-to-day basis without our being particularly aware of it. We discussed this process in Chapter 1. The choice of method of delivery is often made according to the needs and preferences of the teacher rather than the needs of learners. This is a pity, because it can lead to much time-wasting for those involved. A better basis would be the choice of opportunities available and the nature, or learning domains, of the material to be learnt.

Learning domains

The nature of the task to be learnt can vary in content and complexity, which can influence the approach to teaching. The following categorisation of learning situations represents a simple way of helping to decide which approach to teaching is likely to be most helpful to the learner.

Understanding

This is usually acquired as knowledge grows, concepts are grasped and, eventually, learners are able to put together the whole picture for themselves. Often described as the 'cognitive domain', understanding may be developed through reading, studying, question and answer and discussion sessions. Highly developed understanding enables the learner to apply the learning by undertaking an analysis of complex cases, deriving solutions and evaluating outcomes.

Skills

Practical skills, sometimes referred to as being in the 'psychomotor domain', are those that usually involve practice in order to acquire full competence. Learning is achieved through instruction and guided practice. This is what we have referred to as training. Instruction may be as short as three or four minutes, and usually takes place during normal working. Adult learners usually find periods of skills training of more than about 15 minutes to be difficult. They generally want to be involved and begin to practise newly learned skills. Other, more complex, skills are employed when dealing with people. These might be colleagues or patients, individuals or groups. Interpersonal skills are of considerable importance in teamwork, including handling conflict, influencing, counselling, and information gathering. They can also enable you to get important information from patients to aid diagnosis. Such skills are more difficult to impart. Demonstration, role-playing and feedback using video can be helpful. Again, guided practice is an effective way of following up initial training. Professionals frequently find it difficult to admit, even to themselves, that they need help in dealing with others. Most of us believe we are good at communicating. Recognising your need is the first stage in learning.

Attitudes

Attitudes are usually described as being in the 'affective domain', and are based on complex sets of values and beliefs. These are acquired throughout life and are dependent on a wide range of influences. The most important influences are usually close contacts such as family, friends and significant work colleagues. 'Role models' are often referred to in the training of professionals. Affective development is partly dependent on the influence of those who impress us during our formative learning stages. Senior colleagues have almost certainly influenced your attitudes to many

aspects of your work, perhaps even your choice of career. You, in turn, will help to shape the attitudes of more junior colleagues. Indeed, you may also help shape the attitudes of some of your senior colleagues. Teaching and training require developed skills. The following text will help you to understand how to do it, but there is no substitute for guided practice. Every time you help others to learn, try to get feedback on your own performance.

Teaching

Teaching is taken to describe pre-arranged situations in which one person delivers learning material to a group, normally as a formal presentation. Such sessions can take place within the hospital or off-site, according to the demands of the learning. They usually concentrate on one-way transfer of information, rather then the passing on of skills. The presentation may be in the form of a tutor-led discussion or a lecture; the latter has been described as an activity during which the notes of the lecturer are transferred to the notebooks of the students, without passing through the minds of either! Good teachers can generally make their presentations interesting and sufficiently relevant to avoid this description.

Teaching is a didactic process which focuses on formal presentations such as lectures, where the communication is mainly one way. Please refer to Chapter 4 of this handbook for a detailed guide to presentation techniques.

The defining characteristic of a teaching session is the expectation (or hope, at least) that the audience will leave with an improved level of understanding of the topic, and perhaps be able to develop their own capability as a result. Your first responsibility, then, is to select, arrange and deliver your material to meet their expectations. It is helpful to start by attempting to define the needs of the audience, rather than first deciding what you want to tell them.

The next responsibility is to find and use ways of making your delivery interesting as well as relevant. Personal skills in delivery can be developed, either through attending a training course, or by practising and getting feedback from reliable members of your audiences. Sensible use of audiovisual aids, careful planning and, when possible, audience participation will help to create effective teaching sessions.

Training

Training or instruction is a two-way process in which the learner is helped to develop their understanding and to practise a skill or set of skills. It is usually only through continuing practice that a satisfactory level of competence is achieved. The focus here is on the development of skills in others. Practical skills are best trained on a one-to-one basis, where the learner can be involved in as much of the procedure as possible.

Each training event should be planned, and the following should be taken into account:

- *current level of capability of the trainee*: this means checking that they are ready for the learning and that it fits with their current needs. By discussing their needs with them it is probable that their motivation to learn will also be increased

- *resources should be available to complete the whole training session*: these include your time, equipment, a room, other participants in the process – e.g. patients and any paperwork that is associated with the activity

- *learning goals or objectives for the session*: these should be agreed with the trainee and stated in measurable terms

- *method of instruction*: this is dealt with in more detail later

- *evaluation*: the criteria for success should have been determined, preferably by agreement with the trainee, before the instruction starts

- *record of completion*: it helps to record the achievement of the learning goals for the learner's logbook

- *support and follow-up*: it is very important that learners are given time to master their new-found skills. They should not be left on their own without support and guidance being available during the early practice stages.

Method of instruction

The most common approach to skills training, and one which has stood the test of time, is the 'four-step' procedure. Most other methods of instruction are a variation on this theme. It helps to break down larger, more complex, tasks into smaller elements. The learner can be shown and can practise each separately before attempting the whole task as one.

1 The trainer performs the task in the normal way with the learner observing. Questions should be saved until after the run-through.

2 The trainer performs the task again while talking through each stage. There are three steps within this one – tell them what you are going to do; tell them while you are doing it; take time to deal with further questions after you have done it.

3 The learner talks through the task while the trainer performs it. This gives the trainer an opportunity to check understanding.

4 The learner performs the task and talks it through at the same time. Consolidation of learning begins at this stage. There is also the opportunity to stop the learner from making a mistake before it occurs. This is obviously critically important in some situations, e.g. in an operating theatre, where the learner would explain each step and get clearance from the trainer before proceeding.

Giving effective feedback is a key part of the training process. This is not always done as well as it should be. The following guidelines for giving feedback will help and they apply to most situations:

- *maintain a positive approach*: be encouraging and supportive

- *be direct*: be specific and deal clearly with particular incidents and examples of behaviour. Avoid being woolly or vague

- *suspend judgement*: it is unhelpful to pronounce judgement but better to say how you see the situation and let the learner make their own evaluation

- *make it actionable*: it is not helpful to give someone feedback about something they cannot change. Useful feedback is that which can lead to a change in behaviour

- *time it well*: to be most effective it needs to be given as soon after the event as practical so it is fresh in the receiver's mind

- remember, also, that praise may be given in front of others, but negative feedback is generally best left until you can deal with it on a one-to-one basis.

It would be an unusual learner who got everything right first time. You should always assume that learners will continue to need your support for some time after the training session is finished. At first this may involve direct supervision. Later they can be left alone to perform the task. Explain how you or some other suitable person can be contacted until the learner feels entirely sure of themselves.

Appraisal

Most doctors think firstly of appraisal as being focused on learners and related to the training process. It is important to be clear about the difference between appraisal and assessment. In simple terms, assessment measures progress based on set criteria and is usually a public process, whereas appraisal is concerned with focusing on the appraisee's development needs. Thus, appraisal may be seen as developmental rather than judgemental. It is normally confidential and should enable the trainee to discuss openly their concerns about their performance and future career plans. A well-conducted trainee appraisal meeting provides an opportunity for the trainee to gain important new concrete experience through interaction with a senior colleague whose opinion is important to the trainee. The appraiser helps the trainee to reflect on experience and also assists in the acquisition and development of understanding of new concepts. It remains for the trainee to go out and test out their learning in their own way, taking action (under the supervision of a senior colleague) and acquiring new experience to reflect on later.

In 2001, appraisal was introduced for all doctors as part of the GMC's revalidation process. It is the responsibility of all NHS employers to provide an appraisal scheme which meets the GMC's requirements and satisfies the employers' responsibility under clinical governance for ensuring clinical performance is monitored, supported and evaluated. It thus contributes to a judgemental decision-making process regarding revalidation.

Trainee doctors are subject to these requirements in common with all other doctors working in the NHS. They are required to maintain a portfolio of evidence of their performance indicators as a basis for their appraisals. They are able to use existing educational processes and documentation, thus no extra effort should be required to maintain the portfolio. It is based on the consultant form which is, in turn, designed around *Good Medical Practice* (GMC, 2001). Details can be found on the Department of Health website www.dh.gov.uk/assetRoot/04/08/03/27/04080327.doc.

Registration arrangements with the GMC changed in April 2005. From this date, doctors practising in the UK are required to hold a license which is subject to five-yearly revalidation. Renewal dates are determined by reference to each doctor's GMC registration number. The major element of evidence of continued fitness to practise is taken to be engagement in an appraisal process being administered in a GMC-approved environment (GMC, 2004). Generally, an approved environment is one where all the requirements of good clinical governance are met and where there are appropriate supervision arrangements for doctors.

360° feedback

Increasing use has been made in recent years of 360°, sometimes known as multirater, feedback systems to aid trainees and other doctors in the collection of evidence about their performance and development needs. These are based on systems that allow colleagues from all aspects of an individual's working life to provide an assessment of their work. The most effective of such schemes are administered by an impartial outsider, and are designed to elicit feedback on observed behaviours rather than personal opinion. They should provide anonymity to respondents, and feedback should be facilitated by a person skilled in helping the recipient make sense of the report. The questionnaires are often completed online, and may thus be very simple to administer. The respondent is asked to score the person, usually on a scale of say 1 to 6, in relation to a number of items relevant to their work performance, such as in the team assessment behaviour (TAB) form used in the foundation years and described later. Medical questionnaires might include such items as:

- uses skill and judgement when undertaking practical procedures

- respects the right of patients to be fully involved in their care decisions

- works effectively in the multidisciplinary team

- shows respect for other people's time by being punctual.

This approach has been used extensively for doctors in some other countries. The validity and reliability of the approach was demonstrated in an extensive study undertaken in Canada (Hall *et al.* 1999).

Assessment

There are two types of assessment which are sometimes assumed to overlap in definition with appraisal. The whole area is confused, and we have tried here to make some sense of the language in use and the aims of the different approaches.

Formative assessment

Feedback on appraisal of performance which is primarily aimed at helping the appraisee to learn and develop is sometimes referred to as formative assessment. The Royal College of Obstetricians and Gynaecologists avoids using the word 'appraisal' – it instead uses the term 'formative assessment' to describe its equivalent to appraisal. This may be contrasted with summative assessment, which seeks to measure ability in order to make an award, or to permit progress over a performance hurdle such as in the annual assessment of specialist registrars. Similar terminology is used by the Royal College of General Practitioners, and elsewhere in healthcare education.

Formative assessment is focused on the learner and educational needs. It attempts to measure skills, behaviours, attitudes or knowledge, and may contain elements of self-assessment. Being assessed should encourage you to seek gaps and inform your educational plans. Finding weakness is positively encouraged, as this offers learning opportunities.

The records of formative assessment are confidential to the parties involved, and are usually held by the learner. The teacher's attitude should be non-judgemental and encourage the learners to explore themes that are unanticipated.

Respect should be shown for the trainee by the contents of their learning plan being agreed through negotiation and openness, not coercion or manipulation.

Summative assessment

'Summative assessment' is the final, or end-of-year, criteria-based assessment introduced by Calman for the specialist registrar grade. In addition to regular appraisal, specialist registrars are assessed each year in accordance with their record of individual (in-training) training assessment (RITA). The regulatory framework is set out in *A Guide to Specialist Registrar Training* (NHSE, 1998). Difficulty sometimes arises for educational supervisors when deciding the extent to which they should regard the appraisal as confidential, particularly when the final RITA assessment report is to be prepared.

Summative assessment also tests for skills, behaviours, attitudes and knowledge, but is regulatory. The methods and criteria are set by examiners on behalf of an assessing body. Examiners themselves will have been trained in summative assessment methods. These need to be valid, reliable, feasible and fair. They can be either peer- or norm/criteria-referenced. For fairness, examinees should have access before the examination to the criteria by which they are being judged.

The aim of summative assessment is to identify those trainees who are not ready for independent practice. The results of summative assessment are not confidential. Outcomes will affect career progression.

Modernising Medical Careers (MMC)

The stated aims of MMC are to improve patient care by delivering modernised and focused career structure for doctors through a major reform of postgraduate medical education. To do this, MMC has established two-year foundation schools that require doctors to demonstrate their abilities and competence against set standards.

Foundation year 1 (F1) and foundation year 2 (F2) make up the two-year foundation programme which all UK medical graduates are required to undertake before progressing to specialty or GP training. These two years effectively replace the PRHO year and the first year of SHO training. Foundation doctors are trained and assessed against specific competences set out in the *Curriculum for the Foundation Years in Post-graduate Education and Training*. This curriculum was agreed with the GMC and the Postgraduate Medical Education and Training Board (PMETB). The PMETB is an independent statutory body which is responsible for overseeing and promoting the development of postgraduate medical education and training for all specialties, including general practice, across the UK. It took over the responsibilities of the Specialist Training Authority of the Medical Royal Colleges and the Joint Committee on Postgraduate Training for General Practice in September 2005.

Specialist and general practice training programmes (run-through training) follow on from the F2 year. Once a doctor is in specialist or general practice training, they will have the opportunity to gain a certificate of completion of training (CCT), subject to satisfactory progress. Each programme has a curriculum, agreed by the PMETB, against which doctors in training are assessed. The number of years that a trainee spends in training will vary from programme to programme. After a doctor receives a CCT, they can enter the specialist or GP register, and can then apply for an appropriate senior medical appointment.

Nationally standardised modes of assessment have been introduced as part of the Modernising Medical Careers foundation years. These include the following assessment tools:

* *multisource feedback (MSF)*: there are two versions, the *mini-peer assessment tool (mini-PAT)* which requires the trainee to nominate eight assessors from among clinical colleagues who fill out questionnaires which, together with the trainee's self-assessment, are electronically collated and fed back through an educational supervisor; and the *team assessment behaviour (TAB)* which is a 360° feedback form completed by ten, mainly clinical, co-workers. This is summarised and fed back by an educational supervisor and included in the trainee's portfolio

* *clinical evaluation exercise (mini-CEX)*: this is a 15-minute snapshot of a doctor/patient interaction. It is designed to assess the clinical

skills, attitudes and behaviours of the trainee. Six of these will be undertaken in each year, with a different observer for each encounter

* *direct observation of procedural skills (DOPS)*: trainees are required to undertake six different procedures under observation. An assessor may be any appropriate clinician who is selected by the trainee

* *case-based discussion (CbD)*: the trainee selects two case records from patients they have recently seen and in whose notes they have made an entry. The assessor selects one of these for discussion with the trainee. The purpose is to assess clinical decision making and the application of medical knowledge in the care of the trainee's own patients.

There are three significant roles identified in the MMC process – these had existed previously under similar titles but often with differing or unclear role descriptions:

* *clinical supervisors* are responsible for teaching and supervising trainees. They:
  – supervise day-to-day clinical and professional practice
  – support the assessment process
  – ensure that trainees are exposed to an appropriate range and mix of clinical experience
  – arrange a work programme to enable the trainee to attend fixed educational sessions.

There must be at least one named clinical supervisor in each training placement

* the *educational supervisor* is the doctor responsible for making sure trainees receive appropriate training and experience. They are also responsible for deciding whether individual placements have been completed. Educational supervisors are involved in teaching and training, and help with professional and personal development in each placement. The educational supervisor is responsible for:
  – undertaking regular formative appraisal
  – providing support in the development of the learning portfolio
  – ensuring trainees understand and engage in assessment
  – being the first point of call for trainees' concerns/issues about training

– ensuring appropriate training opportunities are available to learn and gain competences
- *the foundation training programme director* (FTPD) is the individual appointed by the deanery and trust to manage and lead a foundation training programme.

Following the foundation programme, specialty training is aimed at developing specialists in a more streamlined way than previously. This is also intended to afford further opportunities for supra-specialisation to allow doctors to adapt their training to accommodate changes in medical technology.

Basic principles of assessment

- All require trust based on fairness and objectivity.

- Each type of assessment requires a different mixture of skills, knowledge and attitudes. Not all doctors will have the necessary skills and training to assess (or appraise) others.

- Doctors at the receiving end may also require training in how to prepare themselves and make the most of the experience.

- Those involved must know what type of process is being carried out.

- If a change from one type to another is required (e.g. when assessment moves into personal counselling), then permission must be sought.

- It should be clear to all parties whether an encounter is confidential or not.

- Some types of interaction do not sit easily together, i.e. summative and formative assessment, although it is inevitable that they will overlap in the course of training.

Although assessment is also part of the educational process it has an element of performance review. It is a process that is open and objective, subject to appeal and designed to inform decisions about career progress.

Managing the appraisal process

The main aim of this section is to provide a basis for successful medical appraisal interviews.

Appraisal is an integral part of specialist registrar training, and has become a mandatory element in the revalidation process. Although the purpose of this book does not specifically require us to cover consultant appraisal for revalidation, the principles and suggested practice outlined below apply equally to most appraisal situations.

Trainee appraisal is essentially a formative process. Although some judgement is involved, it is normally intended that the trainee should be developed, rather than assessed. Appraisal is intended to be part of the educational process. Kolb *et al.* (1984) proposed a model of learning which we explored in Chapter 1 (*see* Figure 1.4, p. 12).

A well-conducted appraisal meeting provides an opportunity for the trainee to gain important new concrete experience through interaction with a senior colleague whose opinion is important to the trainee. The appraiser helps the trainee to reflect on experience, and also assists in the acquisition and development of understanding of new concepts. It remains for the trainee to go out and test out the learning in their own way, taking risks (under the supervision of a senior colleague) and acquiring new experience to reflect on later.

Appraisal can:

- help identify educational needs at an early stage

- assist in the skills of self-reflection and self-appraisal that will be needed throughout a trainee's career

- enable learning opportunities that will be helpful to the trainee to be provided quickly

- provide a mechanism for reviewing progress and identifying problems in time for remedial action to be taken

- provide a mechanism for giving feedback on the quality of training provided

- make training more efficient and effective.

Appraisal meetings should take place at the beginning, halfway through, and at the end of the post. The first meeting sets up the training agreement, which describes the learning objectives and confirms the support needed by the trainee during their time in the post. It is important that the trainee comes properly prepared for this meeting, and guidelines for this are given below.

The second meeting is primarily concerned with reviewing progress, designing new learning opportunities if they are required, and revising learning goals. The final meeting again reviews the trainee's experience, assists the trainee to reflect on experience gained, and helps to make sense of the complexities of the learning process. It will also, if required, address career-related issues. Appraisers should seek feedback from their trainees on the training and appraisal process at the end of every appraisal meeting.

Preparation for the appraisal meeting

As we indicated earlier, in your current role you may, at different times, be both appraiser and appraisee. First, we address the process for the appraisee.

Preparation: the trainee

You should be aware that the success of the appraisal meeting depends on adequate preparation by both parties. The list under 'Preparing the agenda' (see p. 117) should help you to determine your most important topics. You should ask yourself the following questions, and take notes to the meeting:

Work performance

- Which areas of the work do you enjoy most?

- Which tasks do you feel you perform the best?

- Which areas do you find most challenging and why?

- How might you have improved your performance?

Skills/abilities

- Reflect on your strengths and weaknesses.

- Which skills do you have that you believe are well developed?

- Identify those skills that need more development.

Learning objectives

- What learning objectives would you like to agree for the coming period of training?

Training

- Are there any specific training courses, or areas of need, which you would like to have addressed in the coming period?

Career

- What are the main career-related issues facing you at present? Are there still key decisions to be made? What help do you need with them?

Preparation: the appraiser

In your work as a specialist registrar and, more significantly, as a consultant you are likely to be called upon to appraise colleagues. We concentrate here on the appraisal of trainees rather than colleagues. The aims of a trainee appraisal meeting are to identify relevant learning goals, to agree and commit to them, to reflect on and make sense of the trainee's past experience, and to agree and record actions based on the discussion. These might be for either the appraiser or trainee to implement.

The following guidelines are intended to enhance the quality of the appraisal for both parties:

- *plan the meeting*: dates and times for all meetings to be held during the post should be determined well in advance

- *the trainee should be helped to prepare for the meeting*: after you have prepared an agenda you should show it to the trainee. The trainee preparation guidelines could be given to the trainee and discussed a few days before the meeting

- *relevant materials*: the curriculum, timetable, job description, rotas, previous appraisal records and notes of feedback from third parties should be collected together and considered before the meeting

- *suitable venue*: a quiet room, guaranteed free from interruptions, should be used. Bleeps and mobile phones must always be switched off or passed to a colleague

- *sufficient time*: there is no 'correct' amount of time to set aside for an appraisal meeting, but it is unlikely that much will be achieved in under half-an-hour. Note that the appraisal must take place in protected time

- *third parties*: discuss the trainee with other consultants, trainees, nurses, midwives, technicians, physiotherapists or others as necessary to gain a rounded picture of the trainee.

Preparing the agenda

It helps if the pattern of the meeting is clear from the beginning for both parties. An agenda should be prepared and shared before the meeting. The following checklist should help you to prepare and conduct the appraisal. Choose from it the items you consider should make up the agenda for the meeting:

- *education*: what, if any, examinations should be in preparation? What courses should be undertaken?

- *academic/research*: is advice necessary on research projects, or are there decisions to be made regarding suitable research designs?

- *clinical experience and skills*: what specified procedures does the curriculum indicate? What levels of understanding and competence are indicated? Is good manual dexterity and hand/eye co-ordination necessary? Is experience of clinical risk management a requirement?

- *knowledge*: what is an appropriate level of clinical knowledge? Is knowledge or use of evidence-based practice a requirement?

- *organisation and planning*: what level of ability to organise their own work and self-organisation are demanded of the trainee? Is active participation in audit an element of the training at this stage?

- *teaching skills*: should the trainee be gaining experience of teaching others and, if so, at what level?

- *career*: should the trainee be helped to make career decisions at this stage? What help may be necessary? Would sharing your own experience be helpful to the trainee?

- *personal skills and attributes*: the wide range of personal skills demanded in the work of a doctor is indicated below. Select those you feel should be discussed with the trainee:
  - *interpersonal communication*: rapport building, listening, empathising, persuading and negotiating skills
  - *decisiveness*: taking responsibility, exerting appropriate authority
  - *teamworking*: co-operating with others, leading as required, seeking guidance
  - *flexibility and resilience*: ability to adapt to rapidly changing circumstances and cope with setbacks
  - *thoroughness*: well-prepared, self-disciplined, punctual and committed to carry tasks through to completion
  - *drive and enthusiasm*: committed to patients and colleagues, motivated to achieve, curious, displaying initiative
  - *self-managed learning*: takes learning opportunities, reflects on experience, seeks guidance and advice
  - *probity*: honest, showing integrity and awareness of ethical dilemmas
- *feedback from the trainee* is usually helpful in enabling you to improve your approach.

Finally, the outcomes of the meeting should be recorded. It helps to remind you to include this stage by noting it in the agenda.

Conducting an appraisal meeting

The pattern of the meeting, partly determined by the level and experience of the trainee, should be dictated by the trainee's needs. Effective appraisal means getting the trainee to identify strengths and areas of need, and to propose ways of meeting the latter. Although guided by the appraiser, a successful meeting will feel as if it has been led by the trainee's priorities.

Confirm the agenda

The agenda should have been determined in advance, with the trainee's help, but it is worthwhile briefly re-establishing the aims and key items for discussion. If a record of the previous appraisal is available, this should be used to inform the discussion at this stage.

Review past performance

Get the trainee talking as soon as possible. Use questions to open up issues and probe to help the trainee to explore their own strengths and weaknesses in the light of their performance. Try to avoid being directive. Allow the trainee to describe their perspective on issues, and help them to reflect by using open and probing questions. Focus on specific aspects of the work. Give positive feedback where possible, particularly as a balance to any comments on less successful aspects of the trainee's work. Giving feedback requires a high level of skill and sensitivity. It demands a careful blend of drawing out the trainee to describe their own strengths and, particularly, weaknesses, and being direct in explaining concerns that you have, and that the trainee does not appear to recognise.

Explore and agree current learning needs

The trainee should have identified key learning needs in advance, but these may need to be modified in the light of the previous discussion. It may also be affected by information you have obtained from third parties in preparation for the meeting. You should remember that the responsibility for the trainee's learning is a joint one. Avoid taking on a list of jobs which could be more suitably undertaken by the trainee. Make brief notes to ensure you can recall critical issues. Reflect on learning objectives agreed for the post.

Agree learning objectives for the next period

These should be 'SMART'. This means they should be:

- *specific*: relate to specific tasks and activities, not general statements about improvement

- *measurable*: it should be possible to assess whether or not it has been achieved

- *attainable*: given the time available, it should be possible for the trainee to achieve the desired outcome

- *realistic*: set within the trainee's capability

- *timed*: the next appraisal date, or earlier, should be agreed as the time for reviewing the achievement of the objective.

Review and record decisions

You may wish to make brief notes throughout the meeting, in order to ensure that all the key points are reviewed at the end. It is vital that a record is kept of the outcome of the meeting. This should be agreed at the end of the meeting, and a copy kept by both parties. It will prove useful at the next meeting and may also form a useful document for the trainee to use as a record of progress in a logbook or portfolio. Doctors should retain records of appraisal meetings for their revalidation folders.

Get feedback on your performance

It is not common for appraisers to welcome informal feedback from the trainee at the end of an appraisal meeting. Indeed, it could prove to be an uncomfortable experience. Nevertheless, if the relationship between the two has developed positively, it can be very helpful for the appraiser to get an immediate indication of the benefits gained by the trainee. Bolder trainees may even give constructive criticism of the training received and any weaknesses perceived by them in the scheme. While this may be difficult, it will help future trainees and give the appraiser greater satisfaction in the long term. Alternatives include written feedback forms, which college tutors often use to route feedback to the Royal College.

Dealing with difficult issues

Confidentiality

There are mixed messages from some sources regarding the confidential nature of the appraisal meeting. Typically, it is suggested that if trainees are to feel free to express concerns about their capability or commitment to a specialty, then the appraiser must indicate that he or she will maintain confidentiality. On the other hand, in some cases the appraiser is also the assessor who is required to complete an assessment, in the case of specialist registrars, for the RITA. The final appraisal of foundation year one trainees is intended as the indicator of suitability for registration. In these and other cases, the appraiser/ assessor is in a difficult situation if confidentiality is an issue. There may also be circumstances when the appraiser feels, in the interests of patient safety, that information about the trainee should be passed on to others. Appraisers should help trainees to recognise that confidentiality is limited by the above conditions, and that they will do all they can to support the trainee, while ensuring that the normal procedures are followed.

Conflict

The management of conflict has been addressed in Chapter 2. Disagreements are bound to arise from time to time and these should be resolved quickly to avoid escalation. Should serious conflict arise between an appraiser and trainee, it serves little purpose to attempt to resolve it since the trainee will always be concerned that fair assessment is compromised. A new appraiser should be found as quickly as possible.

Serious personal problems

Difficulties in appraisal may arise due to the serious nature of personal problems that afflict some trainees from time to time. It is important that the appraiser takes responsibility for ensuring the trainee receives suitable support in these circumstances. They should not, however, assume responsibility for taking on a counselling role or becoming personally burdened with the trainee's situation.

Further advice on counselling is given below. Occupational health officers or personnel departments can usually assist in such circumstances.

Lack of personal insight

Occasionally, trainees seem to lack the ability to see their own weaknesses as others see them. This can be particularly true where there is a lack of interpersonal skill. It may also be that trainees are not able to see their lack of progress in developing clinical competence and judgement. It is important to distinguish between those who really are unaware of the negative impact they create, or the concerns of other staff at the inadequacy of their clinical practice, and those who refuse to admit to weakness in order to

protect themselves from negative consequences. In the latter case, it is important to help the trainee to recognise the value of talking about their problems, since it may lead to better career decisions if they are struggling with the demands of the specialty in which they are working. Once again, the most helpful way to do this is to use open and probing questions focused on specific examples of their performance to get them to confront the problem. Those trainees who truly are unable to see their weakness, even after supportive questioning and gentle challenge, will only perhaps come to terms with their situation when they fail an assessment. It is crucial that the clinical tutor, and perhaps the postgraduate dean, is made aware of such problems at as early a stage in training as possible.

Revalidation

It is relevant to touch briefly on revalidation here, although further details are given in the following chapter. Appraisal provides a basis for determining education and development plans. It also contributes to the revalidation process. The revalidation folder contains information on how well the doctor is practising, and evidence of continuing professional development. Professional development portfolios are designed by the medical Royal Colleges and maintained by all doctors. These provide some of the evidence on which appraisal is based. Any concerns regarding a doctor's fitness to practise should have been be raised long before appraisal. There should be no surprises at the revalidation stage. Thus, appraisal for revalidation is essentially similar to trainee appraisal. The major part addresses all aspects of performance and will relate to:

- good clinical care
- maintaining good practice
- relationship with patients
- working with colleagues
- teaching and training
- probity
- health (source: GMC, 2001).

Preparation for appraisal relies heavily on the appraisee, who should have collected information about their performance from a range of sources, including:

- patients, e.g. through a patient survey

- immediate colleagues such as partners or other professionals, e.g. through a peer-associate questionnaire

- managers, where appropriate

- colleagues who refer to, or accept referrals from, the doctor

- the doctor, e.g. through a self-assessment questionnaire.

It may be that 360° feedback is available, in which case this is likely to provide the simplest and most reliable means of collecting information.

Supporting and advising others

Mentoring

In Greek mythology in Homer's *Odyssey*, Odysseus appointed Mentor as advisor to the young Telemachus. The dictionary defines 'mentor' as 'experienced and trusted advisor'. The use of mentors has become fairly widespread throughout the NHS over recent years. The term started to appear in management literature in the 1970s. Mentors are individuals who enter into a special working relationship with another person, usually a more junior colleague, to act as their advisor, counsellor and even role model.

It often involves a senior keeping an interest in the development of a protégé through a significant aspect of his or her career. Mentors may be asked to adopt a high-flier on a course or provide advice or assistance to a young professional. The role may be informal, where a senior takes an active interest in the career development of a trainee, and could also be regarded as developing a support network. The core capabilities have been identified as self-awareness (understanding self); behavioural awareness (understanding others); professional insight; sense of proportion and good humour; communication competence; conceptual modelling; commitment to own continued learning; a strong interest in developing others; building and maintaining relationships; and goal clarity (Foster-Turner, 2005).

Mentoring demands a close professional relationship between individuals. It involves a long-term supportive relationship involving assessment, career guidance and often counselling. Mentors need a wide range of assessment, appraisal and counselling skills. Mentors are usually more senior individuals, chosen for their perceived wisdom by the learner, but can also be peers in a group.

Counselling

Doctors, often without extensive psychological training, are from time to time called on to deal with troubled people, sometimes patients and sometimes colleagues. Although not professional counsellors, they are often regarded as well suited (or the nearest available) to address the woes of others.

The aim of a one-to-one interaction may be to solve a serious personal problem faced by someone who has brought it to you on the assumption that you will be able to help. Common sense demands that, if you judge the problem to be beyond your capability, you should direct the person to someone more suited to advise them. Frequently, however, it may be within your power to help someone resolve their problem by merely acting as a sounding board. This does not, however, involve playing a passive role.

The aims of such counselling may include:

- clarifying problem issues

- facilitating problem solving

- encouraging insight.

It will not include:

- curing mental health problems

- relieving drug or alcohol dependency

- removing all suffering

- solving social or political problems.

Common factors in an effective approach will usually involve:

- listening

- encouraging

- exploring
- following the lead given by the client.

The most critical of these is listening, which is covered in detail below.

Personal counselling

The contents of personal counselling are confidential. They generally deal with personal, social, family, cultural or spiritual issues which are affecting performance at work or life generally. It should only be carried out when explicitly agreed by the individuals concerned.

Carrying out personal counselling requires training in counselling skills. Thus counselling should only be carried out within the limits of the individual's training, and they should recognise when to refer on to a more experienced or more highly trained counsellor. Nevertheless, basic-level counselling can be a valuable attribute of many doctors who interact with trainees.

Counselling is non-judgemental, except when the law is broken. Personal counselling may lead to a referral to psychiatric help, or individual, group or family therapy.

Career counselling

Career counselling uses methods to assess attitudes, values, personal attributes, skills and knowledge to inform a career choice. This may be necessary for doctors (and medical students) at or before crossroads in their careers. Career counselling requires the counsellor to have counselling skills, a wide range of knowledge of medical careers, and ready access to career information and the consequences of each choice. There is a danger of career counselling developing into persuasion followed by patronage, leading to unfairness and potentially poor career choice. *Modernising Medical Careers* has led to the introduction of more structured approaches to early career advice. Also, Anita Houghton (2005) has written a useful book for those interested in reflecting on their personal career preferences.

Career guidance

Career guidance differs from career counselling in that the individual is advised about their chosen career pathway. Guidance usually requires someone to have a detailed knowledge of that particular career pathway, and may include assessment of the stage of training reached.

Note: career counselling and career guidance are sometimes confused and used interchangeably. It is important that it is clear whether the process is about making career choice between a variety of careers, or dealing with an already chosen career.

Effective listening

We spend half our working lives in situations in which we are supposed to be listening. For most of this time we are doing anything but listening. We might be hearing what is being said, but our minds are often distracted by other thoughts, and our behaviour sends signals to the other person indicating this fact. Effective (or active) listening is a developed skill and one worth acquiring. Effective listening benefits include:

- gaining a better understanding of what people feel and what is happening
- improved working relationships
- reduced conflict
- new ideas and perspectives on issues.

Guidelines for effective listening

- Prepare yourself to listen by putting your own ideas on hold while you concentrate.
- Avoid distractions from visitors, interruptions, telephone calls, the window etc.
- Listen to the whole message – content, tone and non-verbal cues.
- Be silent, attentive and interested.
- Be receptive and keep an open mind.
- Allow the speaker to finish.
- Take notes where appropriate.
- Respect confidences and build trust.
- Clarify and summarise.
- Reflect feelings to encourage the speaker to be open.

Giving feedback

If you ask people to reflect on some of the more significant aspects of their personal development they will often talk about people who have given them direct and pertinent information about themselves. This personal help can be useful, but sometimes people are hurt by the feedback they receive. So we need to explore ways of giving feedback which enable the person to be stronger as a result. These guidelines may help you give and receive feedback in the most constructive way. You may have to work at it to be effective, but the skills developed will not only be a valuable management asset but can influence and improve your own personal life.

Poorly performing colleagues

Difficulties may arise in an individual's life that affect their performance. These may include personal problems, under-performance, health-related issues (both physical and mental), stress, problems outside of medicine, such as family difficulties or illness, and disciplinary matters. Increasingly, a more systematic and structured approach to appraisal and assessment is beginning to pick some doctors up, at an earlier stage, as they are beginning to run into problems.

Such problems may usually be divided into four main areas:

- personal conduct
- professional conduct
- competence and performance issues
- health and sickness issues.

Early identification of the problem is often critical. Recognition that a colleague is performing below an acceptable professional standard brings with it a heavy responsibility. Patients and other colleagues depend on the professionalism of all those around them. The first step is to seek clarification and not to jump to conclusions based only on one version of events. It is helpful to seek answers to the following questions:

- what is the real problem?

- why has this happened?
- what can we do about it?
- can we get back on course?

Many problems can be resolved at local level, rather than involving all the processes described below. However the principles of finding out and using facts and not opinions, constructive feedback, setting targets for improvement and following these through will hopefully work well in most cases.

The role of the employer

Employers have procedures laid down for discipline, performance and sickness issues. Human resource specialists can usually provide helpful advice regarding procedural and legal matters – it is important to recognise the value of checking up before taking action.

Personal conduct issues

Extreme examples of such problems include theft, fraud, assault on another member of staff, vandalism, rudeness, bullying, racial and sexual harassment, downloading pornography from a computer in the library, and attitude problems in relation to colleagues, other staff and patients. The trust (as the employer) will take the lead under its approved disciplinary procedures.

Professional conduct issues

Examples of such problems include research misconduct, failure to take consent properly, prescribing issues, improper relationships with patients, improper certification issues (such as the signing of cremation forms, sickness certification, passport forms), and breach of confidentiality. In the case of trainees, the employing trust will take the lead under its disciplinary procedures and also inform the deanery in writing at the earliest stage. The deanery will provide an input into such a disciplinary process via the clinical tutor, the GP trainer, the chair of the specialty training committee or regional advisor (for specialist registrars) or other member of the deanery. Any decision to involve the GMC is a very serious one for the doctor involved, and this will be a joint decision between the trust (or other employer) and the deanery.

Competence and performance issues

Examples of such problems include a single serious mistake, or poor results clinically, possibly found as a result of audit, poor timekeeping, poor communication skills, poor consultation skills and repeated failure to attend educational events. Local disciplinary procedures may be employed or, for trainees, this type of problem may be dealt with through the educational framework. The educational supervisor and clinical tutor will take a lead in some of these problems. Postgraduate deaneries may also provide further expert assessment and remedial training in such areas of communication and consultation skills.

An isolated serious mistake could happen to anyone. Many doctors have been in this situation at some time in their careers. It does not necessarily reflect the overall competence of the doctor concerned (National Patient Safety Agency (NPSA), 2005). Such a mistake may even lead to a formal inquiry. It is important that the local deanery be kept informed. Counselling and pastoral support should be available, as such an event can be highly stressful for all concerned. In the past, such a doctor may often have been suspended. The chief medical officer has asked trusts to try not to suspend doctors in such circumstances, but consider using the possibility of a referral to the National Clinical Assessment Service (NCAS).

If the doctor's performance is consistently poor, even though all educational measures have been tried to put things right, then it may on occasions be necessary to inform the GMC. Obviously this is not a decision to be taken lightly, or on the spur of the moment. Such a referral may have momentous and unpredictable consequences for the doctor concerned. In the case of a trainee, this will again need to be a joint decision between the trust and the deanery.

Health and sickness issues

All doctors have a responsibility to ensure that their health does not adversely affect the care that they provide to patients. Circumstances arise, however, particularly in cases of mental health and addictive illness, in which the individual's insight into the need for help and treatment is diminished. In such circumstances, a doctor's close colleagues have a duty to take action, in the interests both of patient care and of the doctor's health. Intervention should be seen both as an ethical responsibility, and also as a caring act. Not to intervene inevitably leads to a deterioration in the doctor's health, and, ultimately, in performance. Indeed doctors are under a professional duty to take steps to protect patients from a risk of harm posed by other health professionals (BMA, 2004).

Every doctor is advised to register with a local general medical practitioner, and consult with their doctor in the first instance when ill. Ill-health and sickness-related absence should be managed through the trust's sickness procedures, and may include their occupational health service. There are GMC guidelines on serious infectious diseases and other health issues, including physical and mental illness that may affect the safety of patients. These need to be consulted, and again the advice of a consultant physician in occupational medicine is essential in such cases. Deaneries can usually enable access for trainees to specialist advice in occupational medicine.

Prevention is better than cure

Regular and constructive day-to-day feedback is one of the best ways to help trainees learn. Regular appraisal and assessments are essential and can do a great deal to identify and help address performance problems before they become serious.

Record maintenance is an important aspect of supervision. Notes should be kept of meetings held to discuss the doctor's adherence to agreed and accepted processes, such as the use of guidelines, furthering their own education, attendance at protected teaching sessions, contribution to research and development activities, audit, and their awareness of their own clinical outcomes. In the absence of written evidence of meetings, the poorly performing doctor may then often claim that they were completely unaware of any problem. Appraisals and assessments must be documented. Keep copies of all assessments and appraisals. Always make notes of performance-related meetings, conversations and so on and keep copies.

The GMC guidance *Good Medical Practice* stresses your duty to protect patients if you believe a colleague's performance or health is a threat. Before taking any action you need to ascertain the facts, and it is often helpful, and certainly sensible, to discuss your concerns with an experienced senior colleague before notifying the employing authority on regulatory body.

The Central Consultants and Specialists Committee (CCSC) has also produced guidance on the actions that consultants should take if they are concerned about the performance of colleagues. They highlight the following:

- act quickly to protect patients

- place clear professional responsibility to take action where there are serious concerns

- the first step may be to discuss with a senior colleague or a colleague in a specialty from another hospital

- consider the use of local informal procedures

- possibly seek advice from the local BMA office

- it may be necessary to bring the matter to the attention of your trust through the medical director, clinical director or even the chief executive.

There are a number of agencies available to help doctors in these situations.

The National Counselling Service for Sick Doctors provides the following contacts:

- *Association of Anaesthetists' Sick Doctor Scheme*: advice for anaesthetists. Tel: 020 7631 1650

- *BMA Counselling Service*: provides 24/7 telephone counselling by qualified counsellors. Tel: 08459 200 169

- *BMA Doctors for Doctors Service*, www. bma.org.uk: provides help for doctors in employment difficulties especially in relation to mental health problems and abuse of alcohol and drugs. The unit provides a signposting service to the area of help that is of most pertinence to the individual doctor's case. Tel: 020 7383 6739

- *British Doctors' and Dentists' Group*: a network of support groups of recovering medical and dental drug and alcohol users. Students are also welcomed. The groups are accessed via the Medical Council on Alcohol. Tel: 020 7487 4445 and *see* website: www. medicouncilalcol.demon.co.uk

- *British International Doctors' Association*: where cultural or linguistic problems may be a contributing factor, doctors can access the health counselling panel. Tel: 0161 456 7828; email: oda@doctors.org.uk

- *Clinicians' Health Intervention Treatment and Support*: promotes a consistent response to substance misuse problems in clinical staff throughout the United Kingdom. Tel: 01335 342144; email: avoca@birdsgrove.freeserve. co.uk

- *Doctors' Support Network and Doctors' Support Line*: self-help organisations for doctors with work difficulties, anxiety, depression, or family problems. Tel: 0870 765 0001; email: lizzie@ dsn.org.uk; websites: www.dsn.org.uk and www.doctorssupportline.org

- *Royal College of Obstetricians and Gynaecologists*: provides mentoring support for fellows and members in difficulties. Tel: 020 7772 6369; email: cdhillon@rcog.org.uk

- Royal Medical Benevolent Fund: provides financial help for sick doctors. Tel: 020 8540 9194; email: seniorcaseworker@rmbf.org; website: www.rmbf.org

- *Sick Doctors' Trust*: a pro-active service, self-help organisation for addicted physicians; provides early intervention and treatment for addiction to alcohol or drugs. Tel: 0870 444 5163; website: www.sick-doctors-trust.co.uk.

Help may often be obtainable from the doctor's GP, medical defence organisation, the NHS occupational health service, the postgraduate deanery and the local medical committee (LMC).

Details of the GMC's role in helping sick doctors can be found at: www.gmc-uk.org.

Key learning points

- *Preparation*: teaching and appraisal are each made more effective if both trainer and trainee come prepared.

- *Agenda*: appraisal meetings should follow an agenda which should be agreed before or at the start of the meeting.

- *Giving feedback*: negative feedback is sometimes made more acceptable if it is preceded by positive remarks about the appraisee's performance. Even better, get them to tell you about the weaker areas of their performance. In any event, make sure they get the message!

- *Setting objectives*: all objectives should meet the criteria of being 'SMART'.

- *Dealing with conflict*: if conflict is not easily resolved, the trainee should be transferred to the responsibility of another trainer.

- *Managing the confidentiality issue*: confidentiality can be crucial in getting the appraisee to open up about weaknesses, but it has to be made clear that behaviour that contravenes GMC or other regulations will lead to disclosure to others.

- *Avoid taking on trainee's problems*: these may be simply to do with training activities. The trainee should carry some responsibility for organising their own learning. Additionally, you should recognise that your role as an appraiser does not make you an expert counsellor. If serious problems are disclosed, refer them to someone who is equipped to help them.

Related reading

- Bennett H, Gatrell J and Packham R (2004) Medical appraisal: collecting evidence of performance through 360° feedback. *Clinician in Management* 12(4):165–71.

- British Medical Association (2003) *Appraisal: a guide for medical practitioners*. BMA, London.
- Bulstrode C and Hunt V (1996) *Educating Consultants*. Oxford University Press, Oxford.
- Department of Health (2003) *Appraisal for Doctors in Training in the NHS*. Department of Health, London.
- Foster-Turner J (1995) *Coaching and Mentoring in Health and Social Care – the Essential Manual for Professionals and Organisations*. Radcliffe Medical Press, Oxford.
- Gatrell J and White T (2000) *Medical Appraisal, Selection and Revalidation*. RSM Press, London.
- General Medical Council (1997) *The New Doctor*. GMC, London
- General Medical Council (2001) *Good Medical Practice*. GMC, London.
- General Medical Council (2004) *Licensing and Revalidation Formal Guidance for Doctors* (Draft). GMC, London.
- Gourlay R (1998) *Dealing with Difficult Staff in the NHS*. Kogan Page, London.
- Hall W, Violato C, Lewkonia R *et al.* (1999) Assessment of physician performance in Alberta: the Physician Achievement Review. *Canadian Medical Association Journal* 161:52–7.
- Houghton A (2005) *Know Yourself – the individual's guide to career development in healthcare*. Radcliffe Medical Press, Oxford.
- Marteau TM, Wynne G, Kaye W and Evans TR (1990) Resuscitation: experience without feedback increases confidence but not skill. *BMJ* 300:849–50.
- NHS Executive (1998) *A Guide to Specialist Registrar Training (The Orange Book)*. Department of Health, London.
- National Patient Safety Agency (2005) *Medical Error – how to avoid it all going wrong and what to do if it does*. NPSA, London.
- Royal College of Surgeons (1996) *Training the Trainers*. Raven Department of Education, The Royal College of Surgeons of England, London.
- Rennie S (2003) *Tossing Salads Too: a users' guide to medical student assessment*. JASME, Edinburgh.
- The Standing Committee on Postgraduate Medical and Dental Education (SCOPME) (1996) *Appraising Doctors and Dentists in Training: a working paper for consultation*. SCOPME, London.

CHAPTER 7

Clinical governance, quality and research

This chapter aims to develop understanding of the role of clinical governance in delivering a quality healthcare service. It explores the role of risk management, clinical audit and research. It also describes current developments in NHS structures and initiatives for improving quality of service.

Current emphasis in the NHS continues to be for a modern, dependable and quality-assured service. Since the mid-1990s, the drive for continuous improvement in quality of care has been underpinned by the implementation and consolidation of clinical governance. Quality is elusive both as a concept and in day-to-day working, but there is nonetheless constant pressure to improve it. This is partly due to the inherent complexity of healthcare and the fact that patients and their families often have only partial insight into what constitutes good or bad treatment. There is continuing debate about the ability of healthcare professionals to self-govern, particularly as the media and public have expressed concern over a few high-profile adverse incidents within NHS organisations. Earlier attempts to overcome some of these concerns included the introduction of medical and clinical audit in the early 1990s. More recently, clinical governance was seen as a system for pulling together a number of initiatives and locating responsibility within healthcare organisations. In essence, clinical governance is a systematic approach to maintaining and improving the quality of patient care. Probably the most widely cited definition is:

A framework through which NHS organisations are accountable for continually improving the quality of their services and safeguarding high

standards of care by creating an environment in which excellence in clinical care will flourish. (Scally and Donaldson, 1998)

The ultimate goal of clinical governance is to change the culture of healthcare provision so that quality improvement becomes routine in clinical practice and the management of the service. Quality comes in different forms. Quality assurance is making sure not only that the right things get done right, but also that the wrong things do not. In clinical practice, audit has been described as a shield of quality. Mistakes matter and, some believe, will always happen. Clinical audit is a process for finding good criteria to work to and, by adhering to them, ensuring continuous improvement in performance.

In this chapter we will cover a number of issues that are linked to quality. According to the Chief Medical Officer (1998) the pursuit of quality can be broken down into three distinct but interrelated strands:

- clinical governance

- enhanced professional self-regulation

- lifelong learning.

Medical research can contribute to improved patient care. Involvement in research can be a powerful aid to learning and understanding. It can also contribute to career development. The research process is also covered in this chapter.

In the 1950s and 1960s it was often assumed that more spending on healthcare would lead to better health. Increased awareness of other determinants of health, such as housing, employment, family and social class positioning has induced a more political approach. Other factors such as the oil crisis of the 1970s, the emergence of previously non-industrial countries as strong economic competitors, the increasing cost of new health technologies, and the growing proportion of the aged population, have led to increased pressure to contain costs. The creation of the NHS internal market as part of the reforms in the late 1980s and early 1990s was accompanied by a plethora of initiatives aimed at improving quality. More recently, quality has become focused on the twin concepts of clinical effectiveness and evidence-based medicine.

Let us consider some of the main issues around quality in healthcare.

What does quality mean in a health service?

The service provided by a healthcare organisation may be excellent, but will not be considered successful unless valued by the patient. The delivery process also has to be excellent. This is difficult in a health service where expectations and requirements of many parties in the system may be very different.

Quality is thus difficult to define and even harder to measure. Yet organisations, including healthcare organisations, strive continuously to measure and improve the quality of their products and services. The Institute of Medicine (2001) defines healthcare quality as 'care to individuals and populations which increases the likelihood of a desired outcome and is consistent with the current state of professional knowledge'. Experts tend to describe three dimensions of quality: structure, process and outcome. Structure comprises organisation of personnel and resources. It could include such items as health and safety. Process describes what is done for patients, and includes the content of care and the skill with which care was executed. Outcome is the end result of care. Is the patient restored to health and

full functional status? Is the patient satisfied with the healthcare services? Some outcomes, like functional status, are difficult to measure. Others, which may be easier to measure, such as mortality, are sometimes difficult to link to a specific process of care. No single dimension alone is sufficient to describe quality.

Working for Patients (Secretary of State for Health, 1989), proposed a set of seven patient-focused factors:

- appropriateness of treatment and care
- achievement of optimum clinical outcome
- clinically recognised procedures to minimise complications and similar preventable events
- an attitude which treats patients with dignity and as individuals
- an environment conducive to patient safety, reassurance and contentment
- speed of response to patients' needs, and minimum inconvenience to them (and their relatives and friends)
- involvement of patients in their own care.

These factors still provide a relevant and fairly simple way determining a quality service to patients.

Quality management

Quality management may be taken to include a number of aspects – including quality control, quality assurance, total quality management (TQM), zero defects and continuous quality improvement (CQI) among many others. There is now more information about how well services perform. Access to internet health information sources such as the Doctor Foster Hospital Guide has raised people's expectations of higher standards of quality in services. According to one of the leading figures in quality management over the past few decades, 'Management is responsible for 94% of quality problems and their first step should be to dismantle the barriers that prevent employees doing a good job' (Deming, 1986).

Implementing quality improvements is a major task requiring commitment of all involved in the delivery of service. Measuring patient satisfaction, while essential, is not the only dimension of quality of care. Professionals have the principal responsibility for defining and maintaining technical standards. Quality has to be built in to the healthcare system – failures cannot be thrown away.

Total quality management (TQM)

Total quality management describes an organisational approach to quality improvement. It emphasises the importance of processes and the involvement of people in continuously monitoring and improving them. The Principles of TQM are said to be:

- quality can and must be managed
- everyone has a customer and is a supplier
- processes, not people, are the problem
- every employee is responsible for quality
- problems must be prevented, not just fixed
- quality must be measured
- quality improvements must be continuous
- the quality standard is defect free
- goals are based on requirements, not negotiated
- management must be involved and lead
- plan and organise for quality improvement.

It can be seen that this approach has to be embedded in the culture of the organisation. It calls for commitment at all levels, and is based on the assumption that processes, or systems, must be attended to as a basis for ensuring a quality of service at the highest level.

Benchmarking

Benchmarking is a process that compares practice and performance across organisations in order to identify ways to improve systems and delivery of care. Its purpose is to provide a basis for:

- understanding how your organisation compares with other organisations

- promoting understanding of the performance gap between organisations
- assisting in the search to find and implement best practice
- helping to identify areas for process improvement.

Its relevance in the NHS is based on the fact that there are many reasonably comparable organisations providing similar services in different parts of the country. This provides an opportunity for assessment of delivery against others. Thus, it is possible to compare outcome measures and set targets for effectiveness. It also offers the opportunity to share value for money improvements both within sites and between other parts of the NHS.

A source of further information is at www.nhsbenchmarking.nhs.uk.

Evidence-based clinical practice (EBCP)

> Evidence based clinical practice is an approach to decision making in which the clinician uses the best evidence available, in consultation with the patient, to decide upon the option which suits that patient best. (Muir Gray, 1997)

Evidenced-based medicine and healthcare are essentially about quality – quality in trying to find studies addressing a question, ensuring that only unbiased studies are included, and distilling that information. There is usually another contributor to quality. This is when the evidence is combined with a doctor's education and experience, insight and knowledge of a patient to make sound decisions. It is the opposite of conjecture-based decision making. Many organisations, journals and electronic databases are dedicated to its pursuit, and encouraging its growth in the NHS. This growth will undoubtedly continue, given financial pressures and the requirements of clinical governance. It has been the main driver for many of the changes in the national healthcare structure.

- *Medline*: PubMed is a service of the United States National Library of Medicine that includes over 16 million citations from Medline and other life science journals for biomedical articles back to the 1950s. PubMed includes links to full text articles and other related resources. It is found at www.ncbi.nlm.nih. gov/entrez/query.fcgi.

- *Cochrane library*: published quarterly on CD ROM. It is part of the Cochrane Centre, itself part of the evidence-based healthcare (EBH) network know as The Cochrane Collaboration. The NHS Centre for Reviews and Dissemination is a sibling organisation and based at York University, which can be accessed at www.york.ac.uk/inst/crd.index.htm.

- *Bandolier:* a monthly journal produced for the NHS Research and Development Directorate. It provides surveys and evaluation and comments on a wide range of conditions and treatments. It can be found at www.jr2.ox.ac. uk/Bandolier.

- *Ovid's Evidenced Based Medicine Reviews*: this database pools EBH literature references from the Cochrane database and Best Evidence, a database containing US effectiveness literature, at www.ovid.com/product/ebmr/ebmr.htm.

- *Centre for Evidence Based Medicine*: this is a valuable resource that provides a range of teaching and learning materials and a toolbox to help to make sense of evidence-based medicine. It can be found at www.cebm. net/index.asp.

- *Department of Primary Health Care*: the department undertakes undergraduate clinical teaching in general practice and conducts research in cardiovascular disease, cancer, infectious disease and diabetes. It can be found at www.primarycare.ox.ac.uk.

- *Centre for Evidence Based Child Health*: run by the Institute for Child Health at Great Ormond Street Hospital for Children, London. It can be found at www.ich.ucl.ac.uk/ich.

- *Institute for Public Health, University of Cambridge*: evaluates interventions and preventive medicine in primary and secondary care. It can be found at www.iph.cam.ac.uk.

- *Centre for Evidence Based Mental Health*: provides information related to EBH in mental health. It can be found at www.psychiatry. ox.ac.uk/cebmh.

NHS quality initiatives

The following organisations and initiatives exist to contribute to the maintenance and improvement of quality in healthcare. Some have been referred to above and elsewhere, but to remind you …

The Healthcare Commission

The Healthcare Commission's legal name is the Commission for Healthcare Audit and Inspection. It is an independent body, set up to promote and drive improvement in the quality of healthcare and public health. It was formed by the Health and Social Care (Community Health and Standards) Act 2003, and launched on 1 April 2004. The Healthcare Commission replaced the work of the Commission for Health Improvement. It also covers the private and voluntary healthcare functions of the National Care Standards Commission, together with those elements of the Audit Commission's work that relate to efficiency, effectiveness and economy of healthcare.

The statutory duties of the Healthcare Commission in England are to:

- assess the management, provision and quality of NHS healthcare and public health services

- review the performance of each NHS trust and award an annual performance rating

- regulate the independent healthcare sector through registration, annual inspection, monitoring complaints and enforcement

- publish information about the state of healthcare

- consider complaints about NHS organisations that the organisations themselves have not resolved

- promote the co-ordination of reviews and assessments carried out by ourselves and others

- carry out investigations of serious failures in the provision of healthcare.

The Healthcare Commission also has certain duties in respect to Wales, mainly relating to national reviews and its annual State of

Healthcare report. However, local inspection and investigation of NHS bodies in Wales rests with the Healthcare Inspectorate Wales, while the Care Standards Inspectorate Wales inspects those organisations providing independent healthcare.

The Healthcare Commission works in close partnership with the Mental Health Act Commission (MHAC), whose role is to ensure that there is adequate and effective protection of patients detained under the Mental Health Act 1983. Under the government's review of legislation on mental health, most of the functions of the MHAC will transfer to the Healthcare Commission, and the MHAC will be abolished some time after April 2007.

The Annual Health Check

The Healthcare Commission is responsible for carrying out independent, authoritative and patient-centred assessments of the performance of each local NHS organisation and awarding an annual rating of that organisation's performance. This system is based upon measuring performance within a framework of national standards and targets set by government. The overall aim is to promote improvements in healthcare. The Annual Health Check replaced the old star rating assessment system for trusts.

The annual health check is designed to establish whether healthcare organisations are achieving core standards, using resources effectively and making and sustaining progress.

Achieving core standards

The Department of Health published *National Standards, Local Action* in July 2004. These comprise a set of 24 essential or 'core' standards that all healthcare organisations in England that treat NHS patients should be achieving immediately, and 13 developmental standards that they should be aiming to achieve in the future.

The standards cover seven 'domains' of activity:

• safety

• care environment and amenities

• clinical and cost-effectiveness

• governance

• patient focus

• accessible and responsive care

• public health.

Use of resources

This aspect of the annual health check looks at how effectively a trust manages its financial resources. All trusts (including PCTs) are assessed annually with the objectives of:

• providing rounded assessments of the financial performance of all NHS trusts

• making use of existing information and avoiding duplication of the work of other regulators.

Assessments differ between foundation and non-foundation secondary and tertiary care trusts and PCTs. Foundation trusts are set up under a different financial framework from other trusts, and have different responsibilities and requirements set in statute. The assessments reflect these differences but have the same purposes – to provide a view of the use of resources at each organisation. The criteria against which assessments are made are published by the Audit Commission.

In order to assess the use of resources by NHS foundation trusts, the Health Commission uses the findings of Monitor (the independent regulator for NHS foundation trusts), using its financial risk ratings as a basis. Monitor is an independent corporate body established under the Health and Social Care (Community Health and Standards) Act 2003. It is responsible for authorising, monitoring and regulating NHS foundation trusts.

Making and sustaining progress: improvement reviews

An improvement review is a review of a particular aspect of healthcare that is applied in every relevant organisation. Its aim is to encourage each organisation taking part to improve the quality of healthcare it provides to patients and the public. It may be a review of a service delivered between different organisations, a population group such as children, or a condition, for instance, diabetes. The Healthcare Commission will identify steps healthcare organisations should take to progress towards meeting standards, and will measure their progress. Each organisation taking part in an improvement review is given an assessment score that contributes to its overall annual rating.

Further information about the Healthcare Commission is available at: www.healthcare-commission.org.

The Institute for Innovation and Improvement

The Institute for Innovation and Improvement is a special health authority which superseded the Modernisation Agency in July 2005. It aims to provide a focus for new ideas, technologies and practices to improve services to patients, users and the public.

Its mission is to support the NHS in accelerating the delivery of world-class health and healthcare for patients and public by encouraging innovation and developing capability at the frontline.

The Institute's priorities are service transformation, technology and product innovation, leadership development and learning. These priorities are set by the Department of Health in consultation with a wide range of stakeholders and are outlined below:

- *technology and product innovation*: The Institute incorporates the National Innovation Centre based at the University of Warwick. It provides an entry point for industry and the NHS to explore and adopt innovative concepts and process new ideas, including and the development of specific products

- *service transformation*: it seeks to lead and commission development and research to build an evidence base of new and best practice in service transformation. It develops methodologies to encourage the adoption of improvement approaches and changes

- *learning*: The Institute works to promote a culture of lifelong learning for all NHS staff by working with NHS organisations and communities to develop learning systems to accelerate organisational and individual growth and change

- *leadership*: the Institute manages a portfolio of leadership development programmes. These include NHS graduate schemes (general management, finance and human resources); Gateway to Leadership; Board Level Development Resources; Breaking Through (for NHS managers from a black or minority ethnic background); the Leadership Qualities Framework.

Further information is available at www.institute.nhs.uk.

National Patient Safety Agency

The National Patient Safety Agency (NPSA) is a special health authority with a wide-ranging quality role within the NHS. It has been estimated that around 10% of patients admitted to the NHS each year are unintentionally harmed in some way, and that half of these incidents may be preventable (Vincent *et al.* 2001). Since April 2005 the NPSA has been responsible for the co-ordination of organisations and individuals in healthcare to investigate and learn from patient safety incidents occurring in the NHS.

The NPSA's work also encompasses safety aspects of hospital design, cleanliness and food and ensuring research is carried out safely through its responsibility for the Central Office for Research Ethics Committees (COREC). The NPSA supports local organisations in addressing their concerns about the performance of individual doctors and dentists through its responsibility for the National Clinical Assessment Service (NCAS). It also manages the contracts with the three confidential enquiries: The National Confidential Enquiry into Patient Outcome and Death (NCEPOD), The Confidential Enquiry into Maternal and Child Health (CEMACH) and The National Confidential Enquiry into Suicide and Homicide by people with mental illness (NCISH).

The NPSA seeks to ensure that all incidents are reported in the first place, to promote an open and fair culture in hospitals and across the health service, and encourage doctors and other staff to report incidents and 'near misses'. A key aim is to encourage staff to report incidents without fear of personal reprimand. It is not responsible for investigating individual cases or complaints. The NPSA has set up a national reporting structure which is aimed at collecting and analysing information from all staff and patients. One interesting example of the output of the NPSA is a publication entitled *Medical Error* (2005). This details personal stories of mistakes made by doctors, many from some of the country's leading figures. The report includes a number of case studies with expert advice, and is aimed at encouraging an open culture in reporting and addressing adverse incidents.

Further information is available at www.npsa. nhs.uk.

The National Clinical Assessment Service (NCAS)

NCAS was formed as a special health authority in April 2001, and was originally called the National Clinical Assessment Authority (NCAA). It became part of the NPSA in April 2005.

NCAS was set up to promote public confidence in doctors and dentists by giving confidential advice and support to NHS organisations on how to manage doctors and dentists whose performance has given cause for concern. If a difficulty becomes apparent, the employer, contracting body or the practitioner can contact NCAS for help. The aim of NCAS is to work with all parties to clarify the concerns and make recommendations to help the practitioner deliver a high-quality and safe service for patients. NCAS covers the NHS in England, Wales and Northern Ireland, and also the prison medical and dental service.

NCAS provides advice, takes referrals and carries out targeted assessments where necessary. It offers a range of services including advice over the phone, through to more detailed and ongoing support such as a full assessment of a practitioner's performance. It is an advisory body, and the referrer retains responsibility for handling the case throughout the process. NCAS also helps NHS organisations improve local management of performance concerns so that difficulties are recognised and addressed before they become more serious problems.

NCAS has working arrangements with a number of partners including the GMC, the General Dental Council (GDC), the Healthcare Commission and the Academy of Medical Royal Colleges.

The 'Back on Track' project was developed by NCAS in collaboration with key stakeholders, to create a national framework to support employers in returning doctors and dentists in primary and secondary to safe professional practice. The framework is intended for use by NCAS, the GMC, the GDC, Royal Colleges, deaneries and employer organisations. Its purpose is to facilitate the return to safe professional practice of practitioners who

have been either subject to a formal clinical assessment or investigation related to performance concerns, or absent or out of practice for a significant period.

Further information is available at www.ncaa. nhs.uk.

The National Confidential Enquiry into Patient Outcome and Death (NCEPOD)

Originally the Confidential Enquiry into Perioperative Deaths (CEPOD), NCEPOD's purpose is to assist in maintaining and improving standards of medical and surgical care by reviewing the management of patients, by undertaking confidential surveys and research, and by publishing and making available the results of their studies. Its work does not involve new or additional treatments or therapies. Studies may be initiated by individuals or organisations by submitting a proposal to NCEPOD. Proposals should be relevant to the current clinical environment and have the potential to contribute original work to the subject.

NCEPOD staff may be invited to visit hospitals and give presentations as part of multidisciplinary meetings such as audit days. This provides an excellent opportunity to discuss the ways in which clinicians participate in morbidity and mortality audit and to examine the ways in which recommendations made by NCEPOD should be addressed within the local setting.

Further information is available at www. ncepod.org.uk.

National Service Frameworks (NSFs)

National Service Frameworks are long-term strategies for improving specific areas of care. *The NHS Plan* (Department of Health, 2000) re-emphasised the role of NSFs as drivers in delivering the Modernisation Agenda. They form one of a range of measures to raise quality and decrease variations in service and were introduced in *The New NHS* (Department of Health, 1997) and *A First Class Service* (Department of Health, 1998). They set national standards with measurable goals within set time frames for a defined service or care group and put in place strategies to support implementation and establish ways to ensure progress within an agreed time scale.

Each NSF is developed with the assistance of an external reference group (ERG) which brings together health professionals, service users and carers, health service managers, partner agencies, and other advocates. The Department of Health supports the ERGs and manages the overall process.

The rolling programme of NSFs, launched in April 1998, covers the following:

Coronary heart disease

The NSF for coronary heart disease was launched in March 2000 and sets 12 standards for improved prevention, diagnosis and treatment, and goals to secure fair access to high-quality services. The standards are to be implemented over a 10-year period.

Cancer

The Calman Hine report (*A Policy Framework for Commissioning Cancer Services*) set out a framework for cancer care provision in 1995. *The NHS Cancer Plan* (September 2000) provides the fullest statement of the government's comprehensive national programme for investment and reform of cancer services in England.

Paediatric intensive care

The NSF for paediatric intensive care was established in 1999.

Mental health

The NSF for mental health was launched in 1999, and is a comprehensive statement on how mental health services will be planned, delivered and monitored until 2009. The NSF lists seven standards that set targets for the mental healthcare of adults aged up to 65 years. These standards span five areas: health promotion and stigma, primary care and access to specialist services, needs of those with severe and enduring mental illness, carers' needs, and suicide reduction.

Older people

The NSF for older people was published on 27 March 2001. It sets new national standards and service models of care across health and social services for all older people, whether they live at home, in residential care or are being cared for in hospital.

Diabetes

A total of 1.3 million people in England suffer from diabetes, and the number is increasing. The diabetes NSF is a concerted effort to make sure these people, wherever they live, receive the same excellent standard of care. Embodied in the NSF is the central value of *The NHS Plan* – that good service is the outcome of genuine partnership between the patient and the provider. The NSF, launched in 1999, should substantially reduce the suffering caused by diabetes.

Long-term conditions

The NSF for long term-conditions was published on 10 March 2005. The aim of the NSF is to improve the lives of the many people who live with neurological and other long-term conditions, by providing them with better health and social care services.

Renal services

Part one of the NSF for renal services sets five standards and identifies 30 markers that will help the NHS and its partners manage demand, increase fairness of access and improve choice and quality in dialysis and kidney transplant services. Part two of the NSF for renal services sets four quality requirements and identifies 23 markers of good practice to help the NHS limit the development and progression of chronic kidney disease, minimise the impact of acute renal failure, and extend palliative care to people dying with kidney failure.

Children

This NSF, published on 15 September 2004, sets standards for children's health and social services, and the interface of those services with education.

National Institute for Health and Clinical Excellence (NICE)

NICE is an independent organisation responsible for providing national guidance on the promotion of good health and the prevention and treatment of ill-health. NICE's role is to provide authoritative advice on the effectiveness of interventions to improve health and reduce health inequalities, and to advise on treatments and best clinical practice. Its role was set out in the 2004 White Paper *Choosing Health: making healthier choices easier*. NICE is made up of a board of health professionals, managers, academics, economists and patient representatives to work on and produce clinical guidelines. The functions of the Health Development Agency (HDA) were transferred to NICE as a result of the Department of Health's 2004 review of its 'arm's length bodies'. The Department of Health commissions NICE to develop clinical guidelines and guidance on public health and technology appraisals.

NICE produces three kinds of guidance:

- *public health*: guidance on the promotion of good health and the prevention of ill-health – for those working in the NHS, local authorities and the wider public and voluntary sector
- *health technologies*: guidance on the use of new and existing medicines, treatments and procedures within the NHS
- *clinical practice*: guidance on the appropriate treatment and care within the NHS of people with specific diseases and conditions.

Once NICE publishes guidance, health professionals and the organisations that employ them are expected to take it fully into account when deciding what treatments to give people. However, NICE guidance is not seen as replacing the knowledge and skills of individual health professionals who treat patients; it is still up to them to make decisions about a particular patient in consultation with the patient and/or their guardian or carer when appropriate.

NHS organisations in England and Wales are required to provide funding for medicines and treatments recommended by NICE in its technology appraisals guidance. The NHS normally has three months from the date of publication of each technology appraisal guidance to provide funding and resources. Local NHS organisations are expected to meet the costs of medicines and treatments recommended by NICE, out of their general annual budgets.

Its website is at www.nice.org.uk.

Health Improvement and Modernisation Programmes (HIMP)

HIMPs are 'the local strategy for improving health and healthcare', drawn up by health authorities in consultation with trusts, primary care groups, and other primary care professionals and patients. They are three-year action plans, developed in each health authority district, aimed at improving the health of the local population. Local authorities also have an input. They began in 1999 and are updated annually. PCTs ensure that the services they provide are commissioned are in tune with the priorities set out in the HIMP.

Critical Appraisal Skills Programme (CASP)

The Critical Appraisal Skills Programme (CASP) is a programme within learning and development at the Public Health Resource Unit. Since 1993, the programme has helped to develop an evidence-based approach in health and social care, working with local, national and international groups. CASP aims to enable individuals to develop the skills to find and make sense of research evidence, helping them to put knowledge into practice. CASP's workshops and resources are in three main areas of work, which are reflected in CASP's three-arrow logo: finding research evidence, appraising research evidence, and acting on research evidence.

CASP's website is at www.prhu.nhs.uk/casp/casp.htm.

Clinical guidelines

Clinical guidelines or protocols often set out treatment pathways and suggest options. An important function is to stop the use of established but unduly hazardous treatments as well as discouraging the use of ineffective and possibly also expensive treatments. They have become a component of clinical governance. NICE has a central role in co-ordinating work on guidelines.

National Clinical Audit Support Programme (NCASP)

NCASP, commissioned by the Healthcare Commission, manages the national clinical audits for heart disease, diabetes and cancer. National clinical audit is a continuous process whereby healthcare professionals review care against agreed standards and make changes, where necessary, to meet those standards. The audit is then repeated to see if changes have been made and if the quality of patient care is improved. The overall aim of clinical audit is to improve patient outcomes by improving professional practice and the general quality of services delivered. The aim is to provide the widest possible access to timely and reliable clinically endorsed audit data, through the delivery of a relevant and robust infrastructure. NHS organisations have a corporate responsibility for clinical quality and performance. NCASP supports NHS partners and professional bodies to fulfil this responsibility through the development of agreed clinical standards and comparative datasets.

Working in collaboration with a range of NHS organisations and professional bodies, NCASP provides an infrastructure for the collation, analysis and feedback of local clinical data to support effective clinical audit across the NHS.

Maintaining Good Medical Practice Guide

This is a booklet published by the GMC and designed to strengthen the process of professional self-regulation. It forms the basis of the GMC's medical appraisal scheme and provides advice on how to maintain good practice and what to do in cases of poor practice, the procedures involved and whom to contact.

Continuing medical education (CME) and continuing professional development (CPD)

Lifelong learning and continuing education are a stated part of the NHS Human Resources Agenda. This states that NHS organisations must provide programmes on education and training and personal and organisational development particularly around clinical governance. CME and CPD support healthcare professionals. There is, for example, a network of postgraduate medical centres based at district general hospitals. The medical Royal Colleges regard encouraging CPD as one of their key responsibilities.

Clinical governance

The main aim of clinical governance is to achieve continuous quality improvement (Som, 2004). Clinical governance is the process by which NHS organisations ensure that clinical activities are carried out to professionally agreed high standards and, by ongoing assessments and reviews, continued improvements are maintained. The Health Act (1999) outlined the legal responsibility of healthcare organisations as follows:

> It is the duty of each Health Authority, Primary Care Trust and NHS Trust to put and keep in place arrangements for the purpose of monitoring and improving the quality of health care which it provides to individuals.

Scally and Donaldson's 1998 definition (above) is intended to embody three key attributes:

- recognisably high standards of care
- transparent responsibility and accountability for those standards
- a constant dynamic of improvement.

The concept has some parallels with the more widely known corporate governance, in that it addresses those structures, systems and processes that assure the quality, accountability and proper management of an organisation's operation and delivery of service. However, clinical governance applies to health and social care organisations, and only those aspects of such organisations that relate to the delivery of care to patients and their carers; it is not concerned with the other business processes of the organisation except in so far as they affect the delivery of care.

Prior to 1999, trust boards had no statutory duty to ensure a particular level of quality. Their principal statutory responsibilities were to ensure proper financial management of the organisation and an acceptable level of patient safety. Maintaining and improving the quality of care was understood to be the responsibility of the relevant clinical professions. From 1999, trust boards assumed a legal responsibility for quality of care that is equal in measure to their other statutory duties. Clinical governance is the mechanism by which that responsibility is discharged.

Trust boards are, therefore, responsible for ensuring that systematic processes are in place for:

- continuous improvement in the quality of professional and clinical services provided by the organisation

- encouraging and guiding the dissemination of good practice

- evaluating, supporting and monitoring clinical practice

- facilitating the rapid detection and open investigation of adverse incidents, and ensuring that lessons are learnt from them.

There are nine areas of clinical governance as defined by the Healthcare Commission:

1 *strategic capacity*: the ability within the trust to monitor and improve the quality of patient care

2 *patient experience*: a patient's experience of the NHS is partly concerned with whether the outcome of their treatment is as good as it could have been, although this can be hard for a patient to judge. Other aspects can be less important to the final outcome, but may be of great importance to patients and their relatives as their diagnosis and treatment progresses

3 *patient involvement*: describes how patients can have a say in their own treatment and how they and patient organisations can have a say in the way that services are provided

4 *clinical risk management*: means having systems to understand, monitor and minimise risks to patients, and to learn from mistakes

5 *clinical audit*: the continual evaluation and measurement by health professionals of their work and the standards they are achieving

6 *staffing and staff management*: covers the recruitment, management and development of staff. It also includes the promotion of good working conditions and effective models of working

7 *education, training and continuing professional development*: covers the support available for staff to be competent in doing their jobs, while developing their skills and the degree to which staff are up to date with developments in their field

8 *research and effectiveness*: doing clinical research and caring for patients in a way that is evidence based

9 *using information*: covers the systems the trust has in place to collect and interpret clinical information and use it to monitor, plan and improve the quality of patient care.

Clinical governance consists of the following service improvement processes:

- *education*: responsibility for CPD of clinicians is shared between the trust and the individual clinician. It is also the professional duty of all clinicians to remain up to date (GMC, 2001)

- *clinical audit* is the systematic review of clinical performance, the refining of clinical practice as a result, and the measurement of performance against agreed standards – a cyclical process of improving the quality of clinical care. In one form or another, audit has been part of good clinical practice for generations. The key component of clinical audit is that performance is reviewed to ensure that what should be done is being done, and if not it provides a framework that enables improvements to be made

- *clinical effectiveness* is a measure of the extent to which a particular intervention works. The measure on its own is useful, but it is enhanced by considering whether the intervention is appropriate and whether it represents value for money. In the modern health service, clinical practice needs to be refined in the light of emerging evidence of effectiveness, but also has to consider aspects of efficiency and safety from the perspective of the individual patient and carers in the wider community

- *risk management* involves consideration of the following components:
  - *risks to patients*: compliance with statutory regulations can help to minimise risks to patients. In addition, patient risks can be minimised by ensuring that systems are

regularly reviewed and questioned – for example, by critical event audit and learning from complaints

– *risks to practitioners*: ensuring that clinicians are immunised against infectious diseases, work in a safe environment and are helped to keep up to date are important parts of quality assurance

– *risks to the organisation*: poor quality is a threat to any organisation. In addition to reducing risks to patients and practitioners, organisations need to reduce their own risks by ensuring high-quality employment practice (including locum procedures and reviews of individual and team perform-ance), a safe environment (including estates and privacy), and well-designed policies on public involvement

- *research and development*: good professional practice has always sought to change in the light of evidence from research. The time lag for introducing such change can be very long, and reducing time lag and associated mor-bidity requires emphasis not only on carrying out research, but also on using and implement-ing such research. Techniques such as critical appraisal of the literature, the development of guidelines, protocols and implementation strategies are all tools for promoting the implementation of research practice

- *openness*: processes which are open to public scrutiny, while respecting individual patient and practitioner confidentiality, and which can be justified openly, are an essential part of quality assurance. Open proceedings and dis-cussion about clinical governance issues should be a feature of the framework.

Common to most descriptions of clinical govern-ance is the concept of an integrated approach to care. This encompasses the overall patient exper-ience including co-ordination of diagnosis, treat-ment and recovery, taking into account the overall environment (Lugon and Secker-Walker, 1999).

Implementing clinical governance

The following systems and mechanisms con-tribute to clinical governance:

- clinical audit

- risk management

- health needs assessment

- evidence-based clinical practice

- patient feedback

- CPD

- accreditation of healthcare providers

- development of clinical leadership skills

- effective management of poorly performing colleagues

- systems to ensure critical incidents are openly investigated and lessons learnt are implemented.

The introduction of clinical governance has implications for individuals and organisations. It places requirements on healthcare organisations, including:

- developing leadership skills among clinicians (*see* Chapter 2)

- developing mechanisms to ensure that change in clinical practice occurs as a result of audit, risk management and complaints findings, thus closing the 'audit loop'

- developing appropriate accountability structures

- working more collaboratively and effectively between primary and secondary care

- developing more effective multidisciplinary working

- building CME and CPD into quality improve-ment programmes

- improving the information infrastructure of the NHS.

Thus, at trust level, the main principles of clinical governance are:

- clear lines of responsibility and accountability for the overall quality of clinical care

- a comprehensive programme of quality im-provement systems (including clinical audit, supporting and applying evidence-based prac-tice, implementing clinical standards and guide-lines, workforce planning and development)

- education and training plans

- clear policies aimed at managing risk

- integrated procedures for all professional groups to identify and remedy poor performance.

Trust chief executives are ultimately responsible to their boards for assuring the quality of services provided. Trust boards frequently set up clinical governance subcommittees, chaired by a clinical professional. A reporting regime requires trust boards to receive monthly quality reports and publish annual quality statements. At directorate level, a clinician supported by management ensures systems are in place for implementing clinical governance. Models vary from trust to trust.

Action

Check the following are in place in your trust:

- quality improvement programmes (e.g. clinical audit)

- leadership skills are developed at clinical team level

- evidence-based practice is in day-to-day use

- evaluated good practice and innovation are disseminated within and outside the organisation

- clinical risk reduction programmes

- adverse events are detected, openly investigated and the lessons learned applied

- lessons for clinical practice are learned from complaints made by patients

- problems of poor clinical performance are recognised early and dealt with to prevent harm to patients

- all professional development programmes reflect the principles of clinical governance

- the quality of data collected to monitor clinical care is itself of a high standard.

Risk management

Risk management adopts a formal and systematic process to identify and analyse risk and take remedial action to reduce or eliminate the risk of harm to patients, staff and the organisation. Both *The New NHS* (Government White Paper, 1997) and *Clinical Governance: quality in the new NHS* (NHSE, 1999) placed clinical risk management as a key component of clinical governance. They required clear policies to be implemented which were aimed at managing risk, and supporting professional staff in identifying and tackling poor performance. The stated aim was to protect patients and NHS resources.

Effective risk management at trust level demands clearly set out systems. Most trusts have committee structures with lines of responsibility for defined areas of risk, such as clinical risk, infection control and medicines management. Additionally, named individuals will carry responsibility for communicating, co-ordinating and facilitating the process of risk management throughout the organisation. Risk assessment is an integral element. This is normally undertaken by using a scoring, or rating, process. Firstly, the likelihood of the risk occurring is assessed on a scale from 1 (rare) to 5 (almost certain). Secondly, the consequences, or impact, of the occurrence are assessed from 1 (negligible) to 5 (extreme). These scores are multiplied to produce a 'risk rating number' between 1 and 25. The trust then determines response procedures based on the calculated rating. For example, a score of 16 or more is likely to require senior executive involvement and priority for funding.

In the year 2004–2005, £502.9 million was paid out by the NHS in connection with clinical negligence claims. This figure includes both damages paid to patients and the legal costs borne by the NHS. In 2003–2004, the comparable figure was £422.5 million. The figures for non-clinical claims are £25.1 million for 2004–2005 and £10.1 million for 2003–2004.

Trusts are normally insured against risk through the Clinical Negligence Scheme for Trusts (CNST). This scheme rewards trusts for compliance with its standards by discounting fees. The scheme is administered by the NHS Litigation Authority (NHSLA), a special health authority with responsibility for handling negligence claims made against NHS bodies in England. There are three different sets of CNST clinical risk management standards:

- *General Clinical Risk Management Standards* (NHSLA, 2005): these standards apply to all member organisations providing acute and specialist hospital services. They assess a trust's approach to managing risks relating to patient care and cover factors such as consent procedures, health records, infection control and staff induction and training

- *Maternity Clinical Risk Standards*: The CNST maternity standards apply to members providing labour ward services. They assess the way risk management activities are organised in these important services, focusing on areas such as communication, clinical care and staffing levels

- *Mental Health and Learning Disability Standards*: these CNST standards apply to mental health and learning disability trusts. Based on the CNST general standards, they have been developed to reflect the risks faced by such trusts.

All CNST standards are divided into three 'levels': one, two and three. Trusts that achieve success at level one in the relevant standards receive a 10% discount on their CNST contributions. Discounts of 20% and 30% are available to those passing the higher levels. Trusts are normally assessed against the CNST standards once every two years, although they may request an earlier assessment if they wish to move up a level. Trusts at level zero will be assessed every year.

Non-clinical risks are covered under the Risk Pooling Schemes for Trusts (RPST). This scheme dates from 1999, and covers employers' liability claims, from straightforward slips and trips in the workplace to serious manual handling, bullying and stress claims. Such claims are subject to excesses and, like CNST, contributions are calculated on an annual basis using actuarial techniques. Discounts are available to those who meet the relevant risk management standards.

In 2005 the NHSLA estimated that its total liabilities (the theoretical cost of paying all outstanding claims immediately, including those relating to incidents which have occurred but have not yet been reported) are £6.89 billion for

clinical claims and £0.11 billion for non-clinical claims.

Most trusts have a senior individual leading on risk management as part of their system of accountability. A small department will receive and analyse reported incidents. These are usually called adverse incident reports (AIRs) and may be completed by any member of staff. These reports are regarded as valuable, not only to encourage openness in dealing with such incidents, but also to identify trends. This is usually achieved by the use of a software package named DATIX after its supplier. This enables the trust to establish root cause analysis and determine trends as a means of managing future risks. Unfortunately, medical staff seldom see AIRs forms as important. In one medium-sized district general hospital the risk management department received 350 reports over a three-month period during 2005. Only one of these came from a member of the medical staff. Incidents such as an unplanned return to theatre, or admission of an inpatient to an intensive treatment unit would be examples where doctors might initiate a report.

Systems embedded in the working of healthcare organisations are seen as the only means of ensuring continuing responsiveness to risk management needs. The alternative is a 'crisis management' approach, dealing with problems as they arise, which adds risk and cost.

The Manchester Patient Safety Framework (MaPSaF)

The MaPSaF is a tool developed to help NHS organisations assess their progress in developing a safety culture and assist in measuring progress towards making patient safety a central focus within their organisation. It is based on a model that assesses five levels of organisational maturity in determining progress towards safe working systems in ten areas including approach to system errors, incident recording, communication about safety issues and team working. It helps to identify areas of particular strength or weakness and thus enables resources to be invested in the most appropriate fashion to best develop the patient safety culture. The MaPSaF was developed at the University of Manchester and is published by the NPSA. Further details are available at: www.npsa.nhs.uk/site/media/documents/1551_MaPSaF_Acute.pdf.

Clinical audit

Clinical audit is an essential and integral part of clinical governance. Medical audit was formally introduced into the NHS in 1989, changing its name to clinical audit in 1993 to reflect a more multidisciplinary approach. It had existed in good clinical practice for many years before that, some have argued, since 1854, when Florence Nightingale demonstrated the impact of her systematic evidence-based methods on patient mortality rates during the Crimean War. Clinical audit is now defined as a quality improvement process that seeks to improve patient care and outcomes through systematic review of care against explicit criteria and the implementation of change. Aspects of the structure, processes, and outcomes of care are selected and systematically evaluated against explicit criteria. Where indicated, changes are implemented at an individual, team, or service level, and further monitoring is used to confirm improvement in healthcare delivery. (NICE, 2002)

Types of audit

- *Standards-based audit*: a cycle which involves defining standards, collecting data to measure current practice against those standards, and implementing any changes deemed necessary.

- *Adverse occurrence screening and critical incident monitoring*: this is often used to peer-review cases which have caused concern, or from which there was an unexpected outcome. The multidisciplinary team discusses individual, anonymous cases to reflect upon the way the team functioned and to learn for the future. In the primary care setting, this is described as a 'significant event audit'.

- *Peer review*: an assessment of the quality of care provided by a clinical team with a view to improving clinical care. Individual cases are discussed by peers to determine, with the benefit of hindsight, whether the best care was given. This is similar to the method described above, but might include interesting or unusual cases rather than problematic ones. Unfortunately, recommendations made from these reviews are often not pursued as there is no systematic method to follow.

- *Patient surveys and focus groups*: these are methods used to obtain users' views about the quality of care they have received. Surveys carried out for their own sake are often meaningless, but when they are undertaken to collect data they can be extremely productive.

The audit process

The clinical audit process (see Figure 7.1) involves identifying an area for service improvement, developing and carrying out an action plan to rectify or improve service provision, and then re-auditing to ensure that these changes have an effect. As the process continues, each cycle aspires to a higher level of quality.

Stage 1: identify the problem or issue

This stage involves the selection of an issue or process to be audited, and is likely to involve comparison with healthcare processes that have been shown to produce best outcomes for patients. Selection of an audit topic is influenced by factors including:

- a search for national standards and guidelines or examples of excellent practice

- problems that have been encountered in practice

- problems raised by colleagues, patients or relatives

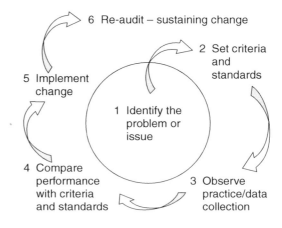

Figure 7.1 The audit process

- identification of potential for improving service delivery

- recommendations by national bodies, such as NICE or the Healthcare Commission.

Stage 2: define criteria and standards

Criteria are explicit statements that define what is being measured and represent elements of care that can be measured objectively. Standards define the aspect of care to be measured, and should always be based on the best available evidence. Decisions regarding the overall purpose of the audit should be written as a series of statements or tasks that the audit will focus on. Collectively, these form the audit criteria.

A *criterion* is a measurable outcome of care, aspect of practice or capacity.

A *standard* is the threshold of the expected compliance for each criterion (these are usually expressed as a percentage).

Stage 3: data collection

Certain details of what is to be audited must be established from the outset. This is to ensure that the data collected are precise, and that only essential information is collected. These details include:

- the user group to be included, with any exceptions noted

- the healthcare professionals involved in the users' care

- the period over which the criteria apply.

Sample sizes for data collection are often a compromise between the statistical validity of the results and pragmatic issues around data collection. Data to be collected may be available in a computerised information system, or in other cases it may be appropriate to collect data manually depending on the outcome being measured. In either case, considerations need to be given to what data will be collected, where the data will be found, and who will collect the data.

Ethical issues must also be considered; the data collected must relate only to the objectives of the audit, and staff and patient confidentiality must be respected – identifiable information must not be used. Any potentially sensitive topics should be discussed with the local research ethics committee.

Stage 4: compare performance with criteria and standards

This involves analysis of the data and comparison with criteria and standards. The final stage of analysis is to conclude how well the standards were met and identify reasons for failure to meet them. Where the standard was not fully met, there may be potential for improvement in care. In practice, where standard results were very close to being met, it might be agreed that any further improvement would be difficult to obtain and that other priorities exist. This decision will depend on the audit area – in some 'life or death'-type cases, it will be important to achieve 100%, in other areas a much lower result might still be considered acceptable

Stage 5: implementing change

Once the results of the audit have been published and discussed, an agreement must be reached about the recommendations for change. Using an action plan to record these recommendations is good practice. This should include who has agreed to do what and by when. Each point needs to be well defined, with an individual named as responsible for it, and an agreed timescale for its completion.

Stage 6: re-audit – sustaining improvements

This stage is sometimes referred to as 'closing the loop'. The audit should be repeated after a suitable period. The same approach to identifying the sample, methods and data analysis should be used to ensure comparability with the original audit. The re-audit should demonstrate any impact created by the changes. This stage is critical to the successful outcome of an audit process – as it verifies whether the changes implemented have had an effect and identifies whether further improvements are required to achieve the standards of healthcare delivery identified in stage 2.

Clinical audit and research

Some quoted differences are:

- research is often deductive and concerned with critical testing

- control groups and validating measures are more likely to be used in research than audit

- audit is often concerned with small-scale problems requiring local solutions

- the scope of research is likely to be different and to reach a wider national/international audience through publication of results in academic journals

- research can provide answers in areas that audit could not tackle, and challenges the efficacy of a particular therapy

- research raises questions about purposes (and the means of achieving them)

- audit evaluates what exists, and takes purposes for granted

- audit ascertains whether the inputs and processes achieve the outcome desired

- audit and research can feed into each other

- audit can give rise to research questions; if the outcomes of audit are not what was intended, research can ask why.

Perhaps the easiest to remember is that research is about finding the right thing to do, and audit is about ensuring you are doing the right thing right!

Clinical audit and education

Some issues and links to consider are that clinical audit is a professional development activity that highlights education needs in terms of audit methods and data analysis. By generating new knowledge, clinical audit can also contribute to postgraduate and undergraduate curricula in the healthcare professions. Education providers can use the knowledge gained through clinical audit to adapt curricula to new requirements, while providing health professionals with advice on research methods.

Audit and professional development

We have already considered that one of the fundamental principles of clinical audit is that it is an educational process as well as being related to the moral and professional accountability for practice. Clinical audit can be seen as a means to develop the team by developing reflective practice.

Audit may also be linked to portfolio learning. Most of the medical Royal Colleges use systems of points for accreditation. These mainly relate to lectures and study days rather than experiential learning, but the potential for the learning that takes place through participation in the audit process can be recognised and accredited as part of any individual's CPD. Records are maintained and kept in the revalidation folder as evidence of involvement in CPD. These approaches are also in accord with principles of adult learning, and generate effective learning.

Audit demands skills in teamwork, identifying problems, process analysis, data collection and management, problem solving, and change-management skills that are not usually a key part of any one key professional's training in healthcare. Thus training and education in clinical audit need to be seen as essential for everyone taking part in audit activities.

Action

Reflect on the credibility and quality of your audit experiences.

The organisation

- Is there a 'supra' trust group to co-ordinate audit?

- How does clinical audit fit with clinical governance in the structure of your trust?

- Is there central co-ordination of quality improvement initiatives?

- Are audit programmes scheduled far enough in advanced to ensure participation by appropriate staff?

- Is there clear responsibility for the development and adoption of external and internal clinical guidelines?

- Are audit and quality management programmes incorporated in the business plan?

Resources

- Is there agreement on how much staff time should be allocated to audit and quality improvement?

- Are audit support staff accessible to all clinical staff in all directorates?

- Is there a mechanism to ensure they are appropriately used?

- Are aggregated data on diagnosis, procedures and diagnostic tests complete, accurate and available for clinical analysis?

- Do staff have access to information on standards, methods and results of relevant projects inside and outside the trust?

- Is there a training budget for audit and quality improvement?

Produce a brief report of a clinical audit you have been involved in and the changes that resulted. Present this to a small group of 4–5 participants who may review the report, listen to your presentation and evaluate the use of the models and their application.

Exercise

- Think of a suitable topic for your next departmental audit, perhaps discussing this with a colleague.

- Find out who is responsible for audit in your department.

- Find out how the audit programme of your department is reported. Is it to the clinical tutor perhaps?

- Obtain a copy of last year's departmental audit report, and consider whether any of the findings have resulted in changes.

Research

Reliable, research-based information is fundamental to the successful implementation of clinical governance. This section provides general guidelines and insight into how to carry out research. It is not a tutorial on how to carry out research. Some suggestions for further reading may be found at the end of the chapter

Engagement in the research fosters characteristics such as logical thought, critical analysis and self-reliance. These are of substantial benefit in clinical practice. Most doctors who have undertaken periods of research would probably agree that they are better doctors for the experience. Research insight enables the interpretation and evaluation of research undertaken by others. It could be argued that all professional practice should be research based and research validated, not only providing patients with quality care and attention, but also ensuring that those commissioning healthcare are getting value in the provision of the services.

When to research

With sufficient time, research can be performed readily. Most doctors research as part of an additional or higher degree, for example, an intercalated BSc, MSc, MD, MS/MCh, MPhil or PhD. The timeframe of these courses varies considerably, and admission to such courses relates to clinical post, experience and interests. Particular attention must also be paid to funding and access to clinical posts upon completion of research.

Undertaking research

You are likely to be influenced by your planned area of specialisation, areas of special interest to you, or questions already under study in the department in which you work. Interest and perceived importance of the topic are necessary in order to maintain motivation. You also need to ask yourself whether you can be unbiased in the chosen topic. There is little point in starting unless you are sure you can complete the project within the available time.

Research is usually divided into 'pure' and 'applied'. Pure research has as its first objective the advancement of knowledge and the understanding of the relations between variables. The researcher may not have any practical intention for the research, only the development of understanding. Because this type of research does not offer any useable outcomes it can be difficult to raise funding. Applied research, on the other hand, is undertaken to solve specific, practical questions. Its purpose is to seek solutions, although it, too, can and often does raise further questions. Thus, the division between the two is seldom clear-cut. The difference between basic and applied research may be said to lie in the time span between research and reasonably foreseeable practical applications.

Research methods

The essential purpose of research is to produce some new knowledge. In medicine, this is likely to involve either exploratory or empirical research.

Exploratory research is conducted because a problem has not been clearly defined. It helps to determine the best research design, data collection method and selection of subjects. Exploratory research often relies on secondary research such as reviewing available literature and/or data, or qualitative approaches such as informal discussions with patients, clinical specialists, managers or other service users. Sometimes more formal methods such as in-depth interviews, focus groups, projective methods, case studies or pilot studies are employed. The results of exploratory research are not necessarily used for decision making, but they can provide significant insight into a situation.

Empirical research attempts to describe accurately the interaction between the researcher's data-collection 'tool' (which may be as simple as the human eye) and the entity being observed. The researcher is expected to calibrate his instrument by applying it to known standard objects, and documenting the results before applying it to unknown objects.

In practice, the accumulation of evidence for or against any particular theory involves planned research design. Design is sometimes determined as much by the researcher's experience and preference, as it is by the nature of the topic being researched. Differences can arise between those who adopt a quantitative, or positivist, model of testing theory, and those who prefer to rely on qualitative methods which are more focused on generating theories and accounts. Positivists treat the social world as something that is external to the social scientist and waiting to be researched. They traditionally seek to minimise intervention in order to produce valid and reliable statistics. Qualitative researchers, on the other hand, believe that the social world is constructed by social agency, and therefore any intervention by a researcher will affect social reality. They traditionally treat intervention as something that is necessary, often arguing that participation in the situation being researched can lead to a better understanding of the social dimension.

Research process

Generally, medical research is likely to follow an established structural process. Though the order of the stages may vary depending on the subject matter and researcher, the following steps are usually part of most formal research, both pure and applied:

- *formulation of the topic*: this may be determined by organisational need, or could arise out of the researcher's experience

- *setting up the hypothesis*: a hypothesis usually refers to a provisional idea whose merit needs evaluation. A hypothesis requires more work by the researcher in order to either confirm or disprove it. In due course, a confirmed hypothesis may become part of a theory, or grow to become a theory itself

- *an operational definition* is a description of something that determines its presence and quantity. It is an exact description of how to derive a value for a characteristic being measured. It includes a precise definition of the characteristic and how, specifically, data collectors are to measure the characteristic. The operational definition is used to remove ambiguity and ensure all data collectors have the same understanding and can independently measure or test for them at will

- *collecting data*: data is the plural of datum. A datum is a statement accepted at face value – a 'given'. A large class of practically important statements are measurements or observations of a variable. They usually are collected as numbers, words, or images

- *analysis of data*: this stage is determined by the topic, the nature of the hypothesis, the approach taken to data collection and the preferences of the researcher. Medical research outcomes are most often based on statistical analysis of data. Such analysis will be challenged if the researcher is unable to demonstrate that systematic bias was avoided in the research process, that the assessment was 'blind' (that the researcher could not have been influenced by any kind of performance bias), and that basic statistical procedures were followed (choice of sample size, duration and completeness of follow-up)

- *conclusion, revising of hypothesis*: a common misunderstanding is that a hypothesis can be proven. Instead, it may only be disproven. The hypothesis may survive several rounds of scientific testing and be widely thought of as true, but this is not the same as it having been proven. It would be better to say that it has yet to be disproved.

Getting published

Publication in academic media is based on peer review before it is made available for a wider audience. Medical specialties generally have their own journals and other outlets for publication. Some journals are interdisciplinary, and publish work from several distinct fields or subfields. The kinds of publications that are accepted as contributions of knowledge or research vary greatly between fields.

Higher, research-based qualifications and publications can be of great value when applying for jobs, particularly in some over-subscribed specialties. They represent not only an interest in improved patient care and scientific understanding, but also a desire to improve personal development. If an academic career beckons, research interests and publications in reputable refereed journals are an essential prerequisite.

Related reading

- Academic Medicine Group (1997) *Guidelines for Clinicians Entering Research*. Royal College of Physicians of London, London.
- Albert T (2000) *Winning the Publications Game. How to write a scientific paper without neglecting your patients* (2e). Radcliffe Medical Press, Oxford.
- Albert T (2000) *A–Z of Medical Writing*. British Medical Journal Books, London.
- *Bandolier* (1999) 6(2):7.
- Commission for Healthcare Audit and Inspection (2005) *Assessment for Improvement – the annual health check: measuring what matters*. Healthcare Commission, London.
- Chandra Vanu Som (2004) Clinical governance: a fresh look at its definition. *Clinical Governance: An International Journal* 9(2): 87–90.
- Crosby PB (1984) *Quality Without Tears: the art of hassle-free management*. McGraw-Hill, New York.
- Deming WE (1986) *Out of the Crisis*. MIT Press, Massachusetts.
- Department of Health (1998) *A First Class Service: quality in the new NHS*. Department of Health, London.
- Department of Health (1999) *Clinical Governance: quality in the new NHS*. Department of Health, London.
- Department of Health (2000) *The NHS Plan: a plan for investment, a plan for reform*. The Stationery Office, London.
- Department of Health (2004) *National Standards, Local Action: Health and Social Care Standards and Planning Framework 2005/6 – 2006/7*. Department of Health, Leeds.
- Department of Health (2006) *Best Research for Best Health – a new national health research strategy*. DH Publications, London.
- Donaldson LJ and Muir Gray JM (1998) Clinical governance: a quality duty for health organisations. *Quality in Health Care* 7 (Suppl):S37–S44.
- General Medical Council (2001) *Good Medical Practice*. GMC, London.
- Institute of Medicine (2001) *Crossing the Quality Chasm: a new health system for the 21st century*. National Academy Press, Washington DC.
- Greenhalgh T (1997) How to read a paper. *BMJ* 315(19 July–6 September).
- Greenhalgh T (2006) *How to Read a Paper – the Basics of Evidence-Based Medicine*. BMJ Books, Oxford.
- Lugon M and Secker-Walker J (1999) *Clinical Governance – Making it Happen*. The Royal Society of Medicine, London.

- Murrell G, Huang C and Ellis H (1999) *Research in Medicine* (2e). Cambridge University Press, Cambridge.
- NCAS (2005) *Back on Track – Restoring Doctors and Dentists to Safe Professional Practice.* NPSA, London.
- NHSE (1999). *Clinical Governance: quality in the new NHS* (HSC 1999/0065). HMSO, London.
- NICE (2002) *Principles for Best Practice in Clinical Audit.* NICE, London.
- NHSLA (2005) *Clinical Negligence Scheme for Trusts – CNST General Clinical Risk Management Standards.* NHSLA, London.
- NPSA (2004) *Making the NHS a Safer Place for Patients.* NPSA, London.
- NPSA (2005) *Medical Error – how to avoid it all going wrong and what to do if it does.* NPSA, London.
- Sackett D L, Rosenberg WMC, Gray JAM and Haynes RB (1996) Evidence-based medicine: what it is and what it isn't. *BMJ* 312:71–2.
- Scally G and Donaldson LJ (1998) Clinical governance and the drive for quality improvement in the new NHS in England. *BMJ* 317: 61–5.
- Secretaries of State for Health (1989) *Working for Patients* (Cm555). HMSO, London.
- Stevens A, Colin-Jones D and Gabbay J (1995) Quick and clean: authoritative health technology assessment for local health care contracting. *Health Trends* 27:37–42.
- Taylor DG (1998) *Improving Health Care.* King's Fund Policy Paper 2. King's Fund, London.
- Vincent, Neale G and Woloshynowich M (2001) Adverse events in british hospitals: preliminary retrospective record review. *BMJ* 332:517–19.
- White A and Gatrell J (1996) Being interviewed. In: A White (ed.) *Textbook of Management for Doctors.* Churchill Livingstone, London.
- White A (1996) Managing meetings. In: A White (ed.) *Textbook of Management for Doctors.* Churchill Livingstone, London.
- www.drfoster.co.uk (accessed 1 May 2006).

CHAPTER 8

Understanding the NHS

The aim of this chapter is to provide an outline of recent reforms and provide a brief outline of the structure of the NHS, both nationally and locally. It also reviews healthcare reforms in a worldwide context, and current thinking about hospitals of the future. Most of the following information can be downloaded from www.dh.gov.uk/PublicationsAndStatistics/fs/en click on 'Statistics' but prepare to be overwhelmed by data. There are also other data sources for some information: for example NHS, BMA and medical college websites, although they do not always agree on statistics.

A statistical picture of the NHS

- 4,604,194 people attended A&E departments in the year 2005–2006.

- Nearly 13 million people attend outpatients every year, and a million patients have ward attendances, which makes a total of nearly 28 million people attending hospitals every day for outpatient treatments.

- There are 3 million day case operations per year, and 3.6 million if day case treatments are included.

- There are nearly 9 million inpatient admissions every year.

- Over 50,000 operations were cancelled in 2005.

- Every day, nearly 700,000 people visit their GP, and about 100,000 visit their dentist.

- Every day, over 1,700 babies are delivered.

- A one-week stay in hospital costs £1,100, and a night in intensive care costs £500.

- Over 559 million prescriptions are dispensed each year, costing over £5 billion and representing 12% of all NHS expenditure.

- During 2005 the estimated annual cost of diet-related illness was £6 billion, of which nearly £500 million was due to obesity.

- In 2007–2008 the NHS budget is predicted to rise to £90.2 billion.

- There are more than 1.33 million staff in the NHS including 117,000 doctors, 397,500 nurses and 128,900 scientists.

- The total number of consultants in England at the end of 2005 was 31,210, an increase of 217 from the previous year.

- The 3-month or more vacancy rate for consultant jobs in trusts for 2004–2005 was 3.3%, a decrease from 4.4% in the previous year.

- The total number of GPs in the NHS at end of 2005 was 31,523 (excluding GP retainers and GP registrars) in England although 25% were part-time.

- In 2003 the number of medical students exceeded 6,000 the highest number ever in the history of the NHS, and 60% up on 1997.

- The official number of patients waiting to be admitted to NHS hospitals in England at the end of March 2006 was 784,500, although other authorities put it at between 814,400 and 826,300.

- Waiting lists for consultations have increased from 248,000 in 1997 to 512,000 in 2005.

- NHS Direct received 240,000 calls and 9,000 visits to its website during the Christmas holiday, 2004.

- 77% of funding comes from general taxation, 12% from the NHS share of national insurance contributions, and 2% from patient charges.

- Just under half of NHS spending goes on acute services. This amounts to about £800 per person per annum.

- The NHS spends £14 billion in Scotland and £7 billion in Wales.

- Over 40% of total hospital and community health services expenditure is for people over 64 years of age, though they represent just 16% of the population.

- About 7.7% of the gross domestic product will be spent on healthcare in 2004–2005, placing the UK sixth out of 22 Organisation for Economic Co-operation and Development (OECD) countries according to 'OECD Internet Health Data 2005'.

- OECD countries are spending record amounts on healthcare, largely due to the rising cost of pharmaceuticals and the diffusion of modern medical technologies.

- The NHS employs nearly 1.3 million people and is Europe's largest organisation and civilian employer.

- Just under 50% of the 1.3 million NHS employees are professionally qualified clinical, scientific, therapeutic or technical staff.

- Staff costs account for two-thirds of all NHS expenditure.

- The national sickness absence level for acute trusts for 2004, the last year for which figures are available, was 4.6%.

- The National Audit Office (NAO) claims that 5000 people die each year from hospital-acquired infections, and that at any one time 9% of patients have a hospital-acquired infection.

- The hospital-acquired infection problem is said to cost the NHS £1 billion a year.

- The estimated costs of adverse events in the NHS is believed to be in excess of £2 billion a year.

- The NHS spends an estimated £30 million a year on recruitment advertising.

- Since 1998, fraud in the NHS has been cut by 54% from £171 million to £78 million.

- Close to 4000 complaints were received by the NHS ombudsperson in 2002–2003, a 50% increase over the previous year.

Problems with the statistics

Conflicts in quoted figures from different authorities appear to be common, and we looked at the reason for this with regard to waiting lists. It is difficult to interpret but it gives a clue to the reason for the variations in published figures. There have always been differences between the official, admitted patient waiting times figures collected, those published by the Department of Health, and the waiting times taken from hospital episode statistics (HES). These appear to be mainly because of the different ways in which the times were calculated.

HES waiting times are worked out as the maximum waiting time; this time is from the date at which the decision is taken to put the patient on a waiting list, until the point at which they are admitted and the treatment takes place. However, the HES waiting times include days when the patient isn't available for treatment, because of illness or holidays, for example. Such days are called suspensions or deferrals from the waiting list.

Before December 2003, all DH official waiting times were worked out as the date that a patient was put on a Trust's waiting list to the date at which they were admitted. Unlike the HES waiting times, they did not include suspensions or deferrals. There were problems with the method for working out official waiting times though, as the definitions for calculating the time when patients were suspended or deferred, were unclear. This led to inconsistencies and local interpretations. There were even suggestions that some trusts were using 'phantom' suspensions to keep patients off waiting lists so that government targets could be met. Another anomaly that arises is that the waiting list time does not include any investigations. So, for example, a patient referred for a replacement hip operation would not start their waiting list time clock until all investigations were completed. The system also gave no way of reflecting the overall waiting time if a patient moved from a waiting list at one trust to a list at another.

In December 2003 a Data Set Change Notice (DSCN 37/2003) was issued. The changes set out in this document attempted to ensure that the Department of Health official waiting times more closely reflect the patients' perceptions of how long they have waited. The DSCN and background documents give the official guidance on this. The new Department of Health official waiting times are worked out from the date at which the patient is placed on a waiting list at any provider, until the date at which the patient is admitted for the treatment. This is regardless of which provider gives the treatment. For example, with their consent, the patient may be moved from the waiting list at one provider to that of another provider, who may be able to treat them more quickly. This might be as a result of the Patient Choice initiative.

The change to the official waiting times doesn't mean that they are calculated as the difference between the date when the patient is added to the waiting list and the operation date. However, if the treatment does not take place, for example if the patient is sent home with a cold, then the waiting time continues to be counted until the date of the admission that does result in the treatment taking place. Patients can be suspended from a waiting list for short periods of time while they are unavailable for admission for social or medical reasons. Also patients may refuse at least two admission dates that they are offered. In this case they are considered to have self-deferred, and the waiting time is then counted from the earliest date offered. The total number of days for periods in which the patient was suspended or was self-deferred can be subtracted from the total waiting time. Patients may also cancel appointments or not turn up on an accepted admission date they had previously accepted. In this case the waiting time is reset to zero, and the clock restarts from the date on which the patient failed to attend. Planned admissions are used where a patient is waiting for treatment for clinical reasons, rather than until resources become available. Such patients are usually excluded from waiting times calculations, although there is no reason why the time waited should not be recorded, as

the time between clinical events could have significance.

Comparing HES and NHS-derived waiting times in theory, it is possible for the HES waiting time to be greater than, equal to, or less than the NHS-derived waiting time. Well, we said it was a complex business, but if you want to try and make sense of it go to www.hesonline.nhs.uk.

The structure of the NHS

We are aware that most doctors in training may not be greatly interested in the structure of the NHS. However, as you approach your consultant post, you will need to have a basic outline of the system if only to be primed for any questions in a consultant interview. We have tried to keep things as basic as possible just to give you an outline.

The NHS still provides care via various routes:

- primary care through family doctors, opticians, dentists and other healthcare professionals

- secondary care through hospitals and ambulance services

- tertiary care through specialist hospitals treating particular types of illness such as cancer

- community care through partnership with local social services departments.

The NHS went through considerable change when Labour entered government in 1997. These changes were set out in the White Paper, *The New NHS*, published in December of that year and accompanied by papers for Scotland, Wales and Northern Ireland. The main commitment was to replace the internal market with a system based on co-operation and partnership. In England this meant essentially two key factors: retaining separation between health authorities and trusts, and replacing GP fundholding with commissioning through PCTs.

The New NHS is based on six principles:

- a national service

- delivery against national standards, and local responsibility

- characterised by partnership, not competition

- efficiency through a rigorous approach to performance and cutting bureaucracy

- moving the focus on to excellence and quality
- rebuilding public confidence in the NHS.

Although co-operation and partnership were stressed, competition did not disappear entirely, as PCTs are still able to choose which NHS trust provides care for their patients. Data published about performance seek to ensure that competition is by comparative results.

So this chapter describes some of the major players in the NHS hierarchy, and how they relate to each other. You need to be aware, however, that details continue to change and where possible we will point you to an appropriate source to update your information. The one continuing feature has been change in the balance between central and local control.

Historical review

This brief historical review is important to know about if you are looking anything about the subject on the internet, as 99% of what appears following a search is out of date and you therefore need to be aware of what has gone before. Up until 1988 hospitals were part of the Department of Health and Social Security (DHSS), but in July 1988 the DHSS was split into two departments: the Department of Health and the Department of Social Security, of which the Department of Health was concerned with care in hospitals, primary care and community health services. As a consequence of the Griffiths Report (1983), there followed a separation of 'policy' from 'management', and the Health Service Supervisory Board was established to advise on the strategic direction of the NHS.

The NHS Management Board was established at the beginning of 1985, and had responsibility for the department's management functions with respect to health authorities, particularly finance and performance review. The NHS Management Board reported to the Health Service Supervisory Board.

In 1989, the NHS Management Board was remodelled to form the NHS Management Executive (NHSME) and the Health Service Supervisory Board was reshaped into the NHS Policy Board, chaired by the Secretary of State.

The NHSME and NHS Policy Board were parallel bodies: the NHS Policy Board dealt with

policy formulation, NHSME with management and policy implementation.

There is a further distinction in function between the Chairman of the NHS Management Board (subsequently Chief Executive of the NHSME), and the Chief Medical Officer for England. The Chief Medical Officer (CMO) acted as an advisor to the government but was also concerned with clinical health issues, whereas the Management Board and NHSME were concerned with NHS management issues.

The division between policy and management was ended in 1995, following the Banks Report in the previous year. Responsibility for all NHS policy matters was transferred to the NHS Executive. (The NHSME consequently dropped the word 'Management' from its title.) (*See* Figure 8.1.)

Central structures

Parliament

The NHS is financed mainly through taxation so it relies on Parliament for its funds, and has to account to Parliament for their use through the Secretary of State for Health, the cabinet member responsible for the service. In addition, Parliament scrutinises the service through debates, MPs' questions to ministers and Select Committees, procedures that mean the government has to publicly explain and defend its policies for the NHS.

Select Committees

Three Select Committees, (the Health Committee, the Public Accounts Committee and the Public Administration Committee) each comprising backbench MPs representing the major parties, are particularly relevant to the NHS. They are all able to summon ministers, civil servants and NHS employees to give oral or written evidence to their inquiries, usually in public. Their reports are published throughout the parliamentary session.

Health Committee

The Health Committee having a maximum of 11 members, examines the expenditure, administration and policy of the Department of Health

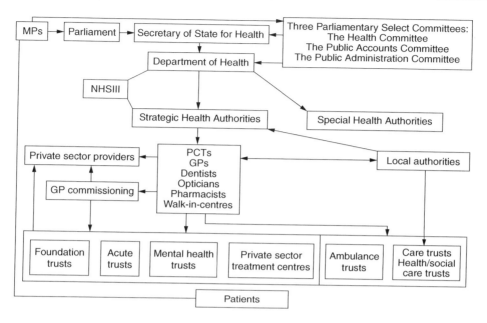

Figure 8.1 The NHS structure: a simplified structure of the NHS in 2006

and its associated bodies. For more information go to www.parliament.uk, 'committees' in left hand column and down to 'health committees'.

Public Accounts Committee

The Public Accounts Committee of 16 members, and traditionally chaired by a member of the opposition is more concerned with ensuring the NHS is operating economically, efficiently and effectively. Its inquiries are based on reports about the service's 'value for money', produced by the Comptroller and Auditor General, who heads the National Audit Office. It tries to draw lessons from past successes and failures that can be applied to the future. For more information *see* either www.parliament.uk/parliamentary_committees/committee_of_public_accounts.cfm or try www.nao.gov.uk.

Public Administration Committee

The Public Administration Committee has 11 members and examines reports from the Health Service Commissioner (better known as the Ombudsman, *see* p. 105).

For more information go to www.parliament.uk, 'committees' in left hand column and down to 'public administration select committee' or try www.ombudsman.org.uk

Health ministers

The Department of Health has six ministers: the Secretary of State, two ministers of state and three parliamentary under-secretaries of state, one of whom is responsible for public health matters and one for social and community services, while the third sits in the House of Lords. The Secretary of State, often referred to as the 'Minister of Health' has overall strategic responsibility for NHS improvement, delivery, reform, finance and resources, while the other ministers each have specific areas of NHS activity assigned to them. The Department for Education and Skills has the lead for children's issues, and works closely with the Department of Health.

The Department of Health

The Department of Health supports the government in improving the health and wellbeing of the population. It is responsible for the NHS, social services and public health. It negotiates levels of NHS funding with the Treasury, and allocates resources to the health service at large.

Setting national standards for the health service has become an important part of its remit. The organisation is divided into three business groups:

- *Health and Social Care Standards and Quality*: this covers international health protection, health and scientific development, research, health improvement programmes, quality and standards, care services, regional public health and a group business team
- *Strategy and Business Development*: this covers four main areas, corporate management and development, communications, user experience and involvement and strategy
- *Health and Social Care Service Delivery*: this covers access, finance and investment, the workforce, international systems and national programme delivery, programmes and performance and a group business team.

The Department of Health is based in London and Leeds. More information can be seen at www.dh.gov.uk.

The Department of Health Board

The Department of Health Board manages the Department of Health's business and priorities. Board members are: the Permanent Secretary and NHS Chief Executive (*see* below), and six directors for delivery, standards and quality (Chief Medical Officer (CMO)), strategy and business development, finance and investment, communications, user experience and involvement (Chief Nursing Officer (CNO)).

The Permanent Secretary and NHS Chief Executive

These two roles were formerly separate but combined in 2000, and are directly responsible to the Secretary of State for the service's management and performance. The Chief Executive's report to the NHS is published in December each year and outlines the service's progress towards meeting key objectives. The NHS Chief Executive produces a weekly bulletin, emailed every Thursday to NHS and council chief executives and directors of social services, containing details of publications, circulars and announcements.

For details *see* www.dh.gov.uk/Publicationsand Statistics, take the shortcut to 'publications' then 'publication policy guidance' and finally select the appropriate report you require.

The Chief Medical Officer and heads of profession

Seven heads of profession currently provide expert knowledge on health and social care:

- Chief Medical Officer
- Chief Nursing Officer
- Chief Dental Officer
- Chief Social Services Inspector
- Chief Health Professions Officer
- Chief Pharmaceutical Officer
- Chief Scientist.

The CMO is the government's principal medical advisor and the professional head of all medical staff in England. The CMO produces an annual independent report on the state of the nation's health. For further information go to www.dh. gov.uk/PublicationsAndStatistics, take shortcut to 'publications' and then shortcut to 'annual reports'.

National Clinical Directors

National Clinical Directors are experts in their field and take the lead in implementing key national clinical priorities. Their roles vary but include chairing taskforces, promoting the work of their specialty, developing clinical networks and advising on clinical quality and governance. There are National Directors for:

- emergency access
- mental health
- children
- heart disease
- primary care
- older people's services
- cancer
- diabetes.

The Modernisation Board

The NHS Modernisation Board was set up to advise the Secretary of State for Health and his ministerial team on implementing *The NHS Plan*. The role of the board is to ensure 'real and speedy progress' in implementing *The NHS Plan*. It aims to smooth obstacles to change and encourage the right people to work together. Members include representatives of professional bodies, medical Royal Colleges and patient groups as well as practising clinicians and NHS managers. It is chaired by the health secretary and also includes the NHS chief executive. *See* www.dh.gov.uk.

The NHS Modernisation Agency to the NHS Institute for Innovation and Improvement

This agency's role had been to support the NHS and its partner organisations in modernising services to meet the needs and convenience of patients. Set up in April 2001, its focus was on improving access, increasing local support, raising standards, and sharing knowledge widely. The agency had sought to make modernisation mainstream, working closely with strategic health authorities. The agency's future role was reviewed as part of the Department of Health's change programme, and in 2005 it was superseded by the NHS Institute for Innovation and Improvement (NHSIII, *see* below). At the same time the NHSU and the NHS Leadership Centre were being dissolved. *See* www.wise.nhs.uk.

The NHS Leadership Centre

This was charged with developing current and future leaders and managers at all levels and from across the professions; its function was taken over by the NHSIII (*see* below).

The NHS Institute for Innovation and Improvement (NHSIII)

Set up in 2005 with an annual budget of £80 million, as a special health authority in England, based on the campus of the University of Warwick, it was given the following roles, to:

* to work closely with clinicians, NHS organisations, patients, the public, academia and industry in the UK and worldwide to identify best practice

* develop the NHS capability for service transformation, technology and product innovation, leadership development and learning

* support the rapid adoption and spread of new ideas by providing guidance on practical change ideas and ways to facilitate local, safe implementation

* promote a culture of innovation and lifelong learning for all NHS staff.

Potential areas of innovation include developing more personalised care for people with long-term conditions, the testing of new procurement models, and ensuring further value from the NHS annual £4 billion training programme for the widest possible range of staff. With the creation of the new NHS Institute, the NHS Modernisation Agency, NHSU and the NHS Leadership Centre were dissolved. All the latest information can be seen at: www.institute.nhs.uk.

Executive agencies

There are executive agencies within the Department of Health responsible for particular business areas, they are:

The Health Protection Agency (HPA)

This is dedicated to protecting people's health and reducing the impact of infectious diseases, chemical hazards, poisons and radiation hazards. In 2003 it was established as a special health authority and its role was to provide an integrated approach to protecting UK public health through the provision of support and advice to the NHS, local authorities, emergency services, other arm's length bodies.

The Department of Health works with three kinds of arm's length bodies (ALBs):

* Executive agencies

* Special Health Authorities

* Non-departmental public bodies.

The three executive agencies have responsibility for particular business areas. The agencies are still part of the Department and accountable to it.

The special health authorities were set up under the NHS Act 1977 to provide a service to the public. They are independent bodies, but can be subject to ministerial direction like other NHS bodies. The non-departmental public bodies have a role in the process of national government, but are not part of government departments. For more information on Arm's Length Bodies within the context of the NHS see www.dh.gov.uk/AboutUs/DeliveringHealthAndSocialCare/OrganisationsThatWorkWithDH/ArmsLengthBodies.

In 2005, the HPA was re-established as a non-departmental public body, replacing the HPA Special HA and the National Radiological Protection Board (NRPB) and with radiation protection as part of health protection incorporated in its remit.

The HPA has a network of about 3000 staff based at three major centres (Colindale, Porton and Chilton) and regionally and locally throughout England. There is a small central office based in London. The Agency works closely with locally based colleagues employed within the devolved administrations.

The Centre for Infections at Colindale is the base for communicable disease surveillance and specialist microbiology. The Centre for Radiation, Chemical and Environmental Hazards is based at Chilton, and the Centre for Emergency Preparedness and Response, focusing on applied microbiological research and emergency response, is based at Porton.

The Medicines and Healthcare Products Regulatory Agency (MHRA)

This agency is responsible for ensuring that medicines and medical devices work, and are acceptably safe. The MHRA combines responsibilities of former medicines control and medical devices agencies including the MDA. No product is entirely risk-free so underpinning their work are fact-based judgements to ensure that the benefits to patients and the public justify the risks. They watch over medicines and devices, and take any necessary action to protect the public promptly if there is a problem. They try to make as much information as possible publicly available. They enable greater access to products, and the timely introduction of innovative treatments and technologies. See www.mhra.gov.uk.

NHS Estates

These provide advice on healthcare buildings and facilities and are now, since 2005, part of the NPSA. More information is available at www.dh.gov.uk.

The NHS Pensions Agency

This administers the NHS pension scheme, with its 1.6 million members. The NHS Pensions Agency is now one of the special health authorities and is the administration centre for NHS Pension Scheme members working in England and Wales, The NHS Injury Benefits Scheme for England and Wales and The NHS Bursary Scheme. For further information go to www.nhspa.gov.uk or www.nhs.uk/England/AuthoritiesTrusts/Special.

The NHS Purchasing and Supply Agency

This advises on procurement policy and strategy, and contracts nationally for products and services critical to the NHS, using its purchasing power to achieve savings. For more information go to www.pasa.doh.gov.uk/.

Non-departmental government bodies

There exist across government, bodies that have been set up when ministers want independent advice without direct influence from Whitehall departments. They fall into three categories:

- *commissions* have a role in national government but are not formally part of any department. They include the
  - Healthcare Commission
  - General Social Care Council
  - Human Fertilisation and Embryology Authority
  - National Radiological Protection Board
- *advisory bodies* of which there are more than 30, and include for example the Expert Advisory Group on AIDS, the Nutrition Forum and the Joint Committee on Vaccination and Immunisation
- *Tribunals* created by legislation and making decisions in specialised fields of law. They are the:
  - Care Standards Tribunal
  - Family Health Services Appeal Authority
  - Mental Health Review Tribunals
  - Registered Homes Tribunal.

Reform and the Department of Health

The Department of Health also engaged in a change programme to reduce its core staff by almost 40% by October 2004, although about half were only to be transferred to arm's-length bodies. This reflected the government's attempt to shift power from Whitehall to frontline health-care staff. The Department of Health's new role was seen as providing strategic leadership to NHS and social care organisations. In addition, as part of the Lyons review of public sector relocation, the Department of Health has proposed moving posts from its arm's-length bodies away from London and the South East by 2008, relocating to Leeds, although its arm's-length bodies would remain in London and the South East.

Strategic health authorities

As part of its *NHS Plan*, the government embarked upon a series of measures aimed at radically reforming the NHS and social care to make the system more patient focused. In April 2002, 28 new larger strategic health authorities (SHAs) were set up to develop strategies for the NHS, replacing NHSE regional offices, and to make sure their local NHS organisations were performing well. In July, 2006 the 28 SHAs were reduced to 10 through mergers. They determine the strategy and performance and manage PCTs and trusts in their area. In the future, their role will increasingly be concerned with financial management of the health economy and ensuring that the commissioning of services meets the needs of the local population. The 10 SHAs manage the NHS locally on behalf of the Department of Health, each covering an average population of over 5 million. Their three key functions are:

- creating a coherent strategic framework
- agreeing annual performance agreements, and performance management of PCTs and NHS trusts
- building capacity and supporting performance improvement.

They develop strategies for capital investment, information management and workforce development. Where problems or conflicts arise between local NHS organisations, SHAs will broker solutions. They foster partnerships with non-NHS bodies, universities and further education institutions, as well as help local authorities to overview and scrutiny committees to monitor the health service. SHAs must ensure consultation on major service reconfigurations.

They manage the NHS locally and are a key link between the Department of Health and the NHS. For more information look at www.nhs.uk/England/AuthoritiesTrusts/Sha.

Special health authorities

Special health authorities provide a service to the whole of England rather than to a local community. They are independent, but can be subject to ministerial direction like other NHS bodies. Each has a unique function and some have remits which extend beyond England. They currently number 19 and include, for example:

- The National Blood Authority
- The NHS Litigation Authority
- The NHS Information Authority
- The Health Education Authority
- The NHS Pensions Agency
- NHS Direct
- The National Institute for Clinical Excellence
- The NHS Counter Fraud and Security Management Service
- The National Patient Safety Agency
- The Mental Health Act Commission
- The Prescription Pricing Authority
- UK Transplant
- NHS Institute for Innovation and Improvement.

Some of the special health authorities are worthy of more detailed mention (*see* below), but to find out more about all the current special health authorities go to www.nhs.uk/England/AuthoritiesTrusts/Special.

NHS Direct

NHS Direct was made a special health authority in April 2004. It is a 24-hour phone line, staffed by nurses, that offers quick access to healthcare advice. NHS Direct nurses will give advice and support on self-treatment or, if further help is needed, will put a patient in touch with the right service. With serious conditions or an emergency, the nurse will give general advice on what to do and will call an ambulance if needed. You can find information and advice about NHS Direct online or by phoning NHS Direct on 0845 4647.

NHS Litigation Authority (NHSLA)

In the past, NHS trusts took out commercial insurance to cover for a wide range of non-clinical risks. The increasing costs of successful clinical negligence claims led to the establishment of the Clinical Negligence Scheme for Trusts (CNST) which is now administered by the NHSLA. More than 80% of NHS trusts insure their clinical risk this way. For more information *see* p. 84 on medical negligence.

The National Patient Safety Agency (NPSA)

The National Patient Safety Agency (NPSA) was formed following the publication of two reports on patient safety in the NHS, *An Organisation with Memory* (2000), and its follow-up *Building a Safer NHS for Patients. Improving medication safety* (2004).

The first report discussed adverse healthcare events that could not be eliminated from complex modern healthcare, and made recommendations designed to ensure that lessons from the past were used to reduce the risk to patients in the future. The cost of adverse events was increasing; there was also a distressing similarity present in some of them. With clinical governance came an opportunity to focus upon the problem. The extent of the serious failures in healthcare was outlined, but the reporting and information systems of the NHS gave an incomplete picture. Very little research on reporting and information systems had been done in the UK. Specific types of adverse events were seen to repeat themselves at intervals, thus demonstrating that lessons could be learned. To make progress four key areas needed addressing and these were detailed in ten recommendations. For further information go to www.dh.gov.uk/.

By extrapolating from a small study in two acute trusts based in London, it was estimated that around 10% (900,000) of patients admitted to NHS hospitals experienced a patient safety incident, and that up to half of these incidents could have been prevented. The study also estimates that 72,000 of these incidents may contribute to the death of patients, although it is unclear what proportion of this number would die as a direct result of the incident. Findings from the US, Australia, New Zealand and Denmark suggested similar levels.

The NPSA was set up not so much to identify things that go wrong in the NHS but to learn from the mistakes, by tracking the scale and frequency of 'patient safety incidents' a generic term used to cover a whole range of events that harm patients. Otherwise called mistakes, accidents, errors or system failures, this information is then used to find solutions to prevent a recurrence. Although it is difficult to estimate the costs of adverse events to the NHS, it is believed to be in excess of £2 billion a year.

The NPSA manages a database on patient safety incidents and safety issues called the National Reporting and Learning System (NRLS) that is used to identify patterns and trends. By examining trends and looking at root causes of incidents, they can prioritise and develop solutions and attempt to minimise the risk of incidents recurring. It does not investigate or comment upon individual incidents. The information held in the database is anonymous and cannot be attributed to an individual healthcare professional or patient. The NPSA is, in effect, providing a safe route for professionals to inform on any issue faced. The NPSA can then try to make the system safer. The data is collected from local reporting systems or by direct input through an internet electronic reporting form, known as the eForm.

Some doctors may not feel comfortable reporting incidents to their local organisations, so they can report directly to the NRLS. The eForm is an electronic reporting form that takes around seven minutes to complete, but it allows you to report independently, confidentially and completely anonymously. To report an incident, go to www.npsa.nhs.uk/staffreports. The NPSA also gathers examples of best practice, recommendations and expertise already in use and shares these more widely. Not only do they involve healthcare staff, but also patients, carers and the public at large in the identification of risks and suggested solutions.

Until the NPSA was set up there was no central national organisation looking at the broad range of patient safety problems happening across the NHS. If a mistake happened only once a year in every trust up and down the UK, a serious problem could be missed because without the NPSA a national picture of these problems was not available. Now there is a clearer picture of the important issues.

Some NPSA projects you may have come across include:

- the 'clean your hands' campaign, which aims to put alcohol gel by each patient's bedside to make it easier for you to keep your hands clean and prevent infection

- standardising the crash call number across the NHS to 2222 so the number is the same wherever you are working

- changing how potassium chloride concentrate is handled and stored to reduce the risk of you administering the wrong dose in error.

The NPSA's definitions of a patient safety incident are:

- any unintended or unexpected incident(s) that could have or did lead to harm for one or more persons receiving NHS-funded healthcare. It can refer to a single incident or a series of related incidents that occur over time

- a prevented patient safety incident is one that had the potential to cause harm but was prevented.

Root Cause Analysis (RCA) is defined as a systematic investigation technique that looks beyond the individuals involved in an incident and seeks to understand the underlying causes and environmental context in which the incident happened. If you are involved in an incident you may be asked to contribute to the RCA investigation. The NRLS is based on the premise that most problems affecting patient safety occur as a result of weaknesses in systems and processes rather than individuals.

Having collated information from data, the NPSA has developed three formats to disseminate its advice and solutions to NHS staff:

- *patient safety alert* requires prompt action to address high-risk safety problems

- *safer practice notice* strongly advises implementing particular recommendations or solutions

- *patient safety information notice* suggests issues or effective techniques that healthcare staff might consider to enhance safety.

They are distributed via the Safety Alert Broadcast System in England, which is an electronic system that sends safety alerts to designated contacts in NHS trusts who are responsible for ensuring the information is disseminated appropriately. They are also sent to NHS organisations in Wales.

In addition there are various regular publications including *Patient Safety Bulletin*. Their website at www.npsa.nhs.uk is kept updated with recent work and announcements. Where appropriate, they may also use national, local and specialist publications to raise awareness as well as attending conferences and events. The NPSA also has links with many medical Royal Colleges and professional organisations to promote their work via their communications channels and networks through college journals or newsletters.

This special health authority also co-ordinates the efforts of all those involved in healthcare to learn from patient safety incidents occurring in the NHS, but from 2005, the NPSA's work also encompasses:

- safety aspects of hospital design

- cleanliness and food (transferred from NHS Estates)

- ensuring research is carried out safely, through its responsibility for the Central Office for Research Ethics Committees (COREC)

- supporting local organisations in addressing their concerns about the performance of individual doctors and dentists, through its responsibility for the National Clinical Assessment Service (NCAS), formerly known as the National Clinical Assessment Authority

- managing the contracts with the three confidential enquiries. This responsibility has been transferred from NICE.

The NPSA covers the work of all the following previously separate areas:

- The National Patient Safety Agency (NPSA)

- The National Clinical Assessment Service (NCAS)

- The Central Office of Research Ethics Committees (COREC)
- The National Confidential Enquiry into Patient Outcome and Death (NCEPOD)
- The Confidential Enquiry into Maternal and Child Health (CEMACH)
- The National Confidential Enquiry into Suicide and Homicide by people with mental illness (NCISH)
- NHS Estates (safety aspects of hospital design, cleanliness, and food).

However they all retain their original websites for further information.

They are also establishing risk registers in hospitals and piloting a risk assessment tool for assessing the level of incident investigation required, and the external reporting requirements to the NPSA, following adverse incidents involving NHS patients.

Primary care

Primary Care Organisations (PCOs) include PCTs in England, the Health and Social Services Boards in Northern Ireland, Local Health Board in Wales and the Primary Care Divisions within Area Health Boards in Scotland. Nine out of ten people are seen in the community. Everyone has the right to be registered with a GP. In addition to providing primary care, GPs also act as 'gatekeepers' to much of the rest of the service, referring patients where appropriate to hospital or specialist treatment. A range of other healthcare professionals also provide primary care services. These include dentists, physiotherapists, opticians, pharmacists, health visitors, midwives, community nurses, occupational therapists and speech therapists.

Primary healthcare teams generally deal with every patient and must cope with many simultaneous demands and pressures. Expectations or treatment goals for groups of people with chronic disease need to be clear, and success or failure of chronic disease treatment often depends on the patient's contribution.

Primary care trusts (PCTs)

PCTs are freestanding, legally established, statutory NHS bodies that are accountable to their strategic health authority. They are responsible for managing health services in a local area, they lead NHS organisations in assessing need, improving health, planning and securing health services in their localities. PCTs provide most community services and develop primary care services, including GPs and dentists in their area. They work with local authorities and other agencies to provide health and social care locally and to make sure the community's needs are met.

PCTs are at the centre of the NHS and get 75% of the NHS budget. As local organisations, they are positioned to understand the needs of their community, and make sure that organisations providing health and social care services are working effectively. For example, PCTs must make sure there are enough services for people in their area and that they are accessible to patients. They must also make sure that all other health services are provided, including hospitals, dentists, opticians, mental health services, NHS walk-in centres, NHS Direct, patient transport (including A&E), population screening, pharmacies and opticians. They are also responsible for getting health and social care systems working together to the benefit of patients. More information about PCTs can be accessed at www.nhs.uk/England/Authorities Trusts/Pct/.

NHS hospitals are available to provide acute and specialist services. PCTs are responsible for planning secondary care. They assess the health needs of the local community and develop plans to improve health and set priorities locally. They then decide which secondary care services to commission to meet public need. They work closely with the providers of the secondary care services that they commission to agree about delivering those services. For more information look at www.nhs.uk/England/ and click on 'about the NHS'.

PCT governing arrangements have established a national approach that provides this balance. Governance arrangements must deliver four key principles:

- primary care professionals in the driving seat
- public accountability
- public involvement
- probity.

At the date of publication of this edition, plans are in place to cut the 302 current PCTs to 100 or fewer by amalgamations and mergers, and commissioning (*see* below) will be transferred to general practices, although this will still be overseen by PCTs.

Practice-led commissioning

The 1997 White Paper *The New NHS* signalled an intention for PCTs to 'extend indicative budgets to individual practices for the full range of services'. This is based on the premise that patient choice will be a driver for quality. Practices will be able to secure a wider range of services, more responsive to patient needs and from which patients can choose. From 2008 the impact of free choice for elective procedures is seen as allowing practices to use their commissioning abilities to identify alternative provision, including in primary care, to give patients greater choice. The introduction of 'payment by results' is expected to mean that where practices are able to provide or commission services locally, as patients choose to use these services, the funds will follow. The system has similarities with GP fundholding, a system considered to have positive aspects but also widely criticised for having serious flaws, one of which was that patients with fundholding GPs were often able to receive treatment faster than those with other GPs, creating a two-tier primary system. PCTs will retain control over budgets, and remain legally responsible for the contracting process, so that any savings made from managing referrals more efficiently will be shared between practices and PCTs, with all savings reinvested into patient care.

The new commissioning scheme is voluntary and, as yet, no targets for its uptake have been published. When a practice requests the right to an 'indicative budget', the sum will be based on historical spend for the previous year. Any initial overspending will be covered by the PCT, but practices will nevertheless be expected to balance their books over a three-year cycle, and those that are unable to do so will be barred from the scheme 'except in exceptional circumstances'.

NHS walk-in centres

NHS Walk-in Centres give fast access to health advice and treatment. They are normally open for seven days each week, from early in the morning until late in the evening. They offer:

- treatment for minor illnesses and injuries
- assessment by an experienced NHS nurse
- advice on how to stay healthy
- information on out-of-hours GP and dental services
- information on local pharmacy services
- information on other local health services.

Secondary care

- Most secondary care is provided by hospitals operating as trusts.
- Around 375 trusts manage more than 98% of all NHS hospitals and community health services.
- There are around 280 major district general hospitals in England.

Secondary care organisations seek to provide a comprehensive service and to meet the needs of patients and their GPs. At tertiary level, services focus on providing specialised service for which they alone may have the skills. Some specialist services are provided at regional and supraregional or national level because of their complexity, cost or level of incidence.

Hospital trusts

NHS trusts provide most secondary care and specialist services in hospitals. Hospitals are managed by NHS trusts (some also known as acute trusts), and also decide on a strategy for how the hospital will develop, so that services improve. Trusts employ most of the NHS workforce. Some trusts are regional or national centres for more specialised care, others are attached to universities and help to train health professionals. Trusts can also provide services in the community, for example through health centres, clinics or in people's homes.

Trusts are independent organisations within the NHS. They may be a single hospital, a group of hospitals, community services provided in health centres and clinics, an ambulance service, or a PCT. There are some 375 NHS trusts in England. Trusts were first established in 1991 under the NHS reforms of the previous year. They are self-governing service providers within the NHS and each has its own trust board comprised of executive and non-executive directors. The chair is appointed by the Secretary of State and they in turn appoint five non-executive directors, bringing expertise and ideas from a range of backgrounds and professions, and providing a link with local communities. The trust board is then responsible for appointing the management board which consists of five executive directors and this must include a:

- chief executive
- medical director
- senior nurse
- finance director.

The major district general hospitals provide services from A&E to the care of elderly people. NHS trusts have full responsibility for operational management. The income they receive comes from contracts negotiated with health authorities and PCTs. In addition to a statutory duty of quality of care they are accountable to the NHS Executive for their statutory duty to break even financially. They also have to work within a framework of HIMPs and contribute to developing these programmes. They are also required to work in partnership with health authorities.

The four most typical models are:

- *acute hospital trusts*: mostly district general hospitals, but some single specialty units also exist
- *integrated service trusts*: providing acute and community services and, in some cases, also mental health services
- *mental health trusts*: sometimes with services for people with learning disabilities
- *primary care trusts*.

Trusts are directly accountable to the Secretary of State via the regional offices of the NHS Executive, which monitor performance. The trust board makes decisions about policy and strategic direction. The statutory basis for the board is contained in the National Health Service Trusts (Membership and Procedure) Regulation 1990 (Statutory Instrument 1990, No 2024). Trusts' statutory powers include:

- setting up their own management structure subject to national requirements regarding the involvement of senior professional staff
- employing staff on terms and conditions set by the trust
- buying and selling property
- borrowing money, within annually agreed limits primarily for capital developments
- entering into NHS and other contracts
- generating income, subject to this not interfering with other obligations.

NHS trusts do not receive direct financial allocations but operate on an income and expenditure basis. Sources of income derive from agreements to provide services for health authorities and primary care organisations; undergraduate medical and dental education; postgraduate medical education; education and training for other healthcare professionals; carrying out medical research; and from other services such as car parking and hospital shops.

NHS foundation trusts

NHS foundation trusts are a new type of organisation, created under the Health and Social Care (Community Health and Standards) Act 2003. They remain part of the NHS but have been freed from direct central government control. They possess three key characteristics that distinguish them from NHS trusts:

- freedom to decide locally how to meet their obligations
- accountability to local people, who can become members and governors
- they are authorised and monitored by Monitor (*see* p. 162) – the independent financial regulator of NHS foundation trusts.

As free-standing legal entities, free from direction by the Secretary of State for Health they can exercise the freedom to:

- retain proceeds from land sales to invest in new services for patients. Land sale receipts from conventional NHS trusts go back to a central Department of Health fund

- decide what they can afford to borrow for investment in services, and to make decisions about future capital investment, instead of receiving a centrally dictated allocation

- use the flexibilities of the new pay system currently being negotiated to modernise the NHS workforce, including developing additional rewards for those staff contributing most.

NHS foundation trusts still operate according to NHS principles and serve NHS patients. Instead of direct line management by the Department of Health, foundation trusts will be held to account through the agreements and cash for performance contracts they negotiate with PCTs and other commissioners, and through independent inspection.

These contracts will reflect national priorities around reduced waiting times and improved clinical outcomes. Those that perform well will benefit from the system of payment by results and patient choice announced in *Delivering the NHS Plan* (2002).

They will be subject to inspection by the Healthcare Commission who will play a key role in assessing performance and in ensuring national standards of service and quality are met. Hence the Healthcare Commission, rather than the Department of Health, will regulate quality in foundation trusts. It will place a premium on greater local accountability and community involvement.

These contracts represent part of a more recent reform programme introduced by the government attempting to introduce two key new ideas:

- *'patient choice'*: giving patients a choice of providers at the referral stage

- *'payment by results'*: a reform of NHS finance whereby activity will be funded at a national tariff, based on average unit cost.

In effect this requires two important cultural shifts as requirements of foundation status:

- customer care

- an entrepreneurial approach.

In respect of the first, it has been suggested that the typical NHS trust structure, based on clinical directorates, might not be the most appropriate for an organisation committed to being patient focused. Patient choice requires NHS foundation trusts to embrace new level of 'patient-friendliness', perhaps related to such mundane issues as car parking (shown to be a key factor in patient choice, behind only waiting times in importance).

As for the second issue of entrepreneurship and running the business, understanding costs is vital to the effective management of those costs and, therefore, financial viability under payment by results. It is thought that current trust accounting systems are inadequate to give the level of detail and sensitivity that is required. If the benefit of removing NHS foundation trusts from central command and control is to be realised, trusts will need to consider afresh what information they need to manage their own performance, and whether their existing systems are suitable. One of the freedoms offered with foundation status, for example, is the ability to establish joint venture companies, and the ability to manage costs to generate a surplus, through the introduction of payment by results. They are required to turn the organisational effort that had been devoted to providing information for 'the centre' and use it to produce information relevant to running autonomous businesses. Until now performance management systems have been designed primarily to collect data for the strategic health authorities or direct to the Department of Health. Clinicians will be encouraged to view their activity in an entrepreneurial way, where surpluses can be generated and recycled for service improvement.

A comprehensive performance assessment carried out in 2002 by the Audit Commission on every major local council in England found that the best performers were consistently superior in three key areas:

- leadership

- performance management

- establishing a positive culture.

An NHS foundation trust's strategy is wider than that of a non-foundation trust. For example, the strategy needs to include the means of generating surpluses, and deciding what to do with them. This changes the whole basis of their financial regime, previously geared to breaking even and carrying less incentive to be efficient, because 'cost equals price'. Patient choice would offer the potential to aim at growth through attracting elective patients from outside the trust's normal geographical area.

Monitor

Monitor is the independent corporate body established under the Health and Social Care (Community Health and Standards) Act 2003. It is the independent regulator of NHS foundation trusts, making sure they are well managed and financially viable. It also plays a key role in authorising applications for foundation trust status.

The authorising process for NHS foundation trusts begins when Monitor receives and considers applications from NHS trusts. If satisfied that certain criteria are met after assessing the applicant and making sure they can live up to their obligations, it authorises them to operate as NHS foundation trusts. The terms of their formal authorisation set out the conditions under which a foundation trust is required to operate, and covers such things as:

- description of the goods and services related to the provision of healthcare that the foundation trust is authorised to provide

- limits on the amount of income that the foundation trust is allowed to earn from private charges

- limits on the amount of money that the foundation trust is allowed to borrow

- financial and statistical information the foundation trust is required to provide.

Monitoring and regulating NHS foundation trusts then continues to be a function of Monitor once NHS foundation trusts are established. It continues to monitor their activities to ensure that they comply with the requirements of their terms of authorisation. Inspection of the performance of a foundation trust against healthcare standards is carried out by the Healthcare Commission, which is required to send Monitor copies of their inspection reports. Monitor then has powers to intervene in the running of a foundation trust in the event of failings in its healthcare standards or other aspects of its activities, which amount to a significant breach in the terms of its authorisation. For more details *see* www.monitor-nhsft. gov.uk/.

Care trusts

Care trusts are organisations that work in both health and social care. They may carry out a range of services, including social care, mental health services or primary care services. Care trusts are set up when NHS and local authorities agree to work closely together, usually where it is felt that a closer relationship between health and social care is needed or would benefit local care services. At the moment there are only a small number of care trusts, though more are planned for the future. More information about care trusts can be found at www.nhs.uk/England/Authorities Trusts/Special.

These new bodies combine aspects of social services, currently provided by local authorities, with health services, provided in the NHS by PCTs. Care trusts are statutory NHS bodies, redesignated as care trusts under Section 45 of the Health and Social Care Act 2001. They build on PCTs, NHS trusts and Health Act flexibilities. They deliver integrated (whole systems) services in a single organisation. NHS and local advisory (LA) health-related functions are delegated to them, not transferred. They are able to commission and/or provide. They are voluntary in the sense that partners can withdraw.

If they are a PCT-based care trust they are able to commission healthcare as well as local authority health-related functions. They also deliver services that the NHS organisation and local authority would normally provide. The introduction of care trusts was seen as an opportunity to deliver improved, integrated health and social care. The process was slow to develop, although it is anticipated that there will be further interest in setting up care trusts in the future.

Mental health trusts

Mental health services can be provided through a GP, other primary care services, or through more specialist care. This includes counselling and other psychological therapies, community and family support, or general health screening. For example, people suffering bereavement, depression, stress or anxiety can get help from primary care or informal community support. If they need more involved support they may be referred for specialist care.

Specialist care is usually provided by mental health trusts or local council social services departments. Services range from psychological therapy to specialised medical and training services for people with severe mental health problems. About two in every thousand people need specialist care for conditions such as severe anxiety problems or psychotic illness. More information about mental health trusts can be obtained at www.nhs.uk/England/Authorities Trusts/MentalHealth.

Trust board members

In addition to the executive directors of the trust board such as the chief executive, medical director, nursing director, and finance director and so on, there are also non-executive directors including one who is chair of the trust.

Non-executive directors in the NHS

There is a statutory duty for trusts and strategic health authorities to have non-executive directors on the board. There are usually five non-executive directors, but there can be up to eight in PCTs and care trusts. They are accountable to the health authority (health board in Scotland) and are expected to work within the spirit of Lord Nolan's (1995) seven principles of public life: selflessness, integrity, objectivity, accountability, openness, honesty and leadership.

Recent guidance defines the four main object-ives of NHS non-executive directors that are also shared with private sector non-executive directors:

- strategy
- performance
- risk
- people

and one additional one for NHS non-executive directors:

- accountability: i.e. ensuring the board acts in the public interest and is accountable to the public for services it provides.

Non-executive directors must outnumber the executive directors on the board (the board chair must be a non-executive director, creating a majority of non-executive directors). In future one non-executive director will be a member of the organisation's patient forum. Membership of the audit, risk management and remuneration committees must include non-executive directors, and the complaints convenor must be a non-executive director. Non-executive directors should not get involved in operational management.

The NHS Appointments Commission makes all non-executive directors' appointments. The inter-view panel consists of three people, including the chair of the organisation and an independent assessor. Selection criteria include the requirement to live or work locally, an interest in healthcare, community commitment, board level contribution, communication skills, strategic thinking and an understanding of public service values. Non-executive directors are appointed for an initial period of four years, renewable subject to satis-factory appraisal, and subscribe to the Codes of Conduct and Accountability for NHS boards. The expected contribution for a chair is three days per week, while other non-executive directors are expected to contribute up to five days per month. The Department of Health and NHS Appointments Commission suggest core non-executive director's duties can be fulfilled in two and a half days.

The person specification drawn up for selection usually includes the following essential qualities:

- live in the area served by the trust
- have a strong personal commitment to the NHS
- demonstrate a commitment to the needs of the local community
- be a good communicator with plenty of common sense
- be committed to the public service values of accountability, probity, openness and equality of opportunity
- demonstrate ability to contribute to the work of the board

- be available for about three days per month

- demonstrate an interest in healthcare issues.

It is also regarded as desirable that they:

- have experience as a carer or user of the NHS

- have experience of serving in the voluntary sector

- have served the local community in local government or some other capacity

- understand or have experience of management in the public, private or voluntary sectors

- offer specialist skills or knowledge relevant to the work of the trust.

Applications are encouraged from all sections of the community, particularly women, people from ethnic minorities and people with disabilities. Political activity should not be a consideration in selection.

Non-executive directors work with four or five other non-executives and the senior trust managers, including the medical director, as equal members of the trust board. They are expected to use their personal skills and experience of the community and the NHS to guide the trust in the following areas:

- developing long-term plans for healthcare in the local community

- best use of its financial resources to help patients

- appointment of the chief executive and other senior managers

- various committees such as the:
  - remuneration committee to ensure fair pay for trust executives
  - audit committee to ensure proper financial procedures
  - committees to review professional conduct and staff discipline matters

- ensuring the trust meets its commitment to the Patient's Charter and other targets

- contributing to the relationship between the trust and the local community and media by representing the board at official occasions

- overseeing the trust's response to complaints from the public

- being involved in hearing appeals by patients detained under the Mental Health Act.

Chairs of NHS trusts

A trust chair must have the same qualities as a non-executive director and, in addition, be able to demonstrate leadership and motivation skills, the ability to think strategically and the ability to understand complex issues. Management experience at a senior level in the public, private or voluntary sectors is seen as a desirable attribute.

The chair is accountable to the Secretary of State for giving leadership to the NHS trust board and to ensure that, through the chief executive, the trust achieves the following:

- provides efficient and effective healthcare and health education services to the community

- collaborates with the other offices of the NHS such as PCTs

- is an executive to implement national and local policies trust

- works with GPs, health authorities, trusts and local authority social services departments to plan and deliver integrated services

- maintains financial viability, using resources effectively, and controls and reports its finances within guidelines issued by the NHS Executive

- meets legal and contractual obligations by carrying out statutory responsibilities with due regard to relevant European Community (EC) directives, requirements of statutory bodies, hazard or safety notices, advice relating to patient, public or staff safety and personal privacy and patient confidentiality

- undertakes, commissions or makes facilities available for research and plays a part in medical education as appropriate, in conjunction with medical schools and research funding bodies

- co-operates and develops links with the community

- promotes actively the values and achievements of the NHS.

It appears, from information obtained from trusts' websites that chairs of trusts may be paid £15–20k per annum depending on the size of the trust.

Action

Consider the background and possible value and input of non-executive directors for your trust.

- Who are the non-executive directors in your trust?

- List any meetings they chair or contribute to.

- What is their background?

- What do you think they might bring to the job?

- What is the chair's leadership style?

- How do they relate to the professionals in the trust?

Clinical directorates or care divisions

A trust's management team is responsible for the operational management and the development of policy within the trust. The management team is made up of the executive directors and the clinical directors of the trust. Clinical directors, (sometimes called clinical services directors, associate directors, etc) are usually consultant medical staff, although they are sometimes a non-medical clinical professional. They are normally accountable to the chief executive or director of operations for the management of patient care and treatment involving clinical staff in the development and management of services. They may share leadership with an operations manager and a lead nurse.

The key elements of the clinical director's role fall under the day-to-day general management headings, and include:

- responsibility for the directorate budget, manpower and staffing

- clinical services including clinical audit and management

- budget management and control

- business and strategic planning

- services planning, service development, strategic development, staff development, business development, and clinical development of the trust.

There are usually several clinical directorates or care divisions within each trust, working alongside others to provide the services required.

Issues for clinical directorates include the development of future patterns of service, medical staffing issues, coping with pressures (particularly in emergency admissions), reorganisations, transfers, mergers, rationalisation and waiting lists.

Action

Draw an organisational chart setting out the location of titles such as chief executive, finance director, human resource director, operations director, medical director, clinical director, director of nursing and others within your trust.

- To whom is the clinical director accountable?

- What is the clinical director responsible for?

- Ask about the difference between operational and strategic management.

- Who decides strategy in your hospital?

- What are the links between the trust strategy and patient care?

It might be helpful to look through the section on key reports and publications in Chapter 9 (p. 176), which gives a brief outline of some of the key legislation and reports in this area.

Other bodies

Public Accounts Committee

This committee scrutinises the way in which money voted by parliament is spent. It is supported by the Comptroller, Auditor General and the National Audit Office. The Chief Executive of the NHS may be called before the Committee to answer questions. For more information go to www.parliament.uk/, then click on 'committees' and 'public accounts committee' and 'formal minutes'.

House of Commons Health Select Committee

This committee complements the work of the Public Accounts Committee and shadows the work of the Department of Health, carrying out inquiries into major health policy issues. This committee follows up reports of the health service commissioner or ombudsman who is responsible for investigating areas of maladministration in the NHS, failure to provide a service and other complaints from the public. *See* Chapter 4 for more detailed information. The Health Committee is appointed by the House of Commons to examine the expenditure, administration and policy of the Department of Health and its associated bodies. Its constitution and powers are set out in House of Commons Standing Order No.152.

The Committee has a maximum of 11 members, and the quorum for any formal proceedings is three. The members of the Committee are appointed by the House and unless discharged remain on the Committee until the next dissolution of Parliament. For further information go to www.parliament.uk/, then click on 'committees' and 'health committees'.

The Audit Commission

This is an independent body set up by Parliament which has a role in auditing the NHS with particular reference to value for money. For further information go to www.audit-commission.gov.uk.

National Institute for Health and Clinical Excellence (NICE)

NICE is the independent organisation responsible for providing national guidance on the promotion of good health and the prevention and treatment of ill-health. In April 2005 NICE joined

with the Health Development Agency to become the new National Institute for Health and Clinical Excellence. Further information can be obtained at www.nice.org.uk, *see* also Chapter 7.

Healthcare Commission

The Healthcare Commission is an independent body, set up to promote and drive improvement in the quality of healthcare and public health. It aims to become an authoritative and trusted source of information. The Healthcare Commission's legal name is the Commission for Healthcare Audit and Inspection (CHAI); it was formed by the Health and Social Care (Community Health and Standards) Act 2003, and launched in April 2004.

It has statutory duties in England to:

- assess the management, provision and quality of NHS healthcare and public health services
- review the performance of each NHS trust and award an annual performance rating
- regulate the independent healthcare sector through registration, annual inspection, monitoring complaints and enforcement
- publish information about the state of healthcare
- consider complaints about NHS organisations that the organisations themselves have not resolved
- promote the co-ordination of reviews and assessments carried out by ourselves and others
- carry out investigations of serious failures in the provision of healthcare.

The Healthcare Commission also has certain separate duties in respect to Wales, mainly relating to national reviews and the annual *State of Healthcare* report. But local inspection and investigation of NHS bodies in Wales rests with the Healthcare Inspectorate Wales, while the Care Standards Inspectorate Wales inspects those organisations providing independent healthcare.

As a public body, the Healthcare Commission also has obligations under the Race Relations (Amendment) Act 2000 and the Human Rights Act 1998, to take active steps to promote respect for human rights and equality of opportunity and good relations between all racial groups.

The Healthcare Commission works in close partnership with the Mental Health Act Commission (MHAC), whose role is to ensure that there is adequate and effective protection of patients detained under the Mental Health Act 1983. Under the government's review of legislation on mental health, it is expected that most of the functions of MHAC will transfer to the Healthcare Commission and that MHAC will be abolished by April 2007. In the meantime, each organisation will maintain its separate statutory responsibilities but work together on a coherent overall programme for the assessment of the provision of care in the field of mental health. For further information *see* www.healthcarecomission.org.uk.

General Medical Council (GMC)

The GMC is a statutory body that is primarily concerned with medical registration and ensuring practising doctors meet certain specified standards. The GMC assesses evidence of continuing education, professional development and standards of performance through the revalidation process. The GMC's website is an important source of information for doctors: www.gmc-uk.org.

Patient and Public Involvement Forums (PPI Forums)

PPI Forums were set up following the NHS Reform and Health Care Professions Act 2002. There are 572 Forums – one for each trust in England. Each Forum needs a minimum of seven members in order to be set up, and the membership reflects the make-up of local communities. They are the local voice of the community on health matters and have a wide range of responsibilities. PPI Forums gather views about the quality of services, monitor service gaps and their impacts, and make suggestions on improving the experience of the user of the service. Their development has been supported by the Commission for Patient and Public Involvement in Health (CPPIH) which is due to be abolished, following which the PPI Forums will be supported by locally based Forum Support Organisations (FSOs). They will also develop closer links with the Healthcare Commission. PPI Forums also have close links

with Patient Advice and Liaison Services (PALS), but Forums have a wider role than PALS. PALS are located within NHS trusts to provide information, advice and support to help patients, families and their carers. PPI Forums focus on all issues which affect health outcomes – including many local authority services, transport, environment and economic issues.

Differences within the UK

The NHS in England

Devolution has had significant implications for the structure and provision of health services across the UK as Wales and Scotland have assumed responsibility for a wide range of services. Westminster has retained UK-wide power only over the following:

- abortion
- human fertilisation
- human genetics
- xenotransplantation
- regulation of medicines.

The NHS in Scotland has a budget of £14 billion and Wales £7 billion. Scotland also has tax varying powers, although Wales has not. Scotland spends 30% more per capita and Wales 15% more, than England.

The NHS in Northern Ireland, Scotland, Wales, The Isle of Man and the Channel Islands have separate independent health service structures and if you are interested they can easily be accessed for details on the internet.

The NHS in Scotland

There have always been differences between the English and Scottish health services, and the variations in approach are reflected in the White Paper for Scotland, *Designed to Care*. The main differences relate to primary care. PCTs came into force in Scotland in April 1999, and are responsible for the full range of services including mental health services. Their organisation reflects the local healthcare co-operatives and voluntary organisations formed by GPs. Scottish

PCTs do not generally commission secondary care, partly due to the fact that there was less interest in fundholding in Scotland. They have, however, developed the Joint Investment Fund (JIF). From July 1999, the Scottish Executive, headed by its First Minister, was responsible and accountable to the Scottish Parliament for the NHS in Scotland. Scottish ministers are accountable to that Parliament for the development and delivery of services. There is a Management Executive with 15 health boards responsible for planning and commissioning hospital and community services as well as managing primary care services. There are 35 trusts, each accountable to the Scottish Minister via the Management Executive.

2004 was a year of change in NHS Scotland; the Scottish Parliament enacted the Primary Medical Services (Scotland) Bill and the NHS Reform (Scotland) Bill. The latter dissolved NHS trusts and integrated the management of acute and primary care services into NHS boards. The reforms aimed to devolve decision making and resources to frontline staff through the establishment of Community Health Partnerships (CHPs).

For more information look at www.show. scot.nhs.uk where you will also find a new expanded NHS Scotland e-Library at www.show.scot. nhs.uk/elibrary providing access to over 4,000 full text electronic journals, over 20 major databases, 200 electronic textbooks and over 1,500 free quality health information websites. It now caters for the work, research, education and personal development needs of the full range of NHS staff. A single username and password, available via online registration, provides access to these resources.

Scotland also has a special health board 'Health Scotland' created in April 2003 by bringing together the Public Health Institute of Scotland (PHIS), www.phis.org.uk, and the Health Education Board for Scotland (HEBS), www.hebs.com. Health Scotland provides a focus for improving health working with the Scottish Executive and other agencies, especially the 15 Scottish NHS boards, but also a broad spectrum of national organisations and educational institutions.

NHS 24 is Scotland's equivalent of England's NHS Direct.

The NHS in Wales

During 1999, all the health responsibilities of the Welsh Office passed to the National Assembly for Wales. There is a Health and Social Services Minister and a director of the NHS Wales Department in the Welsh Assembly Government. NHS Wales is split between the NHS Service sector and the NHS Wales Department, which is the civil service department responsible for the NHS in Wales. Wales also has its own Chief Medical Officer for Wales and Head of the Office of the Chief Medical Officer in the Welsh Assembly Government.

The Assembly is led by the First Secretary, with the Department for Health being the responsibility of the under-secretary. The NHS in Wales is headed by a director, who is supported by a Chief Medical Officer for Wales.

The NHS in Wales spent some £4.2 billion in 2004–2005. It is Wales' largest employer, with over 81 000 staff, representing more than 7% of the Welsh workforce. As in England, the NHS in Wales provides primary care through GPs (there are almost 1900 in Wales) and secondary, tertiary and community care by NHS trusts. There are 14 NHS trusts in Wales, including one all-Wales ambulance trust. Between them, the trusts manage 135 hospitals and some 15,000 beds. Half a million people, one-sixth of the population, will have a hospital stay in any given year.

The Welsh Assembly Government is responsible for policy direction and for allocating funds to the NHS in Wales to 22 local health boards (LHBs), which assess health services, their populations' need and then pay hospital trusts, family doctors, dentists and so on to provide those services. Each LHB has a decision-making board which is made up of local doctors, a nurse, and other health professionals, members of the local council and voluntary organisations, and others to represent the voice of patients. They also have a small executive team to put the decisions into action and provide services for the public.

The LHBs cover exactly the same areas as the 22 local authorities in Wales. This allows much closer working between the NHS and the local councils, which is useful for planning to tackle long-term problems with health. Indeed, the LHBs and local councils have a statutory duty to work together – in partnership with other local organisations – to produce strategies for improving health and social care for the people living in their area. Although LHBs plan and pay for most hospital and family health services, there are a few specialised services which are better planned across the whole of Wales. These are the responsibility of a new organisation, the Health Commission Wales (Specialised Services), which was created in April 2003.

A single organisation for the whole of Wales, the National Public Health Service gives advice and guidance to LHBs on a range of issues such as disease protection and control as well as child protection.

There are three regional offices of the National Assembly based in Mid, North and South East Wales. These regional offices support improved joint working at local levels between LHBs, local authorities and trusts, monitoring the development of local health, social care and well-being strategies. They have a specific role in ensuring that Assembly initiatives are carried out.

For more information on the NHS in Wales go to www.wales.nhs.uk.

The NHS in Northern Ireland

There are currently four area boards in Northern Ireland responsible for assessing the needs of their respective populations and commissioning services to meet those needs. They are charged with the establishment of key objectives to meet the health and social needs of their population and the development of policies and priorities to meet those objectives.

In 2005, a reorganisation of Northern Ireland's Health and Personal Social Services (HPSS), was announced as part of the Review of Public Administration (RPA). It would reduce the 19 trusts and four boards whose running costs exceeded £155 million per year.

Core structures would move from 47 organisations to 18, including a smaller government department, a strategic health and social services authority to replace the four boards and take on some functions currently with the department, and the 18 trusts reduced to five by 2007 but keeping the ambulance service as a separate trust.

There would be seven local commissioning bodies, led by patients and driven by GPs and primary healthcare professionals, taking on some roles from the four boards, and some roles from the 15 local health and social care groups, which will be abolished. Finally a Patient and Client Council would replace the existing four Health and Social Services Councils.

More information is available at www.nics.gov.uk and www.healthandcareni.co.uk.

NHS Isle of Man

The provision of the National Health Service on the Island is set out in the NHS Act 2001. For further information go to www.gov.im/dhss/health.

Types of care

In addition to primary and secondary care there is one other classification of care provided that you may be aware of:

Community care

The NHS spends about £5 billion annually on medicines and around 10,000 pharmacies dispense over 559 million prescriptions annually. Over 80% of these are dispensed free of charge. The NHS also plays an important role in providing community care services to meet the needs of the elderly, those with disabilities, the mentally ill and other frail or vulnerable members of society. Social service departments of local councils take the lead role for community care, and the NHS is responsible for working with them to ensure the effective planning and delivery of community care services. This involves contributing to the assessment of people's needs for community care, and liaising over hospital discharge for those requiring continuing support, as well as delivering services.

Since the introduction of community care reforms in 1993, the lead responsibility for community care has rested with social service departments. Working closely with the NHS, housing authorities and other agencies, they are responsible for planning, co-ordinating and assessing individual need for community care services. The aim of the community care reforms was to ensure that services are more effectively tailored to meet the needs and preferences of individuals. While not appropriate in every case, the emphasis is on supporting people in their own homes or in homely community settings where feasible and sensible. Care trusts (*see* p. 162) have been introduced in some areas across the country, and are expected to develop further in the future.

The NHS makes an important contribution to meeting needs for community care. For instance, district nurses provide 2.3 million episodes of care annually, and over one million chiropody sessions are carried out in the home. Recent guidance has confirmed and clarified the NHS's responsibilities for meeting continuing health-care needs, and all health authorities have been required to publish local policies and eligibility criteria for continuing healthcare, giving details of local services.

Shared care

Shared care is not about a relationship between one doctor and one patient. Rather, it is about multiple relationships to treat a disease or con-dition, involving contributions from the patient and a range of healthcare providers. The objective of healthcare is to achieve a satisfactory clinical outcome within available resources. Increasingly, healthcare professionals work as teams. Surgical and medical teams have different needs; the latter in particular may not only be multidisciplinary but also distributed between primary and second-ary healthcare. Conditions which are relatively common and susceptible to timely appropriate interventions are often managed by fragmented and unco-ordinated services. Such conditions tend to require primary care services, specialised secondary care services and, sometimes, highly specialised secondary care, and a few require highly specialised tertiary care.

Integrated care

PCTs and health authorities have a responsibility for ensuring that patients within the area have a service that meets their needs. A major challenge is commissioning for a service that is met by a variety of providers in primary care, in the community, in local trusts and some in more distant regional centres. Developments in the provision of diabetic services provide a useful example of emerging approaches which include:

- diabetes centre representatives (medical, nursing and relevant professions allied to medicine)

- primary care representatives (medical and nursing)

- community representatives (medical, nursing and relevant professions allied to medicine)

- a director of public health or manager

- patient representatives

- specialist representatives as required.

Integrated care is a logical way to approach the management of chronic diseases. Models vary according to local needs and cultures.

Some notes on recent changes and reforms

Shifting the Balance of Power

Shifting the Balance of Power is the name for the programme of changes that are reforming the way the NHS works. The aim is to design a service centred on patients, which puts them first. Its aim is to be faster, more convenient and offer patients more choice. The main feature of the change has been to give locally based PCTs the role of running the NHS and improving health in their areas. This has also meant creating new strategic health authorities which cover larger areas and have a more strategic role. You can find out more about these NHS reforms at www. dh.gov.uk/PublicationsAndStatistics/Publications/ PublicationsPolicyAndGuidance/.

Choose and Book

Choose and Book is a new service that allows patients to choose their hospital or clinic and book an appointment. It was introduced across England from the summer of 2004. It will eventually be available to all patients. When patients and their GP agree the need to see a consultant, the GP will advise about the clinically appropriate services from which the patient may then go on to choose. They will be able to choose from at least four hospitals or clinics and also the date and time of their appointment and book it on the spot while in the GP's surgery, or later on the phone or via the internet at a time that is most convenient to them. Local SHAs agreed with local hospital trusts and PCTs the programme for local implementation to meet the timetable.

Patients could also access information about healthcare providers by calling the Choose and Book Appointments Line or visiting www.nhs.uk. The information would help them decide their choice of provider. GPs and practice staff can also access this information using Choose and Book. They can also access the same information by calling the Appointments Line on 0845 850 1150. This number is available to NHS staff only, and is different from the number available to patients.

Patients can book their appointment by calling the Appointments Line, using the internet or in the GP practice, but also by calling the hospital booking staff for the service to which the patient wishes to be booked. Training and support was available to NHS staff using the new service. It was claimed that Choose and Book was a big step towards an NHS that offers patients more opportunities to shape their care. For more details go to www.chooseandbook.nhs.uk/.

The NHS Improvement Plan

The NHS Improvement Plan was published in June 2004 and sets out the way in which the NHS needs to change in order to become patient led, moving away from a centrally directed system. It therefore established the National Leadership Network for Health and Social Care to play a key role in taking forward the work, collecting feedback and shaping the way we implement change. The overall change is closely allied with social care, the publication of a Green Paper, linked to the *Choosing Health* White Paper, and requires joint working with local authorities, other parts of government, the voluntary sector and private agencies. Claiming that the past five years have been about building capacity and capability, it stated that the next will be about improving quality, giving the very best value for money and using the new capacity and capability to build a truly patient-led service.

Community matrons

In 2005, the Chief Nursing Officer set out how nurses will help deliver care to patients with long-term conditions, by outlining a blueprint of a new role enabling them to give one-to-one support to patients with long-term conditions. Guidance set out the role of community matrons:

- develop a personal care plan with the patient, carers, relatives and other health professionals based on a full assessment of their needs

- keep in touch and monitor the condition of the patients regularly, though home visits or telephone calls

- work in partnership with the patient's GP, sharing information and planning together.

Earlier the Health Secretary had announced a major overhaul in the way health and social care services would deliver care to the millions with long-term conditions, including diabetes, asthma, and arthritis, to improve health and quality of life, prevent premature death, and reduce the number of times they have emergency visits to hospital. The government committed to having 3,000 NHS community matrons delivering specialist care across the country by March 2007.

Healthcare reforms

Before leaving government and the NHS reforms, it might be helpful to consider healthcare in a global context. In the quest for improved efficiency, policy makers worldwide have introduced a range of healthcare reforms which seek to contain costs, increase efficiency and raise standards. There are no quick-fix solutions to the challenges faced by healthcare systems in developed countries. The experiences of five different countries have been reviewed, chosen for their different systems of finance and delivery. In Holland and Germany, social insurance is the predominant method of funding, with a mixed economy of public and private providers. The UK and Sweden pay for healthcare mainly out of taxation, with a large measure of public ownership of hospitals and public employment of staff. The US relies mainly on private funding and provision, using competition to increase efficiency and promote choice for patients.

Four approaches to reform can be identified and these might be useful ideas to review should you be asked your views about healthcare reforms at interviews.

1 '*Big bang reform*' is introduced in a short period of time and driven through by a government committed to its implementation. This has occurred in the UK, Israel and New Zealand.

2 '*Incremental reform*' tends to be a lengthy process with key proposals not being implemented

after a period of ten years. This has occurred in Holland and Germany.

3 *'Bottom-up reform'* consists of number of national policy initiatives set by local councils, as in Sweden.

4 *'Reform without reform'* covers rapid changes occurring continuously despite the defeat of central plans, as in the US and, partly, Sweden.

The way in which reforms are implemented is also interesting. It may be as a broad outline with the detail added at a later stage, as with the recent NHS reforms. Generally in other countries too the implementation stage is important. Key aspects of the original proposal may be adapted at a decentralised level and the content and direction of the reforms shaped locally. Policies can also create politics. For example, policies developed in one period can give rise to a set of relationships between organisations and interested parties in the healthcare system, which in turn shapes the development of future policies.

The NHS of the future

During the pilot stages of the first edition of this book we were frequently asked to include a section on the future of the NHS. We claim no crystal ball and have no more insight than any other person working in healthcare. The glib answer is to state that you (the intended readers) are the future, but to fulfil our promise to take notice of all comments at the pilot stages of earlier editions we have set out some of the developments that are on the horizon and could well develop in the future. However, for every new Secretary of State for Health there will be new initiatives and change.

If you feel that change is a new issue, you need look no further than *The Principles and Practice of Medicine* by William Osler (1895) who wrote over 100 years ago, 'Everywhere the old order changes and happy those who change with it'.

There exist technological forces for change, such as minimally invasive therapies, diagnostic scanning techniques, microchip technology, advances in biotechnical diagnostic testing and more finely targeted drugs, together with new drug delivery systems and, perhaps, routine genetic therapy.

Social changes must be taken into account in both the domestic and working environment.

Cultural shift caused by societal, individual, political or professional change has tended to decentralise power and influence, and increased user involvement in policy making leads to different expectations of healthcare.

Resource developments in primary care create further pressure for change in the structure of provision.

Increasing patient expectations and patient autonomy, together with the information revolution that allows individuals greater access to global information, will be drivers for change in the responsiveness of professionals.

There is also rising demand due to ageing as well as medical advances.

One recent medical advance is 'telemedicine' where a patient consults the doctor from home via a video link, which incorporates special sensors to relay vital signs. One can also imagine robotic surgeons controlled by experts on the other side of the world operating on patients within the next decade.

The telephone can be used to monitor the heart, as patients are now able to send a 30-second recording for analysis by a doctor. Follow-up telephone consultations at pre-agreed times to discuss progress mean that patients don't have to journey to the outpatients department, and the results of one such example in rheumatology have already been published. Certain specialties such as rheumatology, dermatology and neurology are more suited to this approach, and some centres are already carrying out postoperative follow-ups, particularly for day surgery patients.

NHS Direct, the telephone helpline, is now firmly established. Staffed by nurses, NHS Direct provides medical advice and reassurance to reduce the number of unnecessary ambulance callouts, hospital attendance and out-of-hours GP callouts. Nursing units with nurses running their own hospitals are another possible future development. Hospices and specialised units for AIDS are already taking medical innovation into new territory. Hospital-at-home schemes already cater for renal dialysis, intravenous therapy and nutrition, respiratory therapy, intensive nursing, rehabilitation therapy and obstetrics.

Not only will the buildings change, but the organisation, staff and management will too. Evidence-based management built on good research evidence and appropriate use of limited resources will require managers to have an understanding of key clinical issues. This will all be part of the development of more methodical approaches to risk management and quality, as enshrined in clinical governance.

The Healthcare Commission has established a rolling programme of reviews of NHS trust performance, ensuring that clinical standards are maintained, and much information can be obtained from their website. NICE publishes guidelines on the most clinically effective and cost-effective treatments and drugs. Clinical pathways are developed for optimal sequencing, and timing of interventions by clinicians, nurses and allied healthcare workers show a firm move towards evidence-based medicine but not 'cook book' medicine. For a review of both, read *Evidence-Based Medicine: what it is and what it isn't* by Sackett *et al.* in an article based on an editorial from the *BMJ* on 13 January 1996 (*BMJ* 1996;312:71–2) or see it at www.cebm.net/ ebm_is_isnt.asp. Hospitals are now required to publish detailed league tables and data, and mortality and morbidity leagues are now beginning to appear.

We may also see a continuing move away from professional self-regulation towards more direct accountability. Indeed, since the previous edition there have been dramatic changes in the GMC's role and the introduction of revalidation for continued registration of all doctors. The careers of consultants will change, as the position will no longer represent the pinnacle for hospital doctors. Having reached consultant level they will have various branches to follow: towards clinical director in service work, teaching, research or management; medical director and even chief executive.

Doctors' roles in management will continue to develop as interested parties demand that doctors fulfil their roles with skill. As Plato said, quoting Protagoras in the fifth century: 'Of all things the measure is man: of things that are, that they are, and of things that are not, that they are not'. Staffing will remain the key, for even with the most sophisticated and technical advances there will always be the need for human contact. There will be staffing changes as well as changes in staff, and until recently it was generally accepted that there were shortages of both doctors and nurses. However, some current reports of unemployment amongst doctors and nurses may cast doubt on that although it may be more a question of what a healthcare system can afford. Adequate staffing levels may, however, be interpreted and reacted to differently by governments, patients

and healthcare professionals. However, the NHS has its own plan for reform and has published what it outlines as the vision of a health service designed around the patient, which covers:

- a new delivery system for the NHS
- changes between health and social services
- changes for NHS doctors, nurses, midwives, therapists and other NHS staff
- changes for patients
- changes in the relationship between the NHS and the private sector.

Medical care practitioners

In 2005 the government began steps to introduce a new breed of medical practitioner, with nurses and other professionals including science graduates being retrained as medical care practitioners. The Department of Health said it was introducing 'ER'-style medicine to Britain. These practitioners will be able to undertake many of the tasks undertaken by GPs and will be regulated by the Health Professions Council. In 2006 a health minister said: 'By introducing new roles we are able to offer patients skilled practitioners who are able to manage the care of patients in primary and secondary care'. They will work in hospitals and primary care, diagnosing patients and prescribing drugs, but not have the same medical qualifications as doctors.

The NHS Plan: a plan for investment, a plan for reform

The document published by The Stationery Office in July 2000 sets out how increased funding and reform aim to redress geographical inequalities, improve service standards, and extend patient choice. Since March 2000 specialist teams have been preparing an NHS plan with the vision of a health service designed around the patient. This vision is outlined at the beginning of this report followed by a look at the NHS now. The report then outlines options for funding healthcare and for investing in NHS facilities and NHS staff. The plan outlines a new delivery system for the NHS as well as changes between health and social services, changes for NHS doctors, for nurses, midwives, therapists and other NHS staff. The plan also outlines changes for patients and in the relationship between the NHS and the private sector. The remainder of the plan sets out strategies for cutting waiting time for treatment and improving health and reducing inequality. Actions for tackling clinical priorities and for services to older people are discussed, and the reform programme outlined.

Patient involvement in the NHS

In a further White Paper published in June 2005 it was announced that a new resource centre would be set up to support the delivery of patient and public involvement (PPI), building on the recent commitment to make PPI part of everyday practice.

It was envisaged that the centre which was expected to be up and running in January 2006 would:

- seek out existing and ongoing PPI best practice and innovation, and communicate it widely through exemplars, advice, guidance and information

- identify gaps in learning and skills and support initiatives to address them

- offer signposting, linkages and networks

- provide guidance to PCT patients' forums to enable them to work together to follow the patient's journey, developing existing good forum practice.

It was stated that 'The centre will support and promote the work of patients' forums, influence the future delivery of patient and public involvement nationally and lead to better delivery of patient-led services by the NHS'.

The future of general hospitals

Some authorities believe that even the future of district general hospitals, the historical backbone of NHS hospital care, is at risk under the government's healthcare reforms. The threat is perceived to come from independent providers together with the public's increasing expectations of choice.

With pressure from limited budgets it seems possible that some services will become uneconomical in hospitals struggling to achieve financial balance, particularly with PFI and PPI 'mortgage' commitments.

A range of strategies for dealing with this is likely. The hospitals could compete aggressively for their market share, but this might not be financially sustainable. An alternative would be to reduce some services and focus on better productivity in areas of competitive advantage. More complex arrangements for the commissioning of care through independent networks of doctors and others professionals seems likely. Another strategy would be for some hospitals to diversify their services for example, into only subacute and primary care. Some already see this beginning to happen.

What seems certain, however, is that district general hospitals will have to compete with other NHS hospitals, NHS treatment centres, independent sector treatment centres, and established private hospitals. It is almost certainly going to destabilise the NHS and need careful management, although the problem might be whether this has been fully thought through yet.

The future of doctors and the profession

In the US, 20 conditions account for 80% of healthcare expenditure and 70% of personal healthcare expenditure on those with chronic conditions, and this has implications for clinical practice and therefore the NHS. It has therefore been suggested that healthcare provision needs to be organised around the needs of those with chronic disabilities, perhaps with more integration of primary, secondary and social care. Sir Cyril Chantler in an a Harveian Oration asked if the traditional divide between GPs and hospital consultants was still helpful in an age of teamwork and flexibility in the NHS, and suggested that it maybe the time has come to discard the term 'consultant' in favour of the word 'specialist'.

Sir Cyril went on to identify three paradoxes at the heart of modern medical practice:

- doctors have never before been able to do so much for patients, yet not since the advent of the NHS have we been so criticised and perhaps so unhappy

- we spend massive amounts on the NHS but continue to be short of resources

- in spite of such spending and the successes of modern medicine, the prevalence of disability and illness continues to rise.

Some of these paradoxes stem from the benefits of medicine itself – people are living with disability whereas before they would have died; the achievements of medicine are leading to greater expectations and the plethora of new drugs and treatments puts more pressure on budgets. Sir Cyril also draws out the need for doctors to take a lead in their organisation of care, while continuing to conduct research, not only in the biomedical field, but also in how better to deliver care to patients.

He concluded that:

We shall need help. Doctors in the NHS are under great pressure, we need more understanding and less criticism, more trust and less regulation. Perhaps the public, government and profession need, as has been suggested, a new concordat that sets out the rights and responsibilities of each and maybe explicitly recognises the limits of what the NHS can provide and what modern medicine can achieve.

Related reading

Beware when reading anything about the NHS structure. We have therefore not recommended any text books in this edition. Things change frequently and anything more than a year old is very likely to be out of date. Our best advice for further information is to visit the websites we have indicated, or carry out internet searches and even with the latter, check the date of writing.

CHAPTER 9

Funding and the NHS

The aim of this chapter is to inform you about national and local NHS funding structures. There are two major differences in this latest edition. Firstly, it has expanded as funding is now more complex, and secondly, some of the figures given below cannot be guaranteed because not only do different authorities sometimes give different figures, but one can occasionally find contradictory figures quoted on official Department of Health websites.

Early funding policies of the NHS were concerned with cost control but lacked processes to achieve equity and efficiency in funding. Governments of the 1980s sought to add efficiency through budgetary squeezes, which culminated in funding problems in the late 1980s. The result was an NHS internal market which promised efficiency by introducing a purchaser–provider split and a system of provider competition in which money would follow the patient.

Current policies are aimed at continued increase in spending on healthcare. According to OECD Health Data for 2005, in 2002–2003 the total expenditure was 7.7% of gross domestic product (GDP). It is claimed it will increase yearly to 8.0%, 8.3%, 8.7%, and 9.0% and by 2007–2008 to 9.4%. One authority claims that with current policy it will be 10.5–11.0% of GDP (around £110 billion) by 2010. Indeed, it has been suggested that British health spending has already exceeded the European average.

It has been suggested that future problems may arise from funding the private finance initiative (PFI) and public private partnership (PPP) outcomes, changes and developments in primary care, preferential contracts to private providers, reintroduction of the internal market, and inflation in medical technology and drug costs. All of these problems put pressure on traditional large hospitals, including foundation hospitals.

As well as the additional funding, the government has reintroduced a system of provider competition in which money is intended to follow the patient. In 2002, the Wanless report (see www.hm-treasury.gov.uk/consultations_and _legislation/wanless/consult_wanless04_final.cfm) stated that the NHS would face ever-growing financial pressure in the coming 10 to 20 years. However, Wanless argued that continuing to fund the health service through general taxation was the most cost-effective and fairest system for the future.

If you would like to compare the UK system with those in other countries then visit www. reform.co.uk and click on 'Healthcare systems' for a summary of the systems in Canada, Denmark, France, Germany, Hungary, Netherlands, Switzerland and USA.

The finances of the NHS

In 2003–2004 the Department of Health achieved financial balance overall across the 600 local NHS bodies, and most individual NHS bodies also achieved financial balance, although the proportion failing to achieve financial balance increased from 12% to 18%. The position deteriorated further in 2004–2005.

The Department of Health has estimated that in 2004–2005 the NHS incurred a small overall deficit. The number of individual parts with significant deficits increased. At least twelve strategic health authorities ended 2004–2005 with a deficit compared with seven the previous year.

A recent Audit Commission report concluded that the basics of financial management at most NHS bodies were sound, but that greater control was needed It stated that nearly half of all acute trusts and PCTs suffered from either 'weak' or 'fairly weak' financial planning. It also said the current financial management of most PCTs was inadequate to meet the challenges, and all board members, executives and non-executives, needed to have greater knowledge and skills to discharge their responsibilities effectively.

At the start of Chapter 8 there is a statistical picture of the NHS. The following data may be added to that list to complete the financial picture of the NHS:

- When the NHS began in 1948 it cost £400 million per year.

- By 2004–2005 the NHS cost £64.9 billion (£74.9 billion if private healthcare expenditure is included).

- By 2007–2008 the NHS cost is projected at £90.2 billion.

- The NHS now spends over £1 million every ten minutes, equivalent to £1,825 per head in 2004–2005.

- Just under half of NHS spending goes on acute services, just over £800 per person per annum.

- The NHS accounts for 17% of all government spending.

- 77% of funding comes from general taxation, 12% from the NHS share of national insurance contributions, and 2% from patient charges.

- Over 40% of total hospital and community health services expenditure is for people over 64 years of age, although they represent just 16% of the population.

- A one-week stay in hospital costs over £1,100, and a night in intensive care costs over £500.

- The NHS spends £14 billion in Scotland and £7 billion in Wales.

Distribution of NHS funds

The NHS is the second largest government spending programme. The following paragraphs provide information about the allocation of NHS funding. In England the funding supports the Department of Health, hospital, community and family health services, and centrally purchased services such as the National Blood Authority. The basis for distributing the total NHS funds varies between England, Wales, Scotland and Northern Ireland.

NHS funding in England

Revenue allocations

Recurrent revenue allocations to PCTs cover hospital and community health services (HCHS), prescribing, primary medical services and HIV/AIDS. The Department of Health announced its 2006–2007 and 2007–2008 allocations totalling £135 billion in February 2005. The Department notifies PCTs of their revenue allocations through a Health Service Circular (HSC).

Capital budgets

For the first time, in 2005–2006, capital budgets have been made available to local health services for three years rather than one year. It is also the first time day-to-day operational capital has been allocated directly to NHS trusts and PCTs.

Capital allocations are made to the NHS in two parts: operational capital is for the purpose of maintaining and enhancing existing capital stock. Strategic capital, which is allocated direct to all SHAs, is for distribution at their own discretion for larger-scale investments.

Other allocations

The Department of Health allocated £4.3 billion to PCTs as part of their primary medical services allocations in 2004–2005 for the delivery of general medical services (GMS), personal medical services (PMS), PCT medical services and alternative providers. This was the first time PCTs received a resource-limited allocation for the commissioning of GMS and PMS services.

Spending reviews

Spending reviews set firm and fixed three-year departmental expenditure limits and, through Public Service Agreements (PSAs, *see* below) define the key improvements that the government and public can expect from these resources. Successive spending reviews have targeted resources at the government's priorities, have matched these resources with reforms, and have set targets for improvements in health services. The spending review for 2004 sets spending plans and PSAs for 2005–2008.

One of the aims in public service reform has been to set the spending review to focus on increasing devolution to the front-line, thereby enabling service providers to respond flexibly to local needs.

Public Service Agreements (PSAs)

Examples of Public Service Agreements (PSAs) are:

- to deliver a maximum wait from GP referral to hospital treatment of 18 weeks by the end of 2008

- to give NHS patients the right to choose from at least four or five different healthcare providers from the end of 2005, and from 2008, from any provider that meets independently inspected NHS standards and can do so within the NHS's national maximum price

- to apply much greater priority to disease prevention

- to tackle health inequalities

- to improve chronic disease management

- to introduce targets to reduce the prevalence of smoking

- to introduce targets to reduce the prevalence of child obesity

- to tackle inequalities in health outcomes.

Payment by results

In the document *Delivering the NHS Plan – next steps on investment, next steps on reform* (Department of Health, 2002, go to www.dh. gov.uk/PublicationsAndStatistics, take shortcut to 'publications', then type into search box 'next steps on investment, next steps on reform'), the idea of incentives for performance or 'payment by results' was introduced (*see* below). In October 2002 the Department of Health issued *Reforming NHS Financial Flows: introducing payment by results* (can be accessed most easily by typing full

title into Google within inverted commas) setting out plans for changes in the way that healthcare providers are paid in the NHS.

These included the linking of the flow of funds to activity, and the adoption of a standard national price tariff (adjusted for local differences in pay and input prices) for most services over the medium term. These changes are planned to be implemented over a five-year period, with ongoing consultation. In the reforms, there is no proposal to change the basic principle of allocating resources (on a needs basis) to PCTs, who are free to purchase care from the most appropriate provider. Rather, given the structure of primary care and new unified budgets for PCTs, it creates incentives at primary care level to take prevention seriously rather than merely expand the volume of hospital referrals. In order to get the best from the extra resources being invested in the NHS, major changes are planned to the way money flows around the NHS, including differentiating between incentives for routine surgery and emergency admissions. Instead of block contracts for hospitals, they will be paid for the elective activity they undertake on a system of payment by results, to offer the right incentives to reward good performance, to support sustainable reductions in waiting times for patients, and to make the best use of available capacity.

Over time the system to improve the commissioning process will be developed by:

- providing patients with timely, comparable, regularly updated information on practices and hospitals updated regularly

- offering choice to patients: choice of GPs, choice of hospitals; choice of consultants, and to ensure that where choice is exercised cash for treatment goes with patients

- setting the price for units of activity allowing the PCT to focus on volume, appropriateness and quality

- offering commissioners and providers the flexibility to use savings and additional resources in a way that benefits staff and patients

- requiring 'open book' relationships between PCTs and NHS trusts.

In 2002–2003, a start was made by testing different ways of moving resources with patients to establish the key principle that providers that fail to deliver lose money to those that can deliver.

Experience of the internal market showed that price competition did not work, particularly for emergency cases that were admitted to the nearest hospital, and merely led to excessive transaction costs. The new Healthcare (or Hospital) Resource Group (HRG) benchmarks will be used to establish a standard tariff for the same treatment, regardless of provider. This is the hospital payment system used by many international healthcare systems.

In the medium term it is proposed to move to a system where all activity is commissioned against a standard tariff using either HRG or some other appropriate measure. Local commissioning would focus on volume, appropriateness and quality, not price, as this would be fixed using regional tariffs to reflect unavoidable differences in costs in different parts of the country. The more efficient providers would be able to retain some or all of any surplus they generated to deploy within their organisation to the benefit of patients and staff. The less efficient providers will be helped to improve their performance and, where necessary, new management could be brought in using the franchising process.

A consultation paper, *Payment by Results: preparing for 2005*, identified the key decisions needed for implementing the payment by results and outlined how it would apply to NHS foundation trusts from April 2004 and to all NHS trusts from April 2005.

The information received in response to this exercise and feedback received from the NHS revealed two issues. Firstly, non-elective and outpatient activity is not stable, incurring big increases in short stay, emergency admissions. This means that a tariff based on last year's practice is not reliable for pricing work next year. Secondly, there are concerns about the consistency of approach by the NHS to the baselining exercise.

As a result it was decided to amend the phasing in of payment by results to include elective care only in 2005–2006. The overall implementation timetable remains unchanged, with 90% of hospital care covered by 2008–2009. In effect a new step is being introduced to the phasing-in with non-electives, outpatients and A&E deferred by one year. This does not affect NHS foundation trusts which already operate payment by results.

Relevant information on the progress of the reform may be accessed at www.dh.gov.uk/Policy AndGuidance/OrganisationPolicy/FinanceAnd Planning/NHSFinancialReforms.

In June 2004 the Audit Commission published a useful booklet *Payment by Results – key risks and questions to consider for trust and PCT managers and non-executives* that can be viewed on the internet at the Audit Commission's website.

Reference costs

NHS reference costs and a national tariff were published in 2004, providing information to help the NHS with payment by results. You can find details at: www.dh.gov.uk/PolicyAndGuidance/ OrganisationPolicy/FinanceAndPlanning/NHS ReferenceCosts.

A national tariff for groups of clinical procedures means NHS organisations are paid much more fairly for the treatment they provide. Money is linked directly to patients, so the more productive and efficient an NHS trust is, the more it should benefit from extra resources. The introduction of payment by results was phased in to allow NHS organisations to adjust to the new costs. It commenced with some NHS foundation trusts in April 2004 and other NHS organisations that started in April 2005, and will become fully operational by 2008.

In the past, the NHS paid above its own usual costs when it purchased extra activity from the independent sector. The payment by results system will also apply to the independent sector, which means that in future these additional costs to the NHS will be reduced. The independent treatment centre programme is helping the NHS by negotiating prices that are near (in some cases nearly 10% below) the comparable NHS tariff.

National tariff

The national tariff was used for commissioning services in 2005–2006. From April 2005 the system covered around half of hospital and community health services spend and for large district general hospitals; typically some 70% of income will be covered by the national tariff.

As a result of consultations and contacts with other countries, some modifications have been made to the tariff which will help to ensure that it is as sensitive as possible, closely reflecting the true cost of service delivery.

2005–2006 saw a significant change, and over the next three years NHS trusts, NHS foundation trusts and PCTs would have been adjusting to the transition to tariff-based payments. However during early 2006 the national tariff was deferred because of concerns that the process would lead to over-commitment of funds.

Healthcare resource groups (HRGs)

With the most recent financial reforms, the NHS is moving to a system where tariffs, or reference costs, for a particular treatment are defined by the resources necessary to carry out that treatment. HRGs are defined as 'a tool for classifying patients into a manageable number of groups of cases that are clinically similar and that require similar levels of healthcare resources for diagnosis, treatment and care'.

HRGs have been developed in the UK by the NHS Information Authority, with input from UK clinicians, to reflect our clinical practice and UK patterns of service delivery. Other countries (US, Australia, the Nordic countries, Austria) have developed similar tools, often called diagnostic-related groups (DRGs). Most OECD and EU countries are now using, or planning to use, case-mix tools in their provider payment systems. When DRGs were first introduced in the US there was a significant shift in the pattern of healthcare delivery.

HRGs inform the NHS system of allocating a cost of a treatment. This enables PCTs to commission healthcare on the basis of fixed 'tariffs', and it is an integral part of the payment by results system. The benefit is that PCTs pay a fixed amount regardless of the provider chosen, thereby eliminating price competition between providers. The PCTs can then choose on the basis of quality and waiting time.

When a similar system was introduced in the US where it was called diagnostic resource groups or DRGs, purchasers could see the total cost of a treatment. They became very aware of the proportion of that cost that was due to hospitalisation. Therefore, in order to save money, they began to opt for the same care package but with a home-based patient. The result was a massive swing to homecare, and the creation of a multibillion dollar homecare industry to deliver a range of high-tech treatments, mainly focused on intravenous therapies such as chemotherapy together with the necessary nursing support.

Concern was expressed in the UK that the introduction of HRGs for complex treatments (where it is difficult for acute trusts to calculate the costs) might result in a loss of money. A £50 million 'rescue fund' was reported to be being set up to help any of the first-wave foundation trusts that got into trouble.

Programme budgeting

Programme budgeting is a retrospective appraisal of resource allocation, broken down into meaningful programmes, with a view to tracking future resource allocation in those same programmes. Instead of seeing investment on the level of a hospital or drug budget, the focus switches to specific health objectives or medical conditions.

In future, as part of a National Programme Budget project, financial information that identifies all PCT expenditure, including primary care services, must be allocated to programmes of care based on the following 23 areas:

- infectious diseases
- cancers and tumours
- blood disorders
- endocrine, nutritional and metabolic problems
- mental health problems
- learning disability problems
- neurological system problems
- eye/vision problems
- hearing problems
- circulation problems (coronary heart disease (CHD))
- respiratory system problems
- dental problems
- gastrointestinal system problems
- skin problems
- musculoskeletal system problems (excludes trauma)
- trauma and injuries (includes burns)
- genitourinary system disorders (except infertility)
- maternity and reproductive health
- neonates
- poisoning
- healthy individuals

- social care needs
- other conditions.

This data collection exercise also applies to SHAs. Spending by SHAs on education and training, through workforce development confederations, is given as a key reason for their inclusion in the collection. A *Programme Budgeting Guidance Manual* was issued in December 2003.

Funding for the NHS in Devolved Parts of the UK

The funding of the various parts of the NHS in the UK is slightly different and can be reviewed on the relevant NHS websites. The NHS in Scotland has also undergone a radical reorganisation, but it remains the single largest budget item for which the Scottish Parliament is responsible. In 2003–2004 it was allocated £5.9 billion by the Scottish Parliament and in addition it received £1.8 billion in national insurance contributions and other charges and other income generation schemes. The budget is distributed as general revenue allocations for hospital and community services, family health services, special health boards and other NHS bodies on delivering national services for the NHS, and the remainder on centrally managed expenditure.

The Accounts Commission for Scotland

This is a statutory independent body that assists the NHS (and local government) in Scotland to achieve high standards of financial stewardship and value for money. The duty of the Auditor General and the Accounts Commission is to check that public money is spent properly, efficiently and effectively. It secures an external audit of all Scottish health service bodies, and reports concerns identified through audit, which are followed up by statutory power where appropriate. Copies of reports can be downloaded from their website.

Capital in the NHS

This was formerly a government funded capital grant, but is now a mixture of two elements: government funding and the PFI, part of the PPP agenda.

Public Private Partnership (PPP) and Private Finance Initiative (PFI)

This was intended to give the NHS (and other public sector organisations) access to private sector skills and expertise, as well as being a source of finance for capital investment. The PFI and PPP initiatives have spawned an industry and a collection of websites and literature that it is not useful to cover in a book such as this.

Briefly, PPP is the umbrella name given to a range of initiatives that involve the private sector in the operation of public services. The PFI is the most frequently used initiative. The key difference between PFI and conventional ways of providing public services is that the public does not own the asset. The public authority makes an annual payment to the private company who provides the building and associated services, rather like a mortgage. A typical PFI project will be owned by a company set up specially to run the scheme. These companies are usually consortia including a building firm, a bank and a facilities management company. While PFI projects can be structured in different ways, there are usually four key elements: design, finance, build and operate.

The PFI scheme encourages private investment in public construction projects such as hospitals. This means that the private companies raise the capital and keep the borrowing off the nation's balance sheet. Having built it, the company then undertakes to run it for at least 25 years (sometimes up to 42 years), providing maintenance and upkeep, although not medical staff, and in return the NHS pays the company an annual rent to cover the interest on the money spent, the cost of maintenance and a profit margin for the company.

Some authorities claim that around £100 billion of PFI and PPP contracts have been entered into by government, although this does not include the revenue commitments. They are attractive to government because they take debt off the government's balance sheets and assist the Treasury in not exceeding the EU rules on debt being no more than 40% of GDP. They are also beneficial in fees and profits for merchant banks, accountants, lawyers and construction companies. However they also commit large amounts of future governments' expenditure.

At the time of writing 24 PFI schemes are completed and operational with a capital spend of £2.1 billion, and another 14 schemes are approved with a value of £3 billion. In addition there are further schemes under negotiation worth a further £12.1 billion. One economist has pointed out that due to PFI the UK's hospital building programme is bigger than the rest of the G8 nations put together. The problem may however be that the commitment to the future 'mortgage payments' may prove a burden, as this alone may represent 20% of a trust's future income.

For a detailed discussion on the subject go to www.parliament.uk/ and under advanced search type in 'IV The Private Finance Initiative' then click on 'Select Committee Reports'.

NHS LIFT

In 2001 the government committed to a programme of sustained investment to reform the NHS in order to produce faster services delivering better health and tackling health inequalities. NHS LIFT (Local Improvement Finance Trust) was a major new initiative from the Department of Health which entered a national joint venture with Partnerships UK plc. Its aim was to develop and encourage a new market for investment in primary care and community-based facilities and services.

The National Audit Office (NAO)

Headed by the Comptroller and Auditor General, the NAO is the external auditor of central government spending in the UK. It was established under the National Audit Act 1983 and its role is to ensure accountability to Parliament and the taxpayer for all moneys voted by Parliament. The Comptroller and Auditor General also has statutory powers to certify a wide range of public sector accounts, and statutory powers to report to Parliament on the economic efficiency and effectiveness with which departments and other bodies have used their resources. The NAO publishes about 50 value for money reports each year, including five covering the work of the Department of Health and the NHSE.

Finances at local level

Trusts obtain most of their income through agreements with health authorities and PCTs.

These agreements set out the treatment or services the trust agrees to provide in return for funding. Agreements can include quality clauses and requirements to meet targets for equal opportunities, respond to complaints and provide information to the public. Trusts have the power to make their own investment decisions and, with their financial freedom, can develop services for patients. The single financial obligation of the trust is to break even.

Financial control within NHS trusts

Members of trust boards have to ensure that the trust:

- publishes a strategic direction document every third year covering the next five year period

- publishes a summary business plan by 31 March each year

- ensures that the annual income and expenditure budget is realistic

- makes adequate provision for inflation

- receives a monthly report showing the financial position with a forecast of the year end position

- organises its management in an effective manner within limits set by the NHS.

Trusts must comply with certain requirements in pricing their services:

- prices must equal costs for NHS agreements

- costs must include depreciation and a 6% return on the value of assets employed

- there must be no cross subsidising between services

- marginal costs can only be charged where unplanned spare capacity exists

- for private contracts, charges should be what the market will bear.

Agenda for Change

Agenda for Change forms the basis of a new pay and reward system within secondary and community care. It aims to provide equal pay for work of equal value for all NHS staff. The NHS Job Evaluation Scheme makes provision for most NHS jobs to be matched to nationally evaluated profiles on the basis of information from job descriptions, person specifications and additional information. National job profiles additionally provide a framework against which to check the consistency of local evaluations. Agenda for Change applies to all directly employed NHS staff except very senior managers and those covered by the Doctors' and Dentists' Pay Review Body. It is difficult to put a reliable figure to the cost of implementation, but many hospitals report it as a main factor in creating financial problems in 2005–2006.

Related reading

The websites listed throughout Chapter 8 will provide the latest information, but please check the date on the articles you may find as there is much that is time expired.

CHAPTER 10

Useful information

The aim of this chapter is to provide you with information about health related Acts of Parliament, Health Service Circulars (HSC), Executive Letters (EL), reports, inquiries, Green Papers, White Papers, Codes of Practice and other guidance notes and publications issued by various bodies such as the GMC, Medical Royal Colleges etc, that you may find useful, instructive or that you may need to know. We have divided it into three sections:

- health-related and other useful Acts of Parliament
- government-inspired reports and inquiries
- Health Circulars and guidance notes on codes and best practice.

Health-related Acts of Parliament and legislation

The following list covers Acts of Parliament, Health Service Circulars and Executive Letters. There has been an enormous output of these documents since the last edition of this book, and although we have tried to be as comprehensive as possible, not everything can be included. Some publications have been omitted as we felt the size of the list had to be reduced. Clearly for any individual doctor some will be totally irrelevant, for example all the mental health papers, while they may be of interest to psychiatrists, will be of no interest to general surgeons or physicians, and papers referring to abortion are only likely to interest those pursuing a career in obstetrics and gynaecology.

Births and Deaths Registration Act 1953

Parents have a legal duty to register the details (child's name, sex, date and place of birth, parents'

name, places of birth, address and father's occupation) of a birth with the local registrar within 42 days. The doctor or midwife normally has a duty to inform the district medical officer of the birth within six hours. Still births (a baby born dead after 24th week of pregnancy) must also be registered. Doctors attending patients during their last illness must sign a death certificate, giving cause of death (to their best knowledge). The certificate must be sent to the registrar. The registrar must inform the coroner of any death that occurs without attendance of a doctor at the last illness, or during an operation, or while the effects of an anaesthetic persist.

Abortion Act 1967

Under the terms of the Abortion Act of 1967, termination is legal up to the 24th week of pregnancy, subject to approval from two doctors. To 'qualify' for an abortion, a woman must prove that having a baby would cause her or her family greater physical or mental damage than not having one. The Act was amended and updated by the Abortion Regulations 1991.

Misuse of Drugs Act 1971

Covers dangerous or otherwise harmful drugs and related matters.

NHS (Venereal Diseases) Regulations 1974

Requires health authorities to take all necessary steps to ensure that information capable of identifying patients with sexually transmitted diseases do so not only for the purpose of treating people with the disease but also for preventing its spread. Such disclosure, furthermore, can only be made to a doctor, or to someone working on a doctor's instruction in connection with treatment or prevention. This allows contact tracing. However it does not allow those working in a genitourinary clinic to inform an insurance company of a patient's sexually transmitted disease – even with the patient's consent. Case notes from genitourinary clinics are kept separate from other hospital records. GPs are not routinely informed of the patient's attendance at such clinics, although the patient may request that the GP is informed.

Health and Safety at Work Act 1974

Details how employers are responsible for employees being kept safe at work, by emphasising the need for assessment of risks and adequate training. But also there is a responsibility on the employee to take reasonable steps to safeguard their own safety and health at work.

Sex Discrimination Act 1975

Makes it illegal for employers, professional bodies and trade unions to discriminate either directly or indirectly on the grounds of sex or marital status, except where marital status or a particular sex can be clearly shown to be a genuine requirement.

Medicines Labelling Regulations 1976

Rules about how medicines should be labelled.

Race Relations Act 1976

Aims to eliminate racial discrimination and to remedy individual grievances. It makes unlawful direct or indirect discrimination on the grounds of race, ethnicity or nationality in the fields of, for example, employment, education or housing.

Medical Act 1983 (as amended by the Professional Performance Act 1995, the European Primary Medical Qualifications Regulations 1996, the NHS (Primary Care) Act 1997, the Medical Act (Amendment) Order 2000, the Medical Act 1983 (Provisional Registration) Regulations 2000, the Medical Act 1983 (Amendment) Order 2002, the National Health Service Reform and Health Care Professionals Act 2002, the European Qualifications (Health Care professions) Regulations 2003 and the European Qualifications (Health & Social Care Professions and Accession of new Member States) Regulations 2004)

Sets up and specifies the role of the GMC and its role in the registration and maintenance of a register of doctors.

Mental Health Act 1983 (MHA)

Provides the statutory framework under which mentally ill patients are detained and cared for in hospital. It includes patient admission (under strict guidelines) for assessment, treatment and emergency detention, and outlines the power of the courts, place of safety orders and consent to treatment. A patient should be made aware of their admission to hospital and has a statutory right of appeal.

Data Protection Act 1984

Brings the UK into line with other Western countries in terms of the rights, duties and obligations of all persons and organisations concerned with computers and computerised data. The Act recognises the specific importance of personal data and an individual citizen's rights. The Act allows individuals right of access to information about themselves that is held on computer.

The Registered Homes Act 1984

Sets standards for the independent healthcare sector; it sets out basic standards for facilities, staffing and procedures of a registered home.

Police and Criminal Evidence Act 1984

Gives the police power to apply to a court for access to records to assist in an investigation.

Public Health (Control of Diseases) Act 1984 (Notifiable Diseases)

A doctor must notify the relevant local authority officer (usually a public health consultant) if he suspects a patient of having a notifiable disease or food poisoning. The following information must be provided (by completing a specific certificate): patient's name, age, sex, address, suspected disease, approximate date of outset and date of admission to hospital (if appropriate).

Access to Medical Reports Act 1988, Access to Health Records Act 1990 or Access to Health Records (Northern Ireland) Order 1993

Gives people right of access to their own health records and provides for the correction of inaccurate information in manually held records. It was repealed by the Data Protection Act 1998.

Road Traffic Act 1988

Gives powers to police to require doctors, on request, to give information that might identify a driver alleged to have committed a traffic offence. This would not normally justify providing clinical information without the patient's consent, or a court order.

Prevention of Terrorism Act (Temporary Provision) Act 1989

All citizens, including doctors, must inform police, as soon as possible, of any information that may help to prevent an act of terrorism, or help in apprehending or prosecuting a terrorist.

The Children Act 1989

Provides the foundation for law on children in Britain. Principles laid down include that, wherever possible, children should be cared for by their own family in a safe and protected environment, that parents still have responsibility for their children not living with them, and that both the parents and the child should be kept informed and involved in decisions about the child's future. The Act requires collaboration between agencies in the provision of services to, and the protection of, children deemed to be in need. It also places responsibilities on local authority social services departments (SSDs) in relation to children in need. The Act emphasises the rights of a child to make informed decisions in relation to her or his own medical care. This has major implications about consent to treatment in children.

Food Safety Act 1990

Specifies appropriate qualifications for food examiners and analysts.

Human Fertilisation and Embryology Act 1990 (as amended by the Human Fertilisation (Disclosure of Information) Act 1992

Makes provisions to license and monitor the performance of fertility treatment clinics, and any research using human embryos. It covers three main activities: any fertility treatment which involves the use of donated eggs or sperm (for example, donor insemination) or embryos created outside the body (IVF – *in vitro* fertilisation); the storage of eggs, sperm and embryos; and research on early human embryos.

The Act was amended in 2000 and 2001, to allow the use of a dead person's sperm in IVF and to allow the creation of embryos for therapeutic cloning research. The Act is currently under further review.

The Human fertilisation and Embryology Authority (HFEA) was created under the Act to oversee the licensing and compliance of treatment clinics and research centres in the UK, and to keep under review all new developments in the field.

National Health Service and Community Care Act 1990 (NHSCCA)

Covers the establishment of NHS trusts, the financing of the practices of medical practitioners, the provision of accommodation and other welfare services by local authorities, and the establishment of the Clinical Standards Advisory Group (CSAG). It has also defined membership of health authorities, established the family health services authorities (FHSA), created the internal market, NHS trusts, GP fundholders and a significant change in community-based care arrangements.

Working Together under the Children Act (1989): a guide to arrangements for the protection of children from abuse, Department of Health 1991

Covers arrangements for cross-agency working on child protection policies and procedures.

Welsh Language Act 1993

Sets out provisions for the use of the Welsh language in healthcare. It requires health authorities and trusts to translate into Welsh all documents, information leaflets and signs.

Mental Health (Patients in the Community) Act 1995

Sets out the requirements for supervised discharge for severely mentally ill people. This Act supplements Section 1(18) of the Mental Health Act 1983.

Carers (Recognition and Services) Act 1995

Covers carers who are either providing, or plan to provide, a substantial amount of care on a regular basis. Under the Act, the carer is entitled to request an assessment, the results of which should be taken into account along with the needs of the patient.

Children's (Northern Ireland) Order 1995

Replaces the provisions of the Children and Young Persons Act (Northern Ireland) 1968 and amends the law relating to illegitimacy and guardianship.

Disability Discrimination Act 1995

The Disability Discrimination Act (DDA) aimed to end the discrimination that many disabled people face. It gave disabled people rights in the areas of employment, access to goods, facilities and services, and buying or renting land or property. The employment rights and first rights of access came into force in 1996 with further rights in 1999, and the remainder in 2004. In addition the Act allowed the government to set minimum standards so that disabled people could use public transport easily. For further information go to www.direct.gov.uk/disability.

Employment Rights Act 1996

About the employment right of employees. It requires that certain terms and conditions must be set out in a single document – this can be a written 'contract of employment' or a 'statement of the main terms and conditions of employment'. The written terms and conditions will contain both contractual and statutory rights, that is, both those protected by law and those negotiated directly between the employer and the employee or representative. The Act has been amended, the last occasion being in 2004.

Audit Commission Act 1998

Set up the Audit Commission and passed legislation enabling it to access information to carry out its functions.

Data Protection Act 1998

About access for patients to their medical records. It updates previous Acts and replaces the Access to Medical Records Act 1990.

All businesses that keep any information on living and identifiable people must comply with the Data Protection Act. The Act applies to computerised personal information and to some structured manual records about people. Some businesses must register under the Act and ensure their information is properly managed, but others only need to observe data-protection principles – enforceable rules of good practice for handling personal information. See www.opsi.gov.uk/ACTS/acts1998/19980029.htm for text and www.dh.gov.uk/PolicyAndGuidance/OrganisationPolicy/RecordsManagement and scroll down to Data Protection Act 1998 for details of how it affects NHS trusts and other health organisations and its application to the NHS in general.

Mental Health Act 1983 – memorandum on Parts I to VI, VIII and X 1998

Designed to assist those who work with the Mental Health Act 1983, this memorandum it offers guidance on the main provisions of the Act. The publication advises on appropriate application of the Act, and clarifies its interpretation with regard to the following areas: admission procedures; consent to treatment; court powers; mental health review tribunals; supervised discharge and aftercare; and supplementary provisions of the Act.

Employment Relations Act 1999

This Act is based on the measures proposed in the White Paper *Fairness at Work*.

Health Act 1999

Under the Health Act 1999, money can be pooled between health bodies and health-related local authority services, and resources and management structures can be integrated. The arrangements, which have been in use since April 2000, allow the joining up of existing services and the development of new, co-ordinated services.

The Race Relations (Amendment) Act 2000

Concerned with outlawing discrimination on the grounds of race in public life. For further details go to www.opsi.gov.uk/ and type race relations act in box.

Health and Social Care Act 2001

Provides regulations for functions of care trusts under partnership arrangements. For more details see www.opsi.gov.uk/, click 'legislation UK', then 'UK Acts', then the year of the Act and you will find them in alphabetical order.

Employment Act 2002

Provides statutory rights to paternity and adoption leave and amended the law on statutory maternity leave and pay. See www.opsi.gov.uk/, click 'legislation UK', then 'UK Acts', then the year of the Act and you will find them in alphabetical order.

NHS Reform and Health Care Professions Act 2002

Established the Commission for Patient and Public Involvement in Health. For more information go to www.opsi.gov.uk/, click 'legislation UK', then 'UK Acts', then the year of the Act and you will find them in alphabetical order.

Health and Social Care (Community Health and Standards) Act 2003

Legislation that allows the government to take forward some of the reforms it outlined in *The NHS Plan* – a plan to 'modernise and rebuild' the health service and 'reshape' the health service from the patient's point of view.

Health (Community Health and Standards) Act 2003

Gives the Commission for Healthcare Audit and Inspection access to fulfil its statutory obligations.

Sex Discrimination Act 1975 (Amendment) Regulations 2003

Made some amendments to the original 1975 Sex Discrimination Act. For further details *see* www.lg-employers.gov.uk/relations/law/discrimination/sex.html.

Assisted Dying for Terminally Ill Bill 2004

This Bill, which sought to legalise physician-assisted suicide (PAS) and euthanasia, was considered by a special select committee of the House of Lords, which reported in April 2005. The committee did not reach a conclusion on the principle of whether PAS or euthanasia should become legal, but identified a number of issues that would need to be overcome before any further attempt to introduce legislation on this issue is made. The Select Committee report was debated in the House of Lords in October 2005. However, the Bill fell when the General Election was called earlier in 2005 and did not progress further. For more details see www.publications.parliament.uk.

Children Bill 2004

The Children Bill represents the biggest ever change in the organisation of children's services. New management models must be developed to support integrated services, and all the key agencies must commit to the service model. Its aim is to prevent abuse and killing of children. It creates an obligation for healthcare providers to safeguard and promote the health and wellbeing of children, to be achieved by undertaking new guidance on doctors' roles and responsibilities in promoting children's rights and contributing to improving their access to good-quality healthcare services. Key aspects are ensuring respect for the privacy and confidentiality of the child, protecting children from harm, and providing children and young people with accessible information. Details can be seen at a number of websites including www.publications.parliament.uk, www.gmc-uk.org or www.nspcc.org.uk.

Freedom of Information Act 2004

Gives the public new rights on information held by approximately 100,000 public authorities. It gives them rights to ask how services are organised and managed, how much they cost and how they can make complaints. The organisation must reply to people's requests within 20 working days. There are exceptions, some absolute such as court records, and some non-absolute such as commercial interests. For more information go to www.informationcommissioner.gov.uk.

Gender Recognition Act 2004

Previously transsexuals were defined by the gender they were born into. This Act allows them to apply for a Gender Recognition Certificate for which doctors may be asked to provide supporting medical evidence.

Human Tissue Bill 2004

This is a Bill to provide a consistent legislative framework for issues relating to whole body donation and the taking, storage and use of human organs and tissue. See www.publications. parliament.uk.

Mental Capacity Bill 2004

People with limited mental capacity will be encouraged to take as many decisions for themselves as possible by this new legislation. The Mental Capacity Bill aims to protect more than two million adults who may be unable to take decisions for themselves. See www.direct.gov.uk.

Mental Health Bill 2004

The Mental Health Bill is part of the government's strategy to improve the provision of mental health services and make them more focused on the needs of the individual. For more details see www.dh.gov.uk.

The Disability Discrimination Act 2005

Amends the Disability Discrimination Act (DDA 1995). For further information go to www.opsi. gov.uk and type 'disability discrimination' in box.

Key health-related reports

This alphabetical list includes Green Papers and White Papers with both their short and official titles where appropriate, official government-initiated health-related reports and inquires.

The short titles of reports are often derived from the name of the person who chaired the group or committee that produced the report. Each entry often provides the item's full title and some brief details. Reports are available via the government, NHS or Department of Health websites.

Agenda for Change 1999–2004

Negotiations began in 1999 when the four Health Departments of England, Scotland, Wales and Northern Ireland published a document called *Agenda for Change*. The document highlighted the need for changes to pay, career structures and conditions of employment of all directly employed staff within the NHS except very senior managers and those covered by the Doctors' and Dentists' Pay Review Body. Talks came to an end in November 2002, and the proposals were published in January 2003. It is said by some authorities to have resulted in huge cost increases for minimal return. The full text of the proposals can be found on the Department of Health website www.dh.gov.uk.

Acheson Report 1988

A report of the Committee of Enquiry into the Future Development of the Public Health Function.

Acheson Report 1998

A report of the independent enquiry carried out under the chairmanship of Sir Donald Acheson into inequalities in health.

Allitt Enquiry 1994 (also known as the Clothier Report)

An independent enquiry relating to deaths and injuries on the children's ward at Grantham and Kesteven General Hospital.

An Organisation with a Memory 2000

A report of an expert group on learning from adverse events in the NHS, chaired by the Chief Medical Officer.

Ashton Report 2000

A review of the Cardiac Unit at the Royal Liverpool Children's Hospital NHS Trust Alder Hey.

Ayling Enquiry 2004

Report of an independent investigation into how the NHS handled allegations about the conduct of GP Clifford Ayling. For full details go to www. dh.gov.uk/ and search for Ayling Enquiry.

Banks Report 1994

Review of the Department of Health.

Barlow Report 1994

Report of the Advisory Group on Osteoporosis.

Bevan Report 1989

A study conducted under the guidance of a steering group of staffing and utilisation of operating theatres.

Beveridge Report 1942

The social insurance and allied services report.

Black Report 1980

Report of a Research Working Group into Inequalities in Health. Revised editions have since been published by Penguin.

Blom Cooper Report 1992

Report (in 2 volumes) of the Committee of Enquiry into Complaints about Ashworth Hospital.

Bonham-Carter Report 1969

Report into functions of the district general hospitals.

Boyd Report 1994

Confidential enquiry into homicides and suicides by mentally ill people.

Bradbeer Report 1954

Report on internal administration of hospitals.

Briggs Report 1972

Report of the Committee on Nursing.

Building a Safer NHS for Patients: improving medication safety 2004

This report explores the causes and frequency of medication errors, highlights drugs and clinical settings that carry particular risks, and identifies models of good practice to reduce risk.

Butler Report 1975

Report of the Committee on Mentally Abnormal Offenders.

Butterworth Report 1994

A review of mental health nursing team working in partnership, as a collaborative approach to care.

Cadbury Report 1992 (and Standards of Business Conduct 1993)

Outlines a code of practice that members of boards have a responsibility to the public to manage services efficiently and effectively with proper regard to corporate governance, i.e. a duty to act honestly and diligently. Concern at the time of its publication over certain managerial conduct in the NHS led to the NHSE issuing guidance entitled *Standards of Business Conduct,* as it was felt that the Cadbury Report was not directly transferable to the NHS.

Caldicott Committee Report 1997

Report on the review of patient-identifiable information.

Calman Report 1991

The report on junior doctors, sometimes referred to as the 'new deal'.

Calman Report 1993

The report of the Working Group on Specialist Medical Training for Hospital Doctors' Training in the Future. It reviewed current specialist training and changes necessary for consistency with EC law. It also identified areas for further review and development. The report reviewed progress with the development of structured and planned training programmes, and noted the potential for the duration of specialist training to be reduced, a single training grade and introduction of Certificate of Completion of Specialist Training (CCST).

Calman-Hine Report 1995

An expert Advisory Group on Cancer to the Chief Medical Officers of England and Wales reporting on a policy framework for commissioning cancer services.

Canterbury Report 1984

A report based on an interdisciplinary workshop conference held at Canterbury in 1983 on coronary heart disease prevention and suggested plans for action.

Cave Report 1921

Two reports, an interim and final report on voluntary hospitals and their services.

Ceri Davies Report 1983

Report of an enquiry into ways of identifying surplus and under-used land and property in the NHS.

CHI Reports 2003

The Commission for health Improvement (CHI) is the independent regulator of NHS performance produces ratings for NHS trusts in England. The first year in which primary care trusts and mental health trusts received star ratings was 2003. The government is responsible for setting the priorities, which in turn determine the indicators relating to key targets. Other indicators designed by CHI and the Department of Health cover a wide range of performance issues, following consultation with the service and other stakeholders.

Children's Green Paper 2003

The report *Every Child Matters* can be downloaded as pdf file at www.everychildmatters.gov.uk and search for 'children's green paper' (it can be easier and faster to do a Google search for the paper and go to the link).

Clinical Monitors and Alarms 1995

Report of the Working Party on Alarms on Clinical Monitors 1995, by the Medical Devices Agency.

Clothier Report 1972

Report of the committee appointed to inquire into the circumstances, and production, which led to the use of contaminated infusion fluids in the Devonport section of Plymouth General Hospital.

Clothier Report 1994

Independent enquiry relating to deaths and injuries on the children's ward at Grantham and Kesteven General Hospital. This is the report of the Allitt Enquiry see above.

Clyde Report 1992

Also know as *The Orkney Enquiry*, this is a report of the Enquiry into the Removal of Children from Orkney in February 1991.

Cogwheel Reports 1967–1974

The first report of the Joint Working Party on the Organisation of Medical Work in Hospitals.

It was followed by a second report and a third report published in 1974.

Collins Report 1992

Also known as *When the Eagles Fly,* this is a report on resettlement of people with learning difficulties from long-stay institutions.

Commission on the Provision of Surgical Services 1988

A report of the Working Party on the Composition of a Surgical Team. It covers general surgery, orthopaedics and otolaryngology.

Court Report 1976

Also called *Fit for the Future,* this is a report of the Committee on Child Health Services.

Cranbrook Report 1959

Report of the Maternity Services Committee.

Crown Report 1989

Report of the Advisory Group on Nurse Prescribing, and followed by a *Final Report of the Review of Prescribing, Supply and Administration of Medicines.*

Cullen Report 1991

Chief Nursing Officers of the UK reporting on *Caring for People: mental handicap nursing.*

Culyer Report 1994

A report to the Minister of Health on supporting research and development in the NHS. It makes a variety of recommendations about the research and development funding systems and related topics in the NHS. An implementation plan was issued by the NHS Executive in April 1995. Ask your library for *Implementing Research and Development in the NHS* EL(96)47.

Cumberlege Report 1986

Report on Neighbourhood Nursing: a focus for care.

Cumberlege Report 1993 (in two volumes)

Report on Changing Childbirth.

Curtis Report 1946

Report of the Care of Children Committee.

Davies Report 1973

Report of the Committee on Hospital Complaints Procedure.

Dawson Report 1920

Interim report on the future provision of medical and allied services.

Developing NHS Direct 1998

A study commissioned by the Operational Research Branch of the NHSE advocating the introduction of the nationwide 24-hour telephone advice line. *See* p. 156 for further details.

Donaldson Report 2001

Report of a census of organs and tissues retained by pathology services in England.

Dowie Reports 1991

A report on patterns of hospital medical staffing. It included a series of nine reports entitled,

Overview, Anaesthetics, General Medicine, General Psychiatry, General Surgery, Obstetrics & Gynaecology, Ophthalmology, Paediatrics, Trauma and Orthopaedic Surgery.

Duthie Report 1988

Guidelines for the Safe and Secure Handling of Medicines.

Ethics of Xenotransplantation 1997

Animal Tissue into Humans: the report of the Advisory Group on the Ethics of Xenotransplantation, it outlines the government's proposed course of action following consideration of the Advisory Group's report by government departments.

Fallon Report 1999

Report of the Committee of Enquiry into the Personality Disorder Unit, Ashworth Special Hospital, with Volume II entitled *Expert Evidence on Personality Disorder.*

Farquharson-Lang Report 1966

A report on administrative practice of hospital boards in Scotland.

Farwell Report 1995

On aseptic dispensing for NHS patients.

Firth Report 1987

Public Support for Residential care: report of a joint central and local government working party.

Forrest Report 1986

Breast cancer screening: report to the health ministers of England, Wales, Scotland and Northern Ireland.

Gillie Report 1963

On the field of work of the family doctor.

Glancy Report 1974

Revised report of the Working Party on Security in NHS Psychiatric Hospitals.

Goodenough Report 1944

Report of the Interdepartmental Committee on Medical Schools.

Green Paper 1968

On administrative structure of the medical and related services in England and Wales.

Green Paper 1970

National Health Service: the future structure of the National Health Service in England.

Green Paper 1986

Primary Health Care: an agenda for discussion.

Green Paper 1991

Health of the Nation: a consultative document for health in England.

Green Paper 1998

Our Healthier Nation Green Paper stressed health-promoting settings were key to a public health improvement strategy – and a commitment was made to develop Health Promoting Hospitals (HPHs). There were also separate Green Papers for Wales 1998, Scotland 1998 and Northern Ireland 1997.

Griffiths Report 1983

Report on the effective use and management of resources in the NHS set up by Sir Norman Fowler, then Secretary of State for Social Services. Consists of a short report in the form of a letter comprising only 24 pages. Ask your library for *DHSS NHS Management Enquiry. Griffiths Report 1983* DA(83)38. HMSO, London.

Griffiths Report 1988

Community Care: agenda for action.

Guillebaud Report 1956

Cost of the National Health Service: Report of the Committee of Enquiry.

Hall Reports

Report of the Joint Working Party on Child Health Surveillance: Health for all Children. Published in four editions commencing in 1989.

Halsbury Report 1974

Report of the Committee of Enquiry into the Pay and Related Conditions of Service of Nurses and Midwives.

Halsbury Report 1975

Report of the Committee of Enquiry into the Pay and Related Conditions of Service of the Professions Supplementary to Medicine and Speech Therapists.

Harding Report 1981

The Primary Health Care Team: Report of a Joint Working Group of the Standing Medical Advisory Committee and the Standing Nursing and Midwifery Advisory Committee.

Harvard Davies Report 1971

The Organisation of Group Practice: report of a sub-committee of the Standing Medical Advisory Committee.

Health Service Ombudsman Report for Wales 2004/5

Can be accessed at www.wales.nhs.uk/documents and typing 'ombudsman's report' into search box.

Heathrow Debate 1994

The Challenges for Nursing and Midwifery in the 21st Century: a report of the Heathrow debate between Chief Nursing Officers of England, Wales, Scotland and Northern Ireland.

Hill Report 1968

Hospital Treatment of Acute Poisoning: report of the joint sub-committee of the Standing Medical Advisory Committees. Central and Scottish Health Councils.

Hinchliffe Report 1959

Final report of the Committee on the Cost of Prescribing.

Hunt Report

Report of the Committee on Hospital Supplies Organisation.

Hunter Report 1972

Report of the Working Party on Medical Administrators.

Ingall Report 1958

Training of District Nurses. Report of the Advisory Committee.

Jay Report 1979 (two volumes)

Report of the Committee of Enquiry into Mental Handicap Nursing and Care.

Judge Report 1985

The Education of Nurses: a new dispensation.

Kennedy Report 2001

Learning from Bristol: the report of the public enquiry into children's heart surgery at the Bristol Royal Infirmary, 1984–1995. The final report has two principal sections. Section one considers paediatric cardiac surgical services in Bristol during the years 1984–1995. Section two responds to the last element of the Enquiry's terms of reference: 'to make recommendations which could help to secure high quality care across the NHS'. The full report can no longer be accessed at www.bristol-enquiry.org.uk/. Instead go to www.ccad.org.uk/ccadweb.nsf/ and click on 'older news' then go to The Kennedy report (from the Bristol Enquiry) and you can download three pdf files of the full report, a summary, and the recommendations.

Kerr Report 2005

A report by The Scottish Executive entitled *The National Framework for NHS Scotland, Building a Health Service Fit for the Future.* It comes in two volumes, the first is basically the report and the second the executive summary. *See* www.show.scot.nhs.uk.

Körner Report 1982

First report of the Steering Group on Health Services Information.

Lewin Report 1970

Organisation and staffing of operating departments.

Limerick Report 1998

Expert Group to investigate cot death theories: *Toxic Gas Hypothesis Final Report.*

Lung Report 1996

British Lung Foundation on Lung Disease: a shadow over the nation's health.

Lycett Green Report 1963

Report of the Committee of Enquiry into the recruitment, training and promotion of administrative and clerical staff in the hospital service.

Making Amends 2003

Report by Sir Liam Donaldson CMO on proposals for reform of clinical negligence system. More information is available on www.dh.gov.uk/cmo.

Mansell Report 1993

Services for People with Learning Disabilities and Challenging Behaviour or Mental Health Needs: report of a project group.

Mant Report 1998

Research and Development in Primary Care: national working group report.

Mayston Report 1969

Working Party on Management Structure in the Local Authority Nursing Services.

McCarthy Report 1976

Making Whitley Work.

McColl Report 1986

Review of Artificial Limb and Appliance Centre Services.

Merrison Report 1975

Report of the Committee of Enquiry into the Regulation of the Medical Profession.

Merrison Report 1979

Royal Commission on the National Health Service.

Monks Report 1988

Report of the Working Group to Examine Workloads in Genitourinary Medicine Clinics.

Montgomery Report 1959

On maternity services in Scotland.

Neale Enquiry 2004

Report of an independent investigation into how the NHS handled allegations about the performance and conduct of ex-consultant obstetrician and gynaecologist Richard Neale For full details go to www.dh.gov.uk/ and search for Neale Enquiry.

Nodder Report 1980

Organisational and Management Problems of Mental Illness Hospitals: report of a working group.

Noel Hall Report 1957

Grading structure of the administrative and clerical staff in the hospital service.

Noel Hall Report 1978

Report of the Working Party on the Hospital Pharmaceutical Service.

Omega File 1984

Adam Smith Institute on Health and Social Services Policy.

Orkney Report 1992

Report of the Enquiry into the Removal of Children from Orkney in February 1991.

Patient's Charter Monitoring Guide: key standards 1996

The guide covers key Patient's Charter standards which need to be monitored nationally, and guidance on monitoring local Patient's Charter rights and standards.

Peach Report 1999

UK Central Council (UKCC) Commission for Nursing and Midwifery and Education on Fitness for Practice. You can access details on www.nmc-uk.org.

Peel Report 1970

Standing Maternity and Midwifery Advisory Committee on Domiciliary Midwifery and Maternity Bed Needs.

Peel Report 1972

On the use of foetuses and foetal material for research.

Pennington Report 1997

Report on the circumstances leading to the 1996 outbreak of an infection with *E. coli* in central

Scotland, the implications for food safety and the lessons to be learned.

Pilkington Report 1960

Royal Commission on Doctors' and Dentists' Remuneration.

Platt Report 1959

Report of a Committee of the Central Health Services Council on the welfare of children in hospital.

Polkinghorne Report 1989

Review of the guidance on the research use of foetuses and foetal material.

Powell Report 1946

Report of the Subcommittee of the Central Health Services Council. The Ministry of Health was appointed to study the pattern of the inpatients' day.

Professor Protti's 7th World View Report on PHRs 2005

This is the seventh report in a series, it describes how the introduction of web-based personal health records (PHR) demonstrates an emerging era in healthcare that will revolutionise communication between patients and clinicians. The important issue for Professor Protti is the key role of patients in taking responsibility for their healthcare.

RAWP Report 1976

Resource Allocation Working Party Sharing resources for Health in England.

Red Book 1992

A statement of fees and allowances payable to general medical practitioners in England and Wales from April 1990.

Redfern Report 2001

Report by Michael Redfern QC on the retention and use of children's organs at the Royal Liverpool Children's Hospital (Alder Hey). The full text of the Report of the Royal Liverpool Children's Enquiry can be seen on www. rlcinquiry.org.uk/.

Reed Report 1992/3

Review of mental health and social services for mentally disordered offenders and others requiring similar services: in five volumes including a final summary report, service needs, finance, staffing and training, the academic and research base and special issues and differing needs.

Reed Report 1994

On services for people with psychiatric disorder and on high security and related psychiatric provision.

Richards Report 1997

Report of an independent task force chaired by Sir Rex Richards of Committee of Vice-Chancellors and Principals of the Universities of the UK on clinical academic careers.

Ritchie Report 2000

Report of the Enquiry into Quality and Practice within the National Health Service arising from the actions of Rodney Ledward.

Rothschild Report 1971

The organisation and management of government research and development.

Rothschild Report 1972

A Framework for Government Research and Development.

Rubery Report 1993

Report of the Chief Medical Officer's Expert Group on the Sleeping Position of Infants and Cot Deaths.

Sainsbury Report 1967

Report of the Committee of Enquiry into the Relationship of the Pharmaceutical Industry with the National Health Service.

Salmon Report 1966

Report of the Committee on Senior Nursing Staff Structure.

Salmon letter

Although not a report it is included here as the most convenient place for insertion. A 'Salmon letter' is a letter which gives organisations under scrutiny by an enquiry advance warning of potential criticisms. For example in 2003 the GMC received a 'Salmon letter' that the Shipman Enquiry was required to write to all organisations that had contributed to the Enquiry to outline areas of potential criticism. It advises the recipient of their rights, including having a lawyer through the whole Enquiry, who would be able to ask questions and to assist in asking questions of other witnesses and cross examining other witnesses.

Schofield Report 1996

University of Manchester, Health Services Management Unit. Project Steering Group on the Future Healthcare Workforce.

Scottish Green Paper 1968

Administrative Reorganisation of the Scottish Health Services.

Seebohm Report 1968

Report by the Committee on Local Authority and Allied Social Service.

Seeing the Wood, Sparing the Trees 1996

Efficiency Scrutiny Report by NHSE about bureaucracy in the NHS and the 'burdens' of paperwork in NHS trusts and health authorities.

Sheldon Report 1971

Report of the Expert Group on Special Care Babies.

Shields Report 1996

Scottish Office, Department of Health. *Working Group on the Roles and Responsibilities of Health Boards 'Commissioning Better Health': report of the short life working group on the roles and responsibilities of health boards.*

Shipman Enquiry 2002–2005

The Shipman Enquiry was chaired by Dame Janet Smith and published six reports. The first was *Death Disguised* published in 2002, the second *The Police Investigation of March 1998* was published in 2003 together with the third report *Death Certification and Investigation of Deaths by Coroners*. The fourth report *The Regulation of Controlled Drugs* was published in 2004 followed later that year by the fifth report *Safeguarding Patients: lessons from the past – proposals for the future*. This considered the handling of complaints against general practitioners (GPs), the raising of concerns about GPs, GMC procedures and its proposal for revalidation of doctors. She made recommendations for change based upon her findings. The sixth report *Shipman: the final report* was published in 2005 and considered how many patients Shipman killed during his career as a junior doctor at Pontefract General

Infirmary between 1970 and 1974. She also considered a small number of cases from Shipman's time in Hyde, which the Enquiry became aware of after the publication of the first report. She also considered the claims by a former inmate at HMP Preston regarding alleged claims by Shipman about the number of patients he had killed. The enquiry has its own website where all the data can be accessed at www.the-shipman-inquiry.org.uk/reports.asp or go to www.dh.gov.uk/cmo and put 'Shipman report' into search box for government responses.

Short Report 1980

Second Report from the Social Services Committee on Perinatal and Neonatal Mortality.

Short Report 1984

Third Report from the Social Services Committee, on Perinatal and Neonatal Mortality, follow up.

Spens Report 1946

Report of the Interdepartmental Committee on the Remuneration of General Practitioners.

Spens Report 1948

Report of the Interdepartmental Committee on the Remuneration of General Dental Practitioners.

Stewart Report 2000

Independent Expert Group on Mobile Phones set up in 1999 and reported in 2000. It can be accessed at www.iegmp.org.uk/

The Doctors' Tale 1995

An Audit Commission report on the work of hospital doctors in England and Wales.

Tilt Report 2000

Report of the review of security at the high security hospitals.

Todd Report 1968

Report of the Royal Commission on Medical Education.

Tomlinson Report 1992

Report of the enquiry into London's health service, medical education and research. This is the latest of a series of reports on the future of London's health services.

Tunbridge Report 1968

Report of the Joint Committee of the Central and Scottish Health Services Councils on the Care of the Health of Hospital Staff.

Turnberg Report 1998

A strategic review of health services in London.

Turner Report 1991

Report of the Expert Working Group enquiring into the hypothesis that toxic gases evolved from chemicals in cot mattress covers and cot mattresses are a cause of sudden infant death syndrome (SIDS).

Utting Report 1991

Children in the Public Care: a review of residential care.

Wagner Report 1988

Residential Care: a positive choice (report of the Independent Review of Residential Care).

Wanless Report 2002

Securing our Future Health: taking a long term view: final report. This can be accessed via www.hm-treasury.gov.uk/.

Wanless Report 2004

Securing Good Health for the Whole Population: final report. This can be accessed via www.hm-treasury.gov.uk/.

Warnock Report 1984

Report of the Committee of Enquiry into Human Fertilisation and Embryology.

Wells Report 1997

Review of cervical screening services at Kent and Canterbury Hospitals Trust.

White Paper 1972

NHS Reorganisation England.

White Paper 1977

Prevention and Health.

White Paper 1981

Growing Older.

White Paper 1987

Promoting Better Health: the government's programme for improving primary health care.

White Paper 1989

Caring for People: community care in the next decade and beyond. Note: a separate White Paper on this topic was published for Northern Ireland: *People First: community care in Northern Ireland for the 1990s.*

White Paper 1989

This is the White Paper *Working for patients* published in 1989, which summarises the last Conservative government's Strategy and Programmes for the Reforms of the NHS. The proposals in the paper were incorporated into the NHS and Community Care Act 1990 (NHSCCA).

White Paper 1991

Primary Care: delivering the future. This sets out a series of measures to develop primary care.

White Paper 1992

Health of the Nation: a strategy for health in England. This suggested that a number of health-promoting settings should be developed, including in hospitals.

White Paper 1996

A Service with Ambitions: establishing mechanisms for assessing the extent to which existing policies for professional development and training support the objectives of the NHS, encourage team working and create effective partnerships to ensure that educational objectives reflect changing patterns of service. It also tries to determine whether better use could be made of budgets to meet the needs of employers, and the concerns of the main professional groups.

White Paper 1996

Choice and Opportunity – Primary Care: delivering the future. This presents a programme for action both nationally and locally, building on recent changes. It considers developing partnerships in primary care, and between primary and secondary care and local authorities. The education and training of primary care professionals, the role of research and development and the importance of clinical audit are then discussed. Proposals are made for the fairer distribution of resources and their effective use. There is also a review of workforce planning and employment opportunities, together with plans for improvements in primary care premises. The final section considers the better organisation of primary care by linking practices together, improved management support and increased use of information technology.

White Paper 1996

Health Related Behaviour: an epidemiological overview. The *Health of the Nation* White Paper in 1992 emphasised the fact that an individual's health is dependent, at least in part, on their own chosen lifestyle. This paper underlines the key role of behaviour, and an understanding of health-related behaviours and the factors that influence them. Behavioural epidemiology is an important public health issue for the future. This provides an overview of the existing knowledge in this area.

White Paper 1997

The New NHS: modern, dependable, forms the basis for a 10-year programme to improve the NHS. It describes the replacement of the internal market by a system of integrated care, and identifies the principles underlying proposed changes. Key tasks for health authorities are defined as an assessment of health needs, including reference to HIMPs, primary care groups (PCGs), NICE and CHI.

White Paper NHS Scotland 1997

The NHS in Scotland's *Designed to Care*. There have always been differences and variations in approach and this is reflected in this White Paper. The main differences relate to primary care. PCTs came into force in Scotland in April 1999.

White Paper 1998

Smoking Kills sets out the government's concerted plan of action to stop people smoking. It notes action already taken by the government on tobacco advertising and taxation. It goes on to present a series of measures for reducing smoking among young people, new cessation services for adults, and action on smoking among pregnant women. It then outlines proposals for abolishing tobacco advertising and promotion, altering public attitudes, preventing tobacco smuggling and supporting research. It describes further proposals for working in partnership with businesses to restrict smoking in public places, places of work and government offices, and for working with other governments at European and global levels.

White Paper 1998

Modernising Social Services: promoting independence, improving protection, raising standards. This White Paper presents the government's plans for modernising social services provision. It states the principles underlying the government's 'third way' in relation to social care.

White Paper NHS Wales 1998

The Welsh Office brought out this equivalent White Paper to the *The New NHS: modern, dependable* applicable to the NHS in Wales.

White Paper 1999

The White Paper *Saving Lives: our healthier nation* was published in 1999 together with *Reducing Health Inequalities and Action Report*. All can be downloaded from the NHS website.

White Paper 1999

On Modernising Government deals with public services and their administration, the civil service, management of change and government policy in these areas.

White Paper 1999

Our Healthier Nation White Paper offered more direction on health-promoting settings.

White Paper 2000

Adoption, a New Approach presents the government's new approach on adoption. It sets out what they will do, including the new legislation they will introduce, to make adoption work more clearly, more consistently, and more fairly.

White Paper 2001

Valuing People: a new strategy for learning disability for the 21st century. This is the first White Paper on learning disability for 30 years and sets out an ambitious and challenging programme of action for improving services. The proposals are based on four key principles: civil rights, independence, choice and inclusion. *Valuing People* takes a lifelong approach, beginning with an integrated approach to services for disabled children and their families, and then providing new opportunities for a full and purposeful adult life. It has cross-government backing and its proposals are intended to result in improvements in education, social services, health, employment, housing and support for people with learning disabilities and their families and carers.

White Paper 2003

Our Inheritance, Our Future – Realising the Potential of Genetics in the NHS. A genetics White Paper published in June 2003 sets out a vision of how genetic techniques could benefit patients via a £50 million three-year plan of implementation. New initiatives include substantial investment in upgrading genetics laboratories; a boost to the genetics workforce and more genetics counsellors, consultants and laboratory scientists; more than £7 million on new initiatives to introduce genetics-based healthcare into mainstream NHS services; a new Genetics Education and Development Centre to spearhead education and training in genetics for all healthcare

staff; new research programmes in pharmaco-genetics, gene therapy and health services research to help turn the science into real patient benefit. This plan will be reviewed in three years' time.

This strategy aims to help put the NHS on a sound footing to cope with future developments in genetic knowledge and technology. The White Paper also sets out the safeguards and controls against inappropriate or unsafe use of developments in genetics. In addition to existing controls on gene therapy and use of genetic test results by insurance companies, the government will introduce new legislation to ban DNA theft: it will become an offence to test someone's DNA without their consent, except for medical or police purposes. The government also recognises the importance of openness and public debate, and will continue to be responsive to new developments and shifts in public attitudes. See also the Department of Health Departmental Report of 2005.

White Paper (Summary) 2004

The previous Genetics White Paper in short summary form.

White Paper 2004

Choosing Health: making healthier choices easier and *to enable the public to set the health agenda for the future.* This White Paper sets out how the health service is being reformed to educate people about their health, help them make the right choices, and focus on the promotion of good health. The key principles involve supporting the public to make them healthier and more informed about choices in regard to their health. The government plans to provide information and practical support to get people motivated and improve emotional wellbeing and access to services, so that healthy choices are easier to make. A further White Paper *Choosing Health FAQ* was published the same year answering some of the questions the public might have about the White Paper.

How health service is being reformed to educate people about their health, helping them make the right choices and focus on the promotion of good health. For further details go to www. dh.gov.uk/PublicationsAndStatistics/Publications/ PublicationsPolicyAndGuidance/, in left hand side go to 'Publications Library'. You can then download papers on various aspects of the 2004 White Paper, such as *Choosing Health: making healthy choices easier; Choosing Health Summaries Pack; Choosing Health: a booklet about plans for improving people's health – an easy-read summary*; and a browseable version of *Choosing Health: making healthy choices easier – Executive Summary*.

White Paper 2004

Actually published by The Council of Europe, this is a White Paper on the human rights of people with mental illness, especially those subject to compulsory detention. The White Paper contains a draft recommendation No.R (83) 2 concerning the legal protection of persons suffering from mental disorder placed as involuntary patients.

White Paper 2005

About Commissioning a Patient-led NHS – Delivering the NHS Improvement Plan. This is a White Paper that follows on from earlier publication of same name, and focuses on how commissioning will develop throughout the whole NHS, with some changes in function for PCTs and SHAs, which in future will concentrate on three main areas, promoting health improvement and reducing inequalities, securing safe and high-quality services for their population, and emergency planning. The document asks SHAs to work with their local health communities to consider roles and responsibilities of organisations in their areas, and sets out criteria for assessing any local proposals for change within a realistic timetable. It also commits to a development process for PCTs and SHAs similar to that for NHS trusts to prepare them fully for their new roles.

White Paper 2005

A *Public Health White Paper.* Action on obesity, sexually transmitted diseases, alcohol abuse and smoking is at the top of the agenda in this White Paper on public health. Key points include an overhaul of sexual health services, so that patients can receive appointments at a genitourinary

(GUM) clinic within 48 hours, and a nationwide chlamydia screening programme to be set up by 2007. Each PCT will have a specialist obesity service, with access to a dietician and advice and support on changing behaviour. The NICE will prepare definitive guidance on prevention, identification and management of treatment of obesity by 2007. It also plans action to ensure that children have the healthiest possible start in life, with all advertising, promotion and sponsorship of unhealthy foods and drinks to be restricted voluntarily.

White Paper 2005

Response to The Health Select Committee Report on Continuing Care. This sets out the government's response to the Health Select Committee's Sixth Report of Session 2004–2005 on NHS continuing care. It sets out clearly the difference between fully funded NHS continuing care, and the registered nursing care contributions.

White Paper 2005

Departmental Report 2005. As a result of the genetics White Paper 2003, the capacity of specialist genetic services had been developed and modernised through increased training places for counsellors and laboratory scientists, and an £18 million investment in new laboratory equipment to modernise and expand laboratory capacity and support reduced waiting times for test results.

It also stated that a NHS Genetics Education and Development Centre had been established to provide a focal point for genetics education and training in the NHS. The Department of Health was also funding a number of pilot projects testing out ways of integrating genetics into other clinical areas; this included coronary heart disease prevention and a collaborative project with Macmillan Cancer Relief to develop services for patients with a family history that puts them at increased risk of developing cancer.

The Department of Health had also supported research to generate new knowledge, including £4 million funding for research into pharmacogenetics for existing common drugs, and £6.5 million for gene therapy for single gene disorders such as cystic fibrosis, haemophilia and muscular dystrophy.

White Paper 2006

Published in January 2006. this was entitled *Our Health, our Care, our Say: a new direction in community services* and claimed a fundamental shift to provide integrated health and social care services in local communities and closer to people's homes. It essentially contains initiatives designed to shift the balance of services from secondary to primary care; to provide more choice and say over the care received in the community, and closer working and co-ordination between health and social care, including improved access to GPs by increasing the choice of practices for everyone and extending opening hours; to provide more support for people with long-term conditions; to develop local partnerships between local authorities and PCTs to produce joint teams and common assessments; and provide a new generation of community hospitals and health centres that provide health and care services in the heart of the community.

It shifts expenditure from spending on hospitals to care closer to home and on preventative services. It also brings some specialties out of the hospital (dermatology, ear, nose and throat (ENT), orthopaedics and gynaecology), with a new generation of community hospitals that would provide diagnostics, minor surgery, outpatient facilities and access to social services in one location. There was also to be a pilot of a new NHS 'life check' to assess people's lifestyle risks, the right steps to take and provide referrals to specialists if needed.

It gives patients a guarantee of registration onto a GP practice list in their locality and simplifies the system, gives incentives to GPs to offer opening times responsive to the needs of patients as well as increasing the quantity and quality of primary care. It promised to treble investment in the Expert Patient Programme, supporting people to self-care by developing an 'information prescription' for people with long-term health and social care needs and for their carers.

The Wilson Report 1994

Entitled *Being Heard,* this is the report of a review committee on NHS complaints procedures.

Winterton Report 1992

House of Commons Health Select Committee Second Report on the Maternity Services. Volume 1: Report together with appendices and the proceedings of the Committee; Volume 2: *The Minutes of Evidence*; and Volume 3: *Appendices to the Minutes of Evidence.*

Woolf Report 1996

Lord Woolf's proposals for reform of the Clinical Negligence Scheme. Interim Report (1995), *Access to Justice* and Final Report 1996.

Zuckerman Report 1968

On hospital scientific and technical services.

Various health-related regulations, guidance notes and codes of conduct and good practice

Health and Safety (First Aid) Regulations 1981

Identify the necessary requirements to ensure first aid can be provided in the workplace.

Ionising Radiations Regulations 1985

Statutory requirements to specify radiological protection measures in medical, hospital and dental work, including researchers. They have been replaced (*see* p. 213). *Safety and Care in the Storage, Handling and Use of Medical Cylinders on Health Authority Premises,* HE1 No. 163 1987. Health equipment information guidelines issued by the Department of Health.

Control of Substances Hazardous to Health Regulations 1988 (COSHH)

Often referred to as the 'COSHH requirements', they are now replaced by new regulations.

Guidelines for the Safe and Secure Handling of Medicines Report 1988

Also known as the Duthie (RB) Report.

Ionising Radiation (Protection of Persons Undergoing Medical Examination or Treatment) Regulations 1988 (SI 1988 No 778)

State that in the interest of persons (or patients) undergoing medical examinations, employers must ensure that their employees (carrying out such examinations with ionising radiation) are qualified and can produce a certificate to that effect. Employers must also keep a record of their employees' training.

Care Programme Approach for People with a Mental Illness Referred to the Specialist Psychiatric Services (HC(90)23)

Sets out the general principles of the Care Programme Approach.

Guidelines for Change in Postgraduate and Continuing Medical Education 1990

A set of guidelines for a model of change in post-basic medical education. See *Guidelines for Change in Postgraduate and Continuing Medical Education* published by Gale and Grant (March 1990). Open University and British Postgraduate Medical Federation, London.

Heads of Agreement on Junior Doctors' Hours 1990, NHS Executive

Usually known as *Junior Doctors – The New Deal*.

Welfare of Children and Young People in Hospital 1991, Department of Health

Covers all aspects of caring for children and young people in hospital.

Changing Childbirth 1992, HMSO

Guidelines for the development of maternity services.

Health and Safety (Display Screen Equipment) Regulations 1992

State the minimum requirements for workstations with display screen equipment activities (in line with EC directive 901770 EEC).

Health of the Nation: a strategy for health in England 1992, HMSO

The first attempt of a government to produce a strategy document aimed at improving the nation's health. Produced as a White Paper it set national targets for disease prevention and health promotion in five areas to be achieved by 2000. These were coronary heart disease, cancers, mental illness, HIV/AIDS and sexual health, and accidents. It identified approaches to include public policies such as food labelling, healthy surroundings, healthy lifestyles and high-quality health services. For this to be achieved, links were necessary with schools, local authorities and voluntary agencies.

Management of Food Services and Food Hygiene in the NHS (England and Wales only), HSG(92)34

All about food handling services in the NHS.

Management of Health and Safety at Work Regulations 1992

These regulations set out broad general duties that apply to almost all work activities. They have been replaced (see new Regulations 1999, p. 213).

Post-Registration Education and Practice for Nurses (PREP) 1992, UKCC

Introduces new legislation for the renewal of registration for nurses, midwives and health visitors, and restructures all specialist post-registration education. It sets out the UKCC's requirements for education and practice following registration.

Strategy for Information Management and Technology (IM&T) in the NHS 1992, NHS Executive

Describes a common way forward for IM&T for all sectors of the health service in England. Information management includes both computer- and paper-based systems.

An Introduction to the NHS in Scotland 1993

A simple explanation of the health services in Scotland, which are slightly different to England and Wales. See Ham C and Haywood S (1993) *An Introduction to the NHS in Scotland.* MDG Library, Scottish Health Service Centre, Edinburgh. Now somewhat dated in the light of subsequent legislation.

Guidance and Ethics for Occupational Physicians 1993, Faculty of Occupational Medicine

Guidance addressing the major ethical questions which face occupational physicians. See new edition dated 2006 (*see* p. 217).

Mental Health Act (1983) Code of Practice 1993, HMSO

Provides guidance on the application of the Mental Health Act, section 118.

Tomorrow's Doctors 1993

This was published in 1993 by the GMC as *Recommendations on Undergraduate Medical Education.* It recommends a revision of the curriculum framework, a core curriculum, special study modules and the regulation of the undergraduate course.

Codes of Conduct and Accountability Guidance 1994, EL(94)40, NHS Executive

Codes concerned with the conduct and account of NHS boards and their members. Standing orders should reflect the guidance that deals mainly with exchequer funds. Areas covered include annual reports, remuneration, terms of service committees, declaration of interests and register of interests.

Collection of Ethnic Group Data for Admitted Patients, EL(94)77

The introduction of ethnic monitoring systems in hospitals became mandatory from April 1995.

Education of Sick Children, HSG(94)24

Covers aspects of providing education to children in hospital.

Ethnic Monitoring of Staff in the NHS: a programme of action, EL(94)12

A programme aimed at achieving the equitable representation of minority ethnic groups at all levels in the NHS, reflecting the ethnic composition of the local population.

Guidance on the Discharge of Mentally Disordered People and their Continuing Care in the Community, HSG(94)27

Covers the discharge of people with a serious mental illness. Risk assessment illness is given extensive coverage.

Introduction of Supervision Registers for Mentally Ill People, HSG(94)5

Covers the requirements of the supervision register, set up to ensure continuity of care for mentally ill people, to identify those people with a severe mental illness who may be a significant risk to themselves or others and to ensure that follow-up is effective.

Maternity Allowance and Statutory Maternity Pay Regulations 1994

Sets out the regulations concerning maternity pay. The details can be viewed at www.opsi.gov.uk/ then type 'maternity pay' in search box.

New Deal: plan for action, EL(94)17

A planned approach for reducing junior doctors' hours.

Social Security Maternity Benefits and Statutory Sick Pay (Amendment) Regulations 1994

Sets out the regulations concerning various amendments to the regulations. The details can be viewed at www.opsi.gov.uk/ then type either 'maternity pay' or 'sick pay' in search box.

The Pre-Registration House Officer Experience: implementing change 1994, COPMED UK Conference of Postgraduate Deans.

A consensus statement from the UK Postgraduate Deans on the PRHO year. It covers standards and responsibilities, working conditions, appropriateness of clinical work, workload, education and training, educational supervision, approval of posts and living conditions.

Advance Statements about Medical Treatment 1995, BMA

Gives guidance on dealing with advance directives.

Assessment of Mental Capacity: guidance for doctors and lawyers 1995, BMA/The Law Society

Gives guidance on assessing a person's capacity to give valid consent.

Building Bridges: a guide to requirements for interagency working for the care and protection of severely mentally ill people 1995, DoH

Describes best practice on caring for the severely mentally ill and the importance of interagency working.

Code of Practice on Openness in the NHS 1995

Aimed at increasing access to information in the NHS. It required trusts and health authorities to make available or publish information about services, targets, standards, results, cost-effectiveness, important changes in service delivery, local health service management and who is responsible, details of public meetings, etc, and access to personal health records.

Developing the Care Programme Approach – Building on Strengths 1995, NHS Training Division

A resource pack, developed by the NHS Training Division, enabling organisations to develop good practice around the care programme approach.

European Specialist Medical Qualifications Order 1995

Requires the GMC to be responsible for publishing a register of specialists that states the individual's specialty.

Hospital Infection Control: guidance on the control of infection in hospitals, HSG(95)10

Contains a number of recommendations for health authorities regarding the surveillance, prevention and control of hospital infection.

Reporting of Injuries, Diseases and Dangerous Occurrences Regulations (RIDDOR) 1995, HMSO

Identifies the injuries, diseases and dangerous substances that must be reported, and the relevant authorities to which they should be reported.

The Patient's Charter 1991 (updated 1995)

An attempt to make public services more responsive to consumers. These were stated as basic rights and expectations as applied to the NHS. They include the following:

The Patient's Charter, HSC(96)43

Updated in April 1995, this expanded charter sets out new rights and standards and aims to reduce waiting times. It also aims to promote the respect of dignity, privacy and patient choice.

The Patient's Charter: a charter for patients in Wales

As above but for Wales.

The Patient's Charter: services for children and young people

Sets out new rights for children and young people.

The Patient's Charter: services for children and young people in Wales

As above, again for Wales.

The Patient's Charter: mental health services

Sets out new rights for users of mental health services.

Towards Evidence-Based Practice: a clinical effectiveness initiative for Wales 1995, Welsh Office

Plans to develop evidence-based practice in Wales.

Baseline IT Security Policy in the NHS in Wales, DGM(96)100, and IT Security Policy in the NHS in Wales, DGM(95)199

Covers issues of security in relation to patient information.

Clinical Negligence and Personal Injury Litigation, EL(96)11

First of a linked series of guidance notes which set out the action required by trusts and health authorities in claims handling.

Communication Skills: learning from patients – a training tool to help doctors reflect on their communication with patients 1996

This report presents the findings of the second stage of a College of Health project to develop a tool that will encourage doctors to think about how well they communicate with patients. Reservations were expressed about the validity of the results, but there was general agreement that the tool could be useful in training junior staff.

Guidance on Supervised Discharge (After-Care under Supervision) and Related Provisions, WHC(96)II and WOC 6196

Covers the discharge of seriously mentally ill people in Wales.

Health and Safety (Consultation with Employees) Regulations 1996

Sets out the requirements for consultation with employees on health and safety issues.

NHS Complaints Procedure, EL(96)19

Arose out of the recommendations of the Wilson Report, *Being Heard*, and came into force on 1 April 1996.

NHS Information Management and Technology Security Manual, HSG(96)15

Sets out guidance on the best information systems security practice to be adopted by the NHS.

NHS Waiting Times: guidelines for good administrative practice 1996

Setting out the Patient's Charter guarantees and standards for waiting times as of April 1995, this guide considers the goal of delivering shorter waiting times with a booked admission date, and maintenance of local clinical priorities. This document updates guidance issued in 1990 to waiting list managers. It gives guidance on when

patients should be added to the list and the systems required to maintain it effectively. Regular reviews of the lists are necessary and the guide sets out review criteria. Procedures for the admission of patients or transfer to alternative providers are also included. It considers the role of accurate information on waiting lists in hospital management, detailing the information required by clinicians, managers and GPs.

Promoting Clinical Effectiveness 1996, NHS Executive

Describes sources of information on clinical effectiveness, suggests ways in which changes to services can be encouraged (based on well-founded information about effectiveness) and describes how changes can be assessed to see whether improvements have resulted.

Protection and Use of Patient Information, HSG(96)18

Guidance on the protection and use of patient information, builds on existing legislation and guidance such as the Data Protection Act and *Code of Practice on Openness in the NHS*.

Protection and Use of Patient Information in the NHS in Wales, DGM(96)43

Covers issues of confidentiality and security.

The New NHS Number: the key to sharing patient information 1996

The New NHS Number attempts to ensure unique and unambiguous identification of each patient. The old *NHS Number*, in 22 different formats, is prone to transcription errors and is unsuitable for computer applications. In order to overcome these shortcomings, the NHS Executive as part of its Information Management and Technology Strategy has devised the new numbering system. This booklet describes how the new NHS number is being introduced with the support of a national implementation team, over a two-year period.

The Patient's Charter Monitoring Guide: key standards, April 1996

The guide covers key Patient's Charter standards that need to be monitored nationally, and guidance on monitoring local Patient's Charter rights and standards.

Code of Practice in the Appointment and Employment of HCHS Locum Doctors 1997

Originates from the recommendations of the Working Group on Locum Doctors, set up in December 1993. All locum appointments should comply with the Code. The main action points for trusts and others using locum agencies are listed. Details are given for the employment of locums: standards and conditions of appointment; references; health declarations; and criminal convictions.

National Lottery White Paper healthy living centres, EL (97)44

The Department of Health and Department of Culture Media and Sport published this paper on the use of Lottery Funds.

Primary Health Care Teams Involving Patients: examples of good practice 1997

This document aims to promote awareness and stimulate thinking about appropriate ways for primary healthcare teams to involve patients.

The NHS Number: putting the NHS number to work 1997

Part of the NHSE Information Management and Technology Strategy has led to the introduction of a new NHS number that will uniquely identify each patient and allow patient information to be readily accessible but with suitable security safeguards. This booklet is intended for NHS staff and explains the benefits of the new NHS number.

A Guide to Specialist Registrar Training 1998 ('The Orange Book'), Department of Health

This is the official and full guide to the appointment, training and assessment of specialist registrars.

An Enquiry into Mentoring 1998

Supporting doctors and dentists at work – an enquiry into mentoring. A SCOPME report.

A Review of Continuing Professional Development in General Practice: a report by the Chief Medical Officer 1998

The report of a multidisciplinary group chaired by the CMO, which set out to review the current state of CPD in general practice, and suggest directions for improvement. The group's main recommendation is that the educational process should be integrated through the creation of a practice professional development plan (PPDP).

Composite Directory of NHS Ethnic Health Unit Projects 1998

The NHS Ethnic Health Unit (EHU) was set up in 1994 to work with ethnic minority community organisations to foster confidence in the NHS among black and minority ethnic people. This publication provides details of the 123 projects funded by the EHU between 1994 and 1997.

Developing NHS Direct 1998

A study commissioned by the Operational Research Branch of the NHS Executive advocating the introduction of the nationwide 24-hour telephone advice line, which extended previous pilot studies in the use of health helplines. This report aimed to identify options for the development of the service and provide guidance to other developments throughout the UK.

General Practice Vacancies: revised selection procedures – a quick reference guide for health authorities on the revised arrangements for dealing with GP practice vacancies 1998

The NHS (Primary Care) Act 1997 set out new procedures for the selection of candidates for general practice vacancies. This document provides health authorities with a reference guide on handling vacancies.

National Specialist Commissioning Advisory Group Annual Report 1997–98

The National Specialist Commissioning Advisory Group (NSCAG) is responsible for managing and developing highly specialised services selected for central purchasing.

Partnership in Action (new opportunities for joint working between health and social services): a discussion document 1998

As part of the White Paper *The New NHS: modern, dependable*, the government made a commitment to encourage more joint working between health and social services. This document sets out plans to make partnerships a reality so that people whose needs span both health and social services have those needs met in the most efficient and cost-effective way.

Public Appointments Annual Report 1998

A second annual report covering public appointments made by and on behalf of the Secretary of State for Health. The report shows those in posts at 1 March 1998 and relates to chairmen and non-executives in the following bodies: executive non-departmental public bodies (ENDPBs); advisory non-departmental public bodies (ANDPBs); health authorities; NHS trusts; special health authorities; and the Dental Practice Board. Appointments to the boards of health authorities and NHS trusts are listed by body and the NHS region in which they are located.

Research and Development: towards an evidence base for health services, public health and social care – information pack 1998

Describes elements of the NHS R&D programme, the Department of Health's policy research programme and related research matters.

Seeking patients' consent: the ethical considerations 1998, GMC

Sets out the principles of good practice that doctors are expected to follow when seeking patients' informed consent to investigations, treatment, screening or research.

Shared Contributions, Shared Benefits: the report of the Working Group on Public Health and Primary Care 1998

This working group was set up by the Department of Health in 1995 with the aim of making practical proposals that would promote better co-operation between public health and primary care. The Primary Care Act 1997 enables health authorities, primary care and public health practitioners to become involved in joint enterprises. The recent White Paper *The New NHS* supports this with the development of PCGs and health action zones (HAZs).

The Early Years 1998 GMC

GMC recommendations on SHO training.

The New NHS Finance Function: modern, dependable. A medium-term development programme 1998

This is a response from the Finance Staff Strategy Group to the government White Paper of the same title. The identified key changes are structural, organisational, functional and external, and the support offered to help individuals manage change will be training, personal development programmes and guidance on good practice.

Control of Substances Hazardous to Health Regulations 1999

Replaces the *Control of Substances Hazardous to Health Regulations 1988*.

Getting Patients Treated: the Waiting List Action Team handbook 1999

A handbook about reducing waiting lists and good practices relating to this in the NHS.

Ionising Radiations Regulations 1999

Statutory requirements to specify radiological protection measures in medical, hospital and dental work, including researchers. Replaces *Ionising Radiations Regulations 1985*.

Management of Health and Safety at Work Regulations 1999

Broad guidelines of regulations that apply to almost all work activities. Replaces the *Management of Health and Safety at Work Regulations 1992*.

Modernising the NHS in London 1999

A progress report on implementing the recommendations of the Turnberg report on London's health services, one year on. These include the building programme, HAZs, NHS Direct, reduced waiting lists and improved co-ordination and integration with other services.

Prescription Cost Analysis, England 1999

Prescription items dispensed in the community in England, listed alphabetically within chemical entity by therapeutic class with cost analysis and statistical data.

Quality and Performance in the NHS: clinical indicators 1999

Data were collected on six clinical quality indicators in the NHS: deaths in hospital within 30 days of surgery by method of admission; emergency admission with a hip fracture; or heart attack; emergency readmission to hospital within 28 days of discharge; returning home after treatment for a stroke within 56 days (aged 50 years plus); and hip fracture within 28 days (aged 65 years plus). Data are given for each area in England, classified using the 11 Office of National Statistics groups, and also by type of hospital (nine types listed). The source data were over 11 million patient episode records (1995–1998).

The Doctor as Teacher 1999, GMC

Sets out the expectations required of those who provide a role model to junior colleagues as well as medical students.

Guidance on Providing Online Public Information about Local Healthcare Services 2000

In August 2000, the NHS Executive issued 10 targets associated with an additional £60 million for investment in information and IT. One relates to the online provision of accurate, standard and timely information on local healthcare services and their performance. Guidance is available on the definitive list of core information to be provided and the way in which it will be collected and published. nhs.uk will host and provide the main portal to the core information which will also be featured and accessed through NHS Direct Online.

Millennium Executive Team Report on Winter 1999/2000

Explains preparations taken for winter throughout the health authorities, covering resources and planning, social care, public information and immunisation programmes. The Report describes the impact of winter 1999/2000 and the consequent demand for services. A list of conclusions and recommendations is given.

The Declaration of Helsinki 2000

The Declaration of Helsinki is the most important international guideline on biomedical research involving humans. Published by the World Medical Association (WMA) it is their best-known policy statement. It was first adopted in 1964 and has been amended five times since, most recently in 2000. Notes of clarification were added to para. 29 in 2002 and to para. 30 in 2004. The current (2004) version is the only official one; all previous versions have been replaced and are only cited for historical purposes. You can access it at www.wma.net/e/ethicsunit/helsinki.htm.

The Vital Connection: an equalities framework for the NHS – working together for quality and equality 2000

A framework for equal opportunities in the NHS is described and a strategy is set out for putting equality aims into action. Actions to be taken by the NHS and other organisations to implement the framework are specified. Priorities for 2000–2004 are listed.

UK Antimicrobial Resistance Strategy and Action Plan 2000

This document identifies surveillance, prudent antimicrobial use and infection control as the key elements to controlling antimicrobial resistance. The strategy and plan specifies eight areas for action. The aims are to minimise morbidity and mortality due to antimicrobial-resistant infection and maintain the effectiveness of antimicrobial agents used in the treatment of humans and animals.

Good Medical Practice 2001, GMC

Describes the principles of good medical practice and standards of competence, care and conduct expected of doctors in all aspects of their professional work.

Health Service Circular. Good Practice in Consent 2001 HSC 2002/023

About good practice in obtaining consent and the NHS Plan commitment to the practice of patient-centred consent.

Health Service Circular. Reintroduction of Matrons 2001 HSC 2001/010

Implementing the NHS Plan for modern matrons and strengthening the role of ward sisters and introducing senior sisters.

Health Service Circular. Violent and Abusive Patients 2001 HSC 2001/018

About withholding treatment from violent and abusive patients in NHS trusts and the NHS zero tolerance zone.

Working Together, Learning Together: a framework for lifelong learning for the NHS 2001

Outlines the lifelong learning strategy for the NHS, a strategic framework setting out a co-ordinated approach to lifelong learning in health-care. It sets the direction for delivering systematic development for all NHS staff.

Doctors for the Future: Standing Medical Advisory Committee advice (2001)

Published by the Department of Health in June, 2006, this was a follow-on discussion from advice in April 2001 about what could enable doctors to have satisfying careers in the future and what changes might be necessary in the ways they work, bearing in mind the apparent shortage of doctors to implement *The NHS Plan*.

First Report of Select Committee on Health: IV The Private Finance Initiative 2002

A useful and informative discussion on 'What is the Private Finance Initiative?' It can be accessed at www.parliament.uk/ and under advanced search type in 'IV The Private Finance Initiative' or 'Select Committee Reports'

Withholding and Withdrawing Life-prolonging Treatments: good practice in decision-making 2002, GMC

Develops the advice given in the GMC booklets *Good Medical Practice* and *Seeking Patients'*

Consent. It sets out the standards of practice expected of doctors when they consider whether to withhold or withdraw life-prolonging treatments. It was the subject of a judicial review focusing on whether the guidance complied with the European Convention on Human Rights that handed down a ruling in July 2004. The GMC appealed and in July 2005 the Court of Appeal upheld and endorsed the GMC guidelines (*see* p. 216).

Building on the best: choice, responsiveness and equity in the NHS 2003, Department of Health

This strategy paper draws out and develops the main themes that emerged from the 'Choice, Responsiveness and Equity' consultation, which closed in November 2003. This document broadly sets out how the government will make NHS services more responsive to patients, by offering more choice across the spectrum of healthcare. Its main aim is to improve patient and user experience and build new partnerships between those who use health and social care and those who work in them.

Health Service Circular. What to do if you are worried a child is being abused 2003 HSC 2003/007

Advice on what to do if you are worried a child is being abused.

Health Service Circular. Protecting Staff and Delivering Services 2003 HSC 2003/001

About implementing the European Working Time Directive for doctors in training

Making Amends – Clinical Negligence Reform 2003

A consultation paper by the CMO sets out proposals for reforming the approach to clinical negligence in the NHS. The aims of these proposals are to ensure that the emphasis of the NHS is directed at preventing harm, reducing risks and ensuring safety.

Choosing Health: making healthy choices easier 2004, Department of Health

This White Paper sets out the key principles for supporting the public to make healthier and more informed choices in relation to their health and how the government will provide information and practical support to get people motivated and improve emotional wellbeing and access to services, so that healthy choices are easier to make.

Confidentiality: protecting and providing information 2004, GMC

Doctors hold information about patients that must not be disclosed without the patient's consent. This booklet gives guidance on the principles of confidentiality, disclosures required by law, the public interest and what to do when the patient cannot give consent such as with children and disclosures after a patient's death. When it can be released you should act promptly.

Delivering the NHS Plan: next steps on investment, next steps on reform 2004 Department of Health

In this document the Secretary of State for Health presented a progress report on The NHS Plan. He detailed what had been achieved to date and the programme of changes yet to come. This document presented a progress report on The NHS Plan up to 2002. Achievements to this point and planned changes to the programme were detailed.

Standards for Better Health 2004

The document establishes the core and developmental standards covering NHS healthcare provided for NHS patients in England.

The NHS Improvement Plan: putting people at the heart of public services 2004, Department of Health

This document sets out the priorities for the NHS between now and 2008. It supports the ongoing commitment to a 10-year process of reform first set out in The NHS Plan.

Creating a patient-led NHS: delivering the NHS Improvement Plan 2005, Department of Health

Explains how the NHS Improvement Plan will be delivered and describes the major changes underway and how some of the biggest changes will be carried forward for a patient-led health service.

GMC Booklet Withholding and Withdrawing Life-prolonging Treatments: good practice in decision-making (judicial review of) 2005

There had been a lot of coverage in the media of a court case involving the GMC booklet on Withholding and Withdrawing Life-Prolonging Treatments: good practice in decision-making. In February 2004 Mr Leslie Burke, who has a progressively disabling brain disease, sought a judicial review of the guidance. Based on his understanding of how it might be applied in managing his care, he believed some aspects of the guidance would be seen as unlawful. The guidance was subject to intense scrutiny by the courts. In July 2005 the appeal court was able to reassure Leslie Burke that his fears about the actions of doctors following the guidance were unfounded. They would not be able to deny him (or patients in a similar position) artificial nutrition and hydration when it was necessary to prolong his life and in the face of his clear wish to receive it. Not only would such denial be against the guidance, it would be unlawful. The court also provided reassurance for patients more generally that the contents of the guidance not only reflect current law, but represent good standards of practice which can protect the interests of patients, whether they are able to make decisions about treatment for themselves or have become incapacitated. The GMC promised to consider what steps it could take to raise public and professional awareness of the contents of the guidance, and to help ensure that good practice is followed across the NHS and other healthcare settings. Copies of the guidance and details about the court ruling can be read online at www.gmc-uk.org.

New Developments in Sexual Health and HIV/AIDS Policy White Paper 2005 Department of Health

Sets out the government's response to the Health Select Committee's Third Report of the Session 2004/2005 on New Developments in Sexual Health and HIV/AIDS Policy. It includes discussion of service improvement; charges for overseas visitors for HIV treatment; chlamydia screening; workforce and training; primary care and sex and relationships education.

Now I feel tall: what a patient-led NHS feels like 2005, Department of Health

Provides examples of good practice showing how the NHS is improving the patient's emotional experience. It outlines the policy context and explains why improving the emotional experience of patients matters. It claims to make the NHS more aware of the importance of improving patients' emotional experience and the relevance of this to creating a patient-led NHS.

The New Doctor: recommendations on general clinical training 2005, GMC

This edition is transitional. It is effective from January 2005 until July 2007 when the legal requirements for PRHO training will change. The current legal requirements for obtaining full regis-

tration will remain in place until then. The main purpose of this document is to ensure that by July 2007 both trainers and PRHOs are aware of the list of competencies that will become necessary to be eligible for full registration.

Guidance and Ethics for Occupational Physicians 2006

Recognised as authoritative by regulatory and legal bodies, this guidance addresses the major ethical questions which face occupational physicians today and will be of interest to other occupational health professionals, general practitioners, lawyers, employers, trades unions and human resources personnel. It is published by the Faculty of Occupational Physicians of RCP and is now in its 6th edition.

UK Chief Medical Officers – Direction for Postgraduate Medical Training 2006

Published in June by the DH Press Office, the four CMOs set out plans for the transition into the next stage of the new postgraduate medical education system. New arrangements for specialist and GP training programmes are being introduced in August 2007. The result of more than three years of discussion with various stakeholders including the medical Royal Colleges, the NHS and the BMA. They form the second stage of the reform of postgraduate medical training, Modernising Medical Careers (MMC) initiative. By going to www.mmc.nhs.uk/pages/home and clicking on MMC publications you can access the following documents:

- Modernising Medical Careers: the Foundation Programme.
- Curriculum for the Foundation Years in Postgraduate Training and Medical Education.
- Operational Framework for Foundation Training.
- Foundation Programme Rough Guide.
- Foundation Learning Portfolio.
- Career Management: An approach for medical schools, deaneries, royal colleges and trusts.

- Workforce Planning Resource Pack.

- Modernising Medical Careers.

- Unfinished Business.

- Choice and Opportunities.

- Modernising Medical Careers – The Next Steps.

National Audit Office and the Audit Commission Report *Financial Management in the NHS 2004–05* published June 2006

The deficit across the NHS as a whole in 2004–05 was the first since 1999–2000. Figures show the deficit worsened for 2005–06. Compared to 2003–04, the number of NHS bodies with deficits increased, and more of these deficits were significant in size, according to Financial Management in the NHS, a joint study by the National Audit Office and the Audit Commission. For full details go to www.nao.org.uk.

Good Doctors, Safer Patients: Proposals to strengthen the system to assure and improve the performance of doctors and to protect the safety of patients published July 2006, Department of Health

Report aiming to create a new approach to promoting and assuring good medical practice and protecting patients from bad practice. The CMO was asked to undertake this review of medical regulation, following Dame Janet Smith's inquiry into the circumstances surrounding the murders committed by Hyde GP, Dr Harold Shipman. It contains 44 recommendations, including devolving some of the powers of the GMC to a local level, changing its structure and function, and creating a new framework for revalidation. For more information go to The NHS National electronic Library for Medicines at www.drug infozone.nhs.uk/home and type 'good doctors safer patients' in the search box. Or, you will find lots of links to it with a Google search.

CHAPTER 11

Glossary and acronyms

The aim of this chapter is to provide you with information on terms and a reference source for acronyms that you may come across and need to know about. It gives:

- a glossary of health service, management, and non-clinical terms, with a few telemedical and computer terms

- useful health service-related acronyms.

Glossary of management, NHS reform, non-clinical and other useful terms

This is a glossary of useful terms along with some definitions. Some are fairly obvious and have been included not just for the sake of completeness but just in case they need clarification. Beware – quite often they are terms that have only a loose connection with their real meaning. You may need to check this out when you hear the expressions, but do not be surprised if the speaker is not aware of the correct meaning. The meaning may also relate to a specific connection. A few terms are attempts that have been made to transfer manufacturing terminology to medical work.

Abduction A form of logical inference, commonly applied in the process of medical diagnosis. Given an observation, abduction generates all known causes. *See also* **deduction**, **induction** and **inference**.

Absenteeism Absence from work not authorised through appropriate channels.

Access rate An estimate of the availability of facilities to people living in an identified locality, irrespective of where they are treated. The measure is stated as discharges and deaths per 1,000 population.

Accident Any unexpected or unforeseen occurrence, especially one that results in injury or damage.

Accident and emergency (A&E) The title given to the hospital department previously termed 'casualty' and now frequently called 'emergency'. The accident and emergency patient may be brought by ambulance or car, or may arrive on foot.

Accident report A written report of an accident. The format of the report is laid down in health and safety legislation.

Accommodation (children) Being provided with accommodation replaces the old voluntary care concept. It refers to a service that the local authority provides for the parents of children in need, and for their children. A child is not in care when they are being provided with accommodation. Nevertheless, the local authority has a number of duties towards children for whom it is providing accommodation, including the duty to discover the child's wishes regarding the provision of accommodation, and to give them proper consideration.

Accountability Being answerable for one's decisions and actions. Accountability cannot be delegated.

Added value A measure of productivity expressed in terms of the financial value of an item as a result of workforce. Often used loosely in the NHS.

Adolescents Young people in the process of moving from childhood to adulthood. Because of their age, adolescents may have special needs as patients.

Adoption Total transfer of parental responsibility from the child's natural parents to the adopters.

Advance directives A document which sets out the wishes of a patient if they are later unable to give or withhold consent for a particular treatment. This is particularly important when the patient's/user's wishes may conflict with clinical judgement.

Advocate An individual acting on behalf of, and in the interests of, patients who may feel unable to represent themselves in their contacts with a healthcare or other facility.

Affidavit Statement in writing and on oath sworn before a person who has the authority to administer it, e.g. a solicitor.

Amenity bed A bed in a single room or small NHS hospital ward for which a patient may be charged a small fixed amount for the hotel part of the cost, but not the cost of treatment, under section 12 of the 1977 NHS Act.

Analysis of expenditure by client group Analysis of expenditure over broad groups of service related to patient care groups, e.g. services for mentally ill people, services mainly for children, and general and acute hospital and maternity services.

- *Functional (objective)*: the object for which the payment has been made – medical staff services, nursing staff services, transport services and so on.
- *Subjective*: according to the nature of the payment, e.g. salaries and wages, travel, drugs, etc.

Annual report A report, written annually, which details progress over the last year and plans for the following year. It includes financial and activity statements.

Apology A sincere expression of regret.

Appeal (Care of Child) Appeals in care proceedings are now to be heard by the High Court or, where applicable, the Court of Appeal. All parties to the proceedings will have equal rights of appeal. On hearing an appeal, the High Court can make such orders as may be necessary to give effect to its decision.

Application In computer technology this is a synonym for a program that carries out a specific type of task. Word processors or spreadsheets are common applications available on personal computers.

Arbitration The process of settling a disagreement between two or more parties by the introduction of an external body or person with authority to make and implement an agreement.

Arden syntax A language created to encode actions within a clinical protocol into a set of situation–action rules for computer interpretation, and also to facilitate exchange between different institutions.

Area Child Protection Committee (ACPC) Based on the boundaries of the local authority, it provides a forum for developing, monitoring and reviewing the local child protection policies, and promoting effective and harmonious co-operation between the various agencies involved. Although there is some variation from area to area, each committee is made up of representatives of the key agencies, who have authority to speak and act on their agency's behalf. ACPCs issue guidelines about procedures, tackle significant issues that arise, offer advice about the conduct of cases in general, make policy and review progress on prevention, and oversee interagency training.

Artificial intelligence (AI) Any artefact, whether embodied solely in computer software or a physical structure like a robot, that exhibits behaviours associated with human intelligence. *See also* **Turing test**.

Artificial intelligence in medicine The application of artificial intelligence methods to solve problems in medicine, e.g. developing expert systems to assist with diagnosis or therapy planning. *See also* **artificial intelligence** and **expert systems**.

Assessment Process by which the capacities and incapacities of people who may require community care are established by social services departments, with appropriate services thereby identified.

Assessment (children) Process of gathering together and evaluating information about a child, its family and circumstances. Its purpose is to determine children's needs, in order to plan for their immediate and long-term care and decide what services and resources must be provided. Child care assessments are usually co-ordinated by social services, but depend on teamwork with other agencies (such as education and health).

Associates Salaried doctors who support principals in hard-pressed areas, such as the London Implementation Zone Education Initiative (LIZEI) area or remote parts of Scotland.

Asynchronous communication Communication between two parties when the exchange does not require both to be an active participant in the conversation at the same time, e.g. sending a letter. *See also* **synchronous communication** and **email**.

Audit Originally the process by which the probity of operations and activities of an organisation was examined (internal audit) and a report on the annual accounts produced (external audit). It is now used more widely, e.g. clinical audit evaluates the effectiveness of clinical activities; and management audit evaluates the effectiveness and efficiency of organisational and management arrangements. It involves the process of setting or adopting standards and measuring performance against those standards, with the aim of identifying both good and bad practice and implementing changes to achieve unmet standards.

Audit Committee A committee of an NHS trust or authority board, comprising non-executive members, which ensures probity in the corporate governance of the organisation. Following *The Cadbury Report*, NHS bodies should have such a body.

Authorised person (children) In relation to care and supervision proceedings, this is a person not from the local authority who is authorised by the Secretary of State to bring proceedings under section 31 of the Children Act 1989. This covers the NSPCC and its officers. Elsewhere in the Act there is a reference to persons who are authorised to carry out specified functions, e.g. to enter and inspect independent schools.

Average daily available beds The average number of staffed beds in each department in which patients are being treated, or could be treated, each day without any changes being made in facilities or staff. Beds borrowed from other departments are included.

Average length of stay The average number of days a bed is occupied by each patient.

Bayes' theorem Theorem used to calculate the relative probability of an event given the probabilities of associated events. It is used to calculate the probability of a disease given the frequencies of symptoms and signs within the disease and within the normal population.

Bed bureau An administrative unit that ensures that patients needing urgent admission are directed to a hospital that will admit them.

Bed days *Available bed days* – the sum of beds available for use each day during a specified period of time. *Occupied bed days* is the sum of the number of beds occupied by patients each day during a specified period of time. This total, divided by the number of discharges and deaths during the same period, gives the average length of stay. *Vacant bed days* is the number obtained when the total of occupied bed days is subtracted from the available bed days.

Bed norm A measure of the bed requirements for a given population, expressed as number of beds per 1,000 people. Bed norms may be used in several different ways: age specific, as in the case of hospital accommodation for the elderly – ten beds per 1,000 aged 65 years and over; or by specialty, as in the case of orthopaedic beds – 0.35 per 1,000.

Bed occupancy The number of beds occupied by patients at a particular time, usually midnight. It may be expressed as a percentage of available beds.

Bed state The number of beds, both occupied and vacant, at a particular time.

Bed turnover The average number of patients using each bed in a given period, such as a year.

Behavioural science The study of individuals and groups in a working environment. Issues may include communication, motivation, organisational structure and organisational change. The science is still being developed and relies on contributions from psychology and sociology.

Benchmarking Defined by the UK Benchmarking Centre (1993) as the continuous, systematic search for best practices, and the implementation that will lead to superior performance.

Benchmarks Benchmarks are sources of information (such as cost, quality outcomes, etc) used as comparators to compare performance between similar organisations or systems.

Booked case An elective admission where the date has been arranged in advance with the patient. Waiting lists should include booked cases.

British Association of Medical Managers (BAMM) Aims to 'support the provision of quality healthcare by improving and supporting the contribution of doctors in management, together with all other activities which contribute to, further, or are ancillary to this principle aim'.

Broadband A type of data transmission in which a single (telephone) wire can carry several channels at once. Cable TV, for example, uses broadband transmission.

Budget A statement of the financial resources made available to a budget holder to provide an agreed level of service over a set period of time.

Business plan A plan setting out the goals of an organisation and identifying the resources and actions needed to achieve them. Usually prepared on an annual basis, the business plan seeks to balance planned activity with income so as to minimise financial risk.

CAFCASS The Children and Family Court Advisory and Support Services set up in 2001. A national non-departmental public body for England, bringing together the services previously provided by:

- The Family Court Welfare Service
- The Guardian ad Litem Services
- The Children's Division of the Official Solicitor.

CAFCASS is independent of the courts, social services, education and health authorities and all similar agencies. For more information *see* www.cafcass.gov.uk/. The operation in Wales has devolved to the National Assembly for Wales and is now CAFCASS Cymru.

Capital asset Land, property, plant or equipment valued at more than £5,000.

Capital Asset Register A list of all the capital assets of an organisation. This contains information required to administer a capital asset replacement programme such as the purchase price, acquisition and replacement date of assets.

Capital Asset Replacement Programme A programme which uses depreciation accounting techniques to spread the cost of the replacement of capital assets.

Capital charges Since 1991, the use/ownership of capital in the NHS has incurred a cost, the capital charge. This was introduced so that NHS capital was no longer regarded as a free good or gift from the state. Capital charges consist of two elements: depreciation and interest on fixed assets. The interest rate currently applied is 6%. NHS trusts retain depreciation charges within the trust and are required to make a target rate of return equivalent to the interest rate.

Capital programme A plan over a period of time (normally five years) showing costs and starting and final dates of schemes of work to be charged to the capital allocation.

Career advice Providing information on career opportunities and training requirements.

Career counselling Discussing career options for which the individual may be most suited.

Care order (children) Order made by the court under Part IV section 31(1)(a) of the Children Act 1989 placing the child in the care of the designated local authority. A care order includes an interim care order except where express provision to the contrary is made.

Care pathway An approach to managing a specific disease or clinical condition that identifies what interventions are required, and sets out the various stages of care through which a patient passes, and the expected outcome of treatment.

Care plan A written statement of community care services to be provided following assessment (q.v.). The document details the care and treatment that a patient receives, and identifies who delivers the care and treatment. This term covers the term 'individual plan' (*see also* **health record**).

Care Programme Approach (CPA) The individual packages of care (care programmes), developed in conjunction with social services, for all patients accepted by the specialist psychiatric services. Care programmes may range from 'minimal' single-worker assessment and monitoring for individuals with less severe mental health and social needs, to complex and multiprofessional assessments and treatment.

Carer A person who regularly helps (without pay) a relative or friend with domestic, physical, emotional or personal care, as a result of illness or disability. This term also incorporates friends, relatives and partners. There are thought to be six million 'informal carers'.

Case-based reasoning An approach to computer reasoning that uses knowledge from a library of similar cases, rather than accessing a knowledge base containing more generalised knowledge, such as a set of rules. *See also* **artificial intelligence** and **expert system**.

Case conference (children) Formal meeting attended by representatives from all the agencies concerned with the child's welfare. This increasingly includes the child's parents (and the Children Act 1989 promotes this practice).

Casemix The mixture of clinical conditions and severity of condition encountered in a particular healthcare setting.

Cash limit A limit imposed by the government on the amount of cash a public body may spend during a given financial year. Separate cash limits may be set for revenue and capital.

Causal reasoning A form of reasoning based on following from cause to effect, in contrast to other methods in which the connection is weaker, such as probabilistic association.

Chairman (chairperson or **chair** is more politically correct) A person who leads or conducts discussions. A chairman's skill and technique may be used in a one-to-one meeting or by indirect communication methods, such as the telephone. **Change agent** A third party, who may be a trained behavioural scientist, and who acts as a catalyst in bringing about change by means of an organisation development programme.

Checklist A means of recording observations relating to fixed criteria; used to check compliance with agreed procedures or standards.

Child A person under the age of 18 years. There is an important exception to this in the case of an application for financial relief by a 'child' who has reached 18 years and is, or will be, receiving education or training.

Child assessment order The order requires any person who can do so to produce the child for an assessment and to comply with the terms of the order.

Child Protection Register Central record of all children in a given area for whom support is being provided via inter-agency planning. Generally, these are children considered to be at risk of abuse or neglect. The register is usually maintained and run by social service departments under the responsibility of a custodian (an experienced social worker able to provide advice to any professional making enquiries about the child). Registration for each child is reviewed every six months.

Child minder Person who looks after one or more children under the age of eight for reward, for more than two hours in any one day.

Children in need A child is in need if: (i) he or she is unlikely to achieve or maintain (or have the opportunity of achieving or maintaining) a reasonable standard of health or development without the provision for him or her of services by a local authority; or (ii) his or her health or development is likely to be significantly impaired (or further impaired) without the provision for him or her of such services; or (iii) he or she is disabled.

Children living away from home Children who are not being looked after by the local authority but are nevertheless living away from home, e.g. children in independent schools. The local authority has a number of duties towards such children, e.g. to take reasonably practicable steps to ensure that their welfare is being adequately safeguarded and promoted.

Choice Giving patients more choice about how, when and where they receive treatment is one cornerstone of the government's health policy. In the context of NHS reforms, this is the overarching policy term given to a range of initiatives within the reform of the NHS designed to act as a driver for efficiency, quality and effectiveness.

Choose and Book Term given to a national framework which sets out to offer patients fully booked appointments for a range of primarily hospital based interventions. NHS organisations will be expected to increase the levels of choice available to patients so that by December 2005, patients who require an elective referral will be offered a choice of four to five hospitals (or suitable alternative providers) and a choice of time and date for their booked appointment, at the time they are referred by their GP or primary care professional.

Clinic session A session held, and not merely scheduled, for, by or on behalf of one consultant, senior hospital medical officer or dental officer. This is now extended to include sessions run by nurses and other clinical staff.

Clinical budgeting The allocation of specific budgets to consultant clinical staff who are responsible for the budget management; a part of management budgeting.

Clinical directorate A unit of management for specific clinical services. A clinical directorate is usually led by a clinical director, who is often a consultant working in that role for a number of

sessions per week. They are supported by a nurse and/or business manager. The extent to which management responsibilities for budgets and staff are devolved to directorates varies.

Clinical guideline An agreed set of steps to be taken in the management of a clinical condition.

Clinical pathway *See* **clinical guideline**.

Clinical protocol *See* **clinical guideline**.

Clinical responsibilities Range of activities for which a clinician is accountable.

Closed beds Beds which have not been used (i.e. closed) for longer than one month for the purpose of redecoration or structural alterations, or because of a shortage of staff, but are scheduled to be reopened at a future date.

Code In medical terminological systems, the unique numerical identifier associated with a medical concept, which may be associated with a variety of terms, all with the same meaning. *See also* **term**.

Cognitive map A process of recording information in related groupings, and intended to assist lateral thinking. *See also* **mind map**.

Cognitive science A multidisciplinary field studying human cognitive processes, including their relationship to technologically embodied models of cognition. *See also* **artificial intelligence**.

Commissioner An organisation or individual involved in purchasing healthcare. *See also* **purchaser**.

Commissioning Relates to the purchasing and contracting of healthcare services. It is a broad term that can cover a range of activities, but in principle a distinction can be drawn between two levels of commissioning. At one level, commissioning can involve service planning and design, through identifying population need; assessing the local priorities; understanding the market; and determining where and how services should be provided and by whom. Secondly, commissioning can involve the daily purchasing of services, through managing contracts and spending budgets.

Commissioning a patient-led NHS The letter and attachments (entitled *Commissioning a Patient-led NHS*) was sent to NHS Chief Executives and others at the end of July 2005. It builds on the *NHS Improvement Plan* and *Creating a Patient-led NHS*. The details contained in the papers relate to the form and function of primary care trusts (PCTs) and strategic health authorities (SHAs) and was designed to begin to address the tension between providing services and commissioning services in PCTs. It was also intended to prompt cost savings of £250m; deliver practice-based commissioning by December 2006 at the latest; and SHAs will be reconfigured to move towards alignment with government office boundaries.

Communication The two-way process of exchanging ideas, thoughts, feelings and facts.

Communication strategy A written statement of objectives for effective communication, and a plan for meeting those objectives. The strategy should be consistent with the business plan.

Community care The assessment and commissioning of health and social care and treatment to patients/clients outside hospital, who have an identified physical or mental illness or disability. It is often more narrowly associated with patients being resettled from institutional care, e.g. from large psychiatric hospitals, or frail, elderly people who previously would have remained in hospital care.

Community Health Councils (CHCs) 'Patient watchdog' bodies established as part of the NHS reorganisation in 1974. Their role included assisting with complaints and visiting NHS premises. The government published *The NHS Plan* for England in 2000 which proposed the abolition of CHCs in England and their replacement by patient and public involvement forums (PPIF) and patient advocate and liaison services (PALS) and established by each NHS trust, including PCTs in England. CHCs have been retained in Wales and Scotland

Community health services These divide into two main groups: patient care in the community – the treatment or care (outside hospital) of patients with identified physical or mental illness or disability; and services to the community – services

of prevention or intervention that are provided to a population, such as immunisation, screening and health promotion.

Complainant A person who expresses dissatisfaction. They may or may not be the patient concerned.

Complaint An expression of dissatisfaction.

Complaints procedure (children) The procedure that a local authority must set up in order to hear representations regarding the provision of services under Part III of the Children Act 1989 from a number of persons, including the child, the parents and 'such other person' as the authority considers has sufficient interest in the child's welfare to warrant his representations being considered by them.

Compliment An expression of approval or satisfaction.

Computer-based patient record See electronic medical record.

Computerised protocol Clinical guideline or protocol stored on a computer system so that it may be easily accessed or manipulated to support the delivery of care. *See also* **clinical guideline**.

Conciliation The process of a lay person assisting two parties in dispute to reach informal agreement through discussion and persuasion, without any legally binding status.

Conciliatory The application of conciliation techniques particularly outside a formal conciliation process.

Concurrent jurisdiction (children) The High Court, a county court and a magistrates' court (family proceedings court) all have jurisdiction to hear proceedings under the Children Act 1989.

Connectionism The study of the theory and application of neural networks. *See also* **neural network**.

Constant prices A mechanism for comparing prices for goods and services over a number of years, which compensates for the distortion introduced by inflation.

Contact order (children) Order requiring the person with whom a child lives, or is to live, to allow the child to visit or stay with the person named in the order.

Continuing education Activities that provide education and training for staff. These may be used to prepare for specialisation or career development as well as facilitating personal development.

Continuing professional development (CPD) Defined as: 'A process of lifelong learning for all individuals and teams which enables professionals to expand and fulfil their potential and which also meets the needs of patients and delivers the health and healthcare priorities of the NHS'.

Contract/agreement A document agreed between providers and purchasers of healthcare, it details activity, financial and quality levels to be achieved.

Contract currencies Agreed units of measurement for contracting, e.g. finished consultant episodes.

Contracts The basis for agreement on the services that should be provided to patients, including specification of quality. *Block contracts* specify facilities to be provided, and may include workload agreements including patient activity targets within an agreed range. *Cost and volume contracts* specify the level of services required by the purchaser. Purchasers can link payment with agreed activity. Provider units will be able to match funding with workload and deploy resources more flexibly. *Cost per case contracts* cover the cost of treatment for specific patients.

Control measures Ways in which risk can be controlled, including physical controls such as locking away drugs and valuable items, and system controls such as restricting access to hazardous areas to specific staff groups.

Convenor A non-executive director of a trust, health authority or health board who decides whether or not to convene an independent panel to review a complaint against an NHS provider.

Corporate Relating to the whole of an organisation, for example the management of an organisation.

Corporate seal A seal used by organisations to certify documents used in legal transactions (such as the sale of land) so as to fulfil legal requirements.

Court welfare officer (children) Officer appointed to provide a report for the court about the child and the child's family situation and background. The court welfare officer will usually be a probation officer.

Criterion A measurable component of performance. A number of criteria need to be met to achieve the desired standard.

Cross functional team A team of people from different disciplines.

Cruse A non-religious UK-based organisation specialising in bereavement. Their helpline 0870 167 1677 with a website www.cruse bereavementcare.org.uk and email: helpline@ crusebereavementcare.org.uk or general email: info@cruse bereavementcare.org.uk.

Cybernetics A name coined by Norbert Weiner in the 1950s to describe the study of feedback control systems and their application. Such systems were seen to exhibit properties associated with human intelligence and robotics, and so were an early contribution to the theory of artificial intelligence.

Cyberspace Popular term (now associated with the internet) which describes the notional information 'space' that is created across computer networks. *See also* **virtual reality**.

Cycle time The time a patient is under treatment (in hospital). Thus, cycle time plus waiting time equals the lead time.

Database A structured repository for data, usually stored on a computer system. The existence of a regular and formal indexing structure permits rapid retrieval of individual elements of the database.

Day care (children) A person that provides day care if they look after one or more children under the age of eight on non-domestic premises for more than two hours in any day.

Day cases Patients who have an investigation, treatment or operation, but are admitted electively and discharged on the same day.

Decision support system General term for any computer application that enhances a human's ability to make decisions.

Decision tree A method of representing knowledge that makes structured decisions in a hierarchical tree-like fashion.

Deduction A method of logical inference. Given a cause, deduction infers all logical effects that might arise as a consequence. *See also* **abduction**, **induction** and **inference**.

Designated person A person within an NHS provider, or a department of an NHS provider, who is delegated responsibility to ensure that complaints are properly resolved locally.

Direct credits The income from the sale of meals to staff, renting accommodation to staff and so on.

Direct discrimination Where someone is treated less favourably purely on grounds of marital status, sex, ethnic origin or similar criteria which do not affect the individual's ability to perform the job (*see also* **indirect discrimination**).

Disabled (children) A child is disabled if 'he or she is blind, deaf or dumb or suffers from a mental disorder of any kind or is substantially and permanently handicapped by illness, injury or congenital deformity or such other disability'.

Disclosure interview (children) Term sometimes used to indicate an interview with a child, conducted as part of the assessment for suspected sexual abuse. It could be misleading (since it implies, in some people's view, undue pressure on the child to 'disclose') and therefore the latest preferred term is 'investigative interview'.

Discrimination May be direct or indirect. For details see separate headings.

Distributed computing Term for computer systems in which data and programs are distributed and shared across different computers on a network.

Dual registered homes Homes for disabled or elderly people, registered as both a residential care home and a nursing home.

Duty to investigate (children) A local authority is under a duty to investigate in a number of situations where they have a 'reasonable cause to suspect that a child who lives, or is found, in [its] area is suffering, or is likely to suffer, significant harm'.

Education supervision order (children) Order which puts a child under the supervision of a designated local education authority.

Education welfare officer (EWO) Social work support to children in the context of their schooling. While EWOs' main focus used to be the enforcement of school attendance, today they perform a wider range of services, including seeking to ensure that children receive adequate and appropriate education and that any special needs are met, and there is more general liaison between local authority education and social services departments.

Educational psychologist A psychology graduate who has had teaching experience and additional vocational training. Educational psychologists perform a range of functions including assessing children's education, psychological and emotional needs, offering therapy and contributing psychological expertise to the process of assessment.

Electronic mail *See* **email**.

Electronic medical record A general term describing computer-based patient record systems. It is sometimes extended to include other functions, such as order entry for medications and tests, among other common functions.

Email, electronic mail A messaging system available on computer networks, providing users with personal mail boxes from which electronic messages can be sent and received.

Emergency admission A patient admitted on the same day that admission is requested.

Emergency protection order (children) That which a court can make if it is satisfied that a child is likely to suffer significant harm, or where enquiries are being made with respect to the child and they are being frustrated by the unreasonable refusal of access to the child.

Epidemiology Study of the distribution and determinants of disease in human populations.

Epistemology The philosophical study of knowledge.

Estates strategy A written statement of objectives relating to estates management and a plan for meeting those objectives. The strategy should be consistent with the business plan.

European Directive A requirement which binds an EU member state, e.g. the one designed to facilitate the free movement of doctors and the mutual recognition of their diplomas, certificates and other evidence of formal qualifications (Council Directive 93/16/EEC).

Evaluation The study of the performance of a service (or element of treatment and care), with the aim of identifying successful and problem areas of activity.

Evidence-based medicine A movement advocating the practice of medicine according to clinical guidelines, developed to reflect best practice as captured from a meta-analysis of the clinical literature. *See also* **clinical guideline**, **meta-analysis** and **protocol**.

Expert system A computer program that contains expert knowledge about a particular problem, often in the form of a set of if–then rules, that is able to solve problems at a level equivalent or greater than human experts. *See also* **artificial intelligence**.

External financing limit (EFL) A cash limit set by the NHSE on net external financing for an NHS trust. A positive external financing limit is set where the agreed capital spending for an NHS trust exceeds income from internally generated resources. A zero external financing limit is set where the agreed capital spending programme for a trust equals internally generated resources. A negative external financing limit is set where the agreed capital spending programme for a trust is less than internally generated resources.

Extracontractual referral (ECR) The term used for referral of an individual for health services that were not covered in contracts that existed between the old system of purchaser and providers of services.

Family centre A child and parents, or other person looking after a child, can attend for occupational and recreational activities, advice, guidance or counselling, and accommodation while receiving such advice, guidance or counselling.

Family panel Panel from which magistrates who sit in the new Family Proceedings Court are selected. These magistrates will have undergone specialist training on the Children Act 1989.

Family Proceedings Court Court at the level of the magistrates' court to hear proceedings under the Children Act 1989. The magistrates will be selected from a new panel, known as the Family Panel, and will be specially trained.

Fieldworker (field social worker) Conducts a range of social work functions in the community and in other settings (e.g. hospitals).

Financial strategy A written statement of objectives relating to financial management and a plan for meeting those objectives. The strategy should be consistent with the business plan.

Financial target (for an NHS trust) A real pre-interest return of 6% on the value of net assets, effectively a return on the average of the opening and closing assets shown in the accounts.

Finished consultant episode (FCE) An episode where the patient has completed a period of care under a consultant and is either discharged or transferred to another consultant. The total number of episodes is a common measure of overall hospital activity.

Firewall A security barrier erected between a public computer network like the internet and a local private computer network.

Flexible training Available for doctors who have 'well-founded individual reasons' for working less than full time. The Department of Health runs two schemes to encourage flexible training for career registrars and senior registrars (PM(79)3). Flexible training for PRHOs and SHOs is available on a personal basis. In addition, a number of regions organise their own flexible training schemes.

Foster carer Provides substitute family care for children. A child looked after by a local authority can be placed with local authority foster carers.

Foundation trusts (FTs) First set up as a result of the Health and Social Care (Community Health and Standards) Act 2003. More hospitals have become foundation trusts since then and all acute NHS trusts will be required to attain FT status by the end of 2008. Although remaining part of the NHS, foundation trusts are subject to reduced control from central government. They differ from traditional NHS trusts in three main ways:

- they possess the freedom to decide locally how to meet their obligations (which can also involve borrowing money from private sources)
- they are accountable, through (mainly elected) governors, to their members, who are drawn from local residents, patients and staff
- they are authorised and monitored by Monitor, the independent regulator of NHS foundation trusts.

Frequently asked questions (FAQ) Common term for information lists available on the internet which have been compiled for newcomers on a particular subject, answering common questions that would otherwise often be asked by submitting email requests to a newsgroup.

Frontline staff The employees of an NHS provider who have direct, face-to-face contact with patients and other NHS users.

Functional department Examples would include X-ray, a ward, theatre, pharmacy, pathology, a clinic or outpatients.

Functional team A team from within a single discipline.

GMS contract On 20 June 2003, GPs accepted a new General Medical Services (GMS) contract, negotiated by the British Medical Association (BMA) and the NHS Confederation. The terms of this contract mean that payments to GPs are more closely related to the quantity and quality of the services they provide.

GP fundholder Term that was used for GP practice with a budget for the purchase of a range of hospital inpatient and outpatient (and certain nursing and paramedical) services. It ceased in April 1999.

Guardian ad litem (GAL) Person appointed by a court to investigate a child's circumstances and to report to the court (*see* CAFCASS).

Guidance (children) Authorities are required to act in accordance with the guidance issued by the Secretary of State. However, guidance does not have the full force of law but is intended as a series of statements of good practice and may be quoted or used in court proceedings.

Hawthorne effect Term used to describe changes in productivity and employee morale as a direct result of management interest in their problems. Improvements may arise before any management action. Originates from a study of the Hawthorne Works, Western Electric Co, USA (1920s).

Hazard assessment procedures The process by which the origins, frequencies, costs and effects of hazards are identified, and strategies adopted to avoid or minimise their effects.

Hazards The potential to cause harm, including ill-health and injury, damage to property, plant, products or the environment, production losses or increased liabilities.

Health and safety policy A plan of action for the health, safety and wellbeing of staff, patients, residents and visitors.

Healthcare resource groups These are codes that signify clinically similar treatments that use common levels of healthcare resource. An information management tool, they have been developed to support 'payment by results'.

Health economy or health community These terms generally refer to all providers, purchasers, and service users within a defined geographical area.

Health gain The improvement of the health status of a community or population. It is sometimes described as 'adding years to life and life to years'.

Health level 7 (HL7) A healthcare-specific communication standard for data exchange between computer applications.

Healthcare professional A person qualified in a health discipline.

Health promotion Enabling individuals and communities to increase control over the determinants of health, and thereby improve their health.

Health record Information about the physical or mental health of someone, which has been made by, or on behalf of, a health professional in connection with the care of that person. This must be kept for a statutory period of time after the patient is discharged from the service. Records will be held in addition to care plans.

Health Service Commissioner (HSC) The ombudsman, appointed by Parliament to protect the rights of users of the NHS; responsible only to Parliament.

Health service price index This index takes the NHS 'shopping basket' of goods and services (it excludes pay of employees) and weighs them according to use. The cost movement of these items is measured each month and the index updated to reflect these changes. It is used by the NHS to measure price movements, and quite often to update allocations and budgets.

Health status A measure of the overall health experience of an individual or a defined population.

Hearing The process of perceiving sound or agreement to having heard a person's statement.

Herzberg's two-factor theory Herzberg maintained on the basis of research studies that in any work there are factors which satisfy and dissatisfy, but they are not necessarily opposites of each other. The latter are to do with conditions of work which he called hygiene or maintenance factors, and the former are achievement, recognition, responsibility and advancement, which he called motivators.

Heuristic A rule of thumb that describes how things are commonly understood, without resorting to deeper or more formal knowledge. *See also* **model-based reasoning**.

HMRL First of a series of hospital medical record forms. It is usually the front sheet of a patient's case notes, and summarises personal, administrative and medical details. It is used for inpatients in all hospitals except those for mental illness and maternity.

Hospice NHS, voluntary or private residential premises for the provision of clinical and nursing care to residents who are terminally ill.

Hospital-acquired infection An infection acquired by a patient during their stay in hospital, which is unconnected with their reason for admission.

Hospital information system (HIS) Typically used to describe hospital computer systems with functions such as patient admission and discharge, order entry for laboratory tests or medications, and billing functions. *See also* **electronic medical record**.

Hospital stay The number of days a patient stays on one hospital site during a hospital provider spell.

Hotel costs The costs of food, heating, maintenance and so on for keeping a patient in hospital, excluding all medical and treatment costs.

Human–computer interaction The study of the psychology and design principles associated with the way humans interact with computer systems.

Human–computer interface The 'view' presented by a program to its user. Often it is literally a visual window that allows a program to be operated; an interface could just as easily be based on the recognition and synthesis of speech or any other medium with which a human is able to sense or manipulate.

Human resource strategy A written statement of human resource objectives and a plan for meeting those objectives. The strategy should be consistent with the business plan.

Hygiene factor The element of work motivation concerned with the environment or context of job, i.e. salary, status and security, etc. To be distinguished from motivators, i.e. achievement recognition. Based on theory of Herzberg. *See* **Herzberg's two-factor theory**.

In care (children) Refers to a child in the care of the local authority by virtue of an order or under an interim order.

Incident An event or occurrence, especially one that leads to problems. An example of this could be an attack on one person by another within a service.

Income and expenditure reports An accountancy tool which describes and analyses the flow of funds into and out of an organisation in order to assess liquidity. They are sometimes known as 'source and application of funds statements' or more commonly 'cash flow statements'.

Independent contractor In primary care, this normally refers to a self-employed professional. The vast majority of GPs are self-employed – unlike hospital doctors who are normally directly employed by the hospital.

Independent review The process of a panel of lay persons reviewing the case of a complaint where the complainant is not satisfied with the results of local resolution by an NHS provider.

Independent visitor (children) A local authority in certain sets of circumstances appoints such a visitor for a child it is looking after. The visitor appointed has the duty of 'visiting, advising and befriending the child'.

Indirect discrimination Where an unjustifiable requirement or condition is applied to the job which has a disproportionately adverse effect on one sex or group. For example, the career and life pattern of women is often different from that of men as a consequence of family responsibilities and child-bearing. Women may be less mobile than men. Another example of indirect discrimination is insisting on a conventional career path.

Individual performance review (IPR) A system of appraisal based on the setting of agreed object-ives and targets between individual employees and their managers, and the extent of the attain-ment of these targets. Normally IPR is linked to development; within the NHS it is often asso-ciated with performance-related pay for senior managers.

Induction A method of logical inference used to suggest relationships from observations. This is the process of generalisation we use to create models of the world. *See also* **abduction**, **deduction** and **inference**.

Induction programme Learning activities designed to enable newly appointed staff to function effectively in a new position.

Industrial tribunals Set up under the Industrial Training Act 1964, they consider cases of unfair dismissal, sex discrimination and disability.

Infant mortality rate The deaths of infants under one year of age per 1,000 live births.

Inference A logical conclusion drawn using one of several methods of reasoning, knowledge and data. *See also* **abduction**, **deduction** and **induction**.

Information superhighway A popular term asso-ciated with the internet, and used to describe its role in the global mass transportation of information.

Information theory Initially developed by Claude Shannon, this describes the amount of data that can be transmitted across a channel given spe-cific encoding techniques and noise in the signal.

Informed consent The legal principle by which a patient is informed about the nature, purpose and likely effects of any treatment proposed, before being asked to consent to accepting it.

Inherent jurisdiction (children) Powers of High Court to make orders to protect a child.

Injunction Order made by the court prohibiting an act or requiring its cessation.

Inpatient A patient who has gone through the full admission procedure and is occupying a bed in a hospital inpatients' department.

Inspiration trap The difficulty faced by a con-ciliator who can identify an obvious and sensible solution to a dispute but must ensure that the parties to the dispute reach the same conclu-sion without identifiable direction from the conciliator.

Integrated Services Digital Network (ISDN) A digital telephone network that is designed to provide channels for voice and data services. The customer must be within about 3.4 miles of the telephone exchange otherwise expensive repeater devices are required

Inter-agency plan (children) Plan devised jointly by the agencies concerned in a child's welfare which co-ordinates the services they provide.

Interim care order (children) Made by court, placing the child in the care of the designated local authority.

International Classification of Disease (ICD-10) Tenth edition published by the World Health Organization (WHO) for the statistical classification of morbidity and mortality. It may be used in conjunction with another classification termed Read coding. Review of the WHO wesite suggests work is underway on ICD-11 and more information about the ICD can be found at www.who.int/research/en/.

Investigative interview (children) Preferred term for an interview conducted with a child as part of an assessment following concerns that the child may have been abused.

Investment appraisal A means of assessing whether expenditure of capital (or revenue) on a project will show a satisfactory rate of return (e.g. lower costs or higher income), either absolutely or when compared with alternative projects.

Job description Contains standard information for staff regarding conditions of service, location(s) of the post, duties of the post, accountability, education and training facilities, appraisal and the salary scale of the post. It should be available and made known to all potential applicants at the earliest possible stage, and should be sent out with every application form. It contains details of accountability, responsibility, formal lines of communication, principal duties, entitlements and performance review. It is a guide for an individual in a specific position within an organisation. *See also* **person specification**.

Joint financing A sum of money taken from the health allocation and then spent on projects which are agreed by a joint consultative committee. Such monies should normally be spent on personal social service projects to reduce demands on NHS services.

Judicial review An order from the divisional court quashing a disputed decision. The divisional court cannot substitute its own decision, but can merely send the matter back to the offending authority for reconsideration.

Key worker The person responsible for co-ordinating the care plan for each individual patient, for monitoring its progress, and for staying in regular contact with the patient and everyone involved. A key worker may be from a variety of different professional or non-professional backgrounds.

Kipling's serving men 'I keep six honest serving men (they taught me all I know). Their names are What and Why and When and How and Where and Who'.

Knowledge acquisition Subspecialty of artificial intelligence, usually associated with developing methods for capturing human knowledge and of converting it into a form that can be used by computer. *See also* **expert system**, **heuristic** and **machine learning**.

Knowledge-based system *See* **expert system**.

Körner data Körner relates to the review of NHS information requirements by the NHS/DHSS steering group on health services information which was chaired by Edith Körner. The group recommended a minimum set of data that should be collected in all districts for management purposes.

Lay A person who is not, and preferably never has been, a professional in the field under dispute or any associated field.

Lead time Time between presentation to GP or perhaps A&E and discharge. Thus the lead time = cycle time + waiting time.

Lecture 50–55 minutes of largely uninterrupted discourse from a teacher with no discussion between students and no student activity other than listening and note taking.

Listening The process of actively hearing, accepting and understanding a verbal communication.

LIFT (local improvement finance trust) Local improvement finance trusts are a method for funding primary care and community care estates' modernisation, similar in some respects to PFI.

The contracts involved in a LIFT scheme are for buildings and maintenance. It is an additional procurement route for developing primary care estates that currently includes the use of conventional public capital, premises built and operated under the national contract for general medical services (GMS), PFI and other public–private partnerships.

Local resolution The process of resolving a complaint against an NHS provider swiftly, at or very near to the point at which the issue complained about actually occurred.

Local voices initiative Encourages gathering of the views and wishes of local people as a contribution to purchasing intelligence (q.v.).

Logical To follow a sound set of rules and tests.

Looked after (children) A child is looked after when in local authority care or is being provided with accommodation by the local authority.

Machine learning Sub-specialty of artificial intelligence concerned with developing methods for software to learn from experience, or to extract knowledge from examples in a database. *See also* **artificial intelligence** and **knowledge acquisition**.

Mailing list A list of email addresses for individuals, used to distribute information to small groups of individuals who may, for example, have shared interests. *See also* **email**.

Major incident (external) A serious external incident which requires the organisation to implement contingency plans or change or suspend some normal functions. An example would be the aftermath of a rail crash.

Major incident (internal) A serious incident occurring within the healthcare facility resulting in the changing or suspension of some normal functions or threatening of the organisation. This requires the drawing up of contingency plans. Examples of this would include the loss of electricity or telecommunications services, or bomb threats.

Makaton symbols A system of symbols used to communicate with some people who have severe learning disabilities.

Management by objectives An approach to management which aims to integrate the organisation's objectives with the individual's objectives.

Management development An approach for ensuring that the organisation meets its current and future needs for effective managers. It would include succession planning, performance appraisal and training.

Manpower planning A method of ensuring that the organisation's human resources can be met now and in the future.

Market forces May be characterised as any system of incentives that rely on market-type mechanisms such as contracts, price or cost to create a desired behaviour from the various participants in that market. For example, competition, fixed or decreasing budget limits, bidding for contracts, and so on may all be seen as market forces.

Matrix management A system of managing in a horizontal as well as a vertical organisation structure. Typically a person reports to two superiors, a department or line manager and a functional or project manager.

Matrix team People from different parts of the organisation and with no line authority.

Mediation The process of resolving a dispute by the intervention of an expert person who closely guides the disputing parties towards agreement.

Mentoring and co-mentoring An ancient process of learning facilitation by mutual professional support, traditionally given by a senior to a junior colleague. In co-mentoring the process of mentoring is non-hierarchical and involves co-mentees helping and supporting each other in learning.

Meta-analysis Pooled statistical analysis of results from several individual statistical analyses of different experiments, searching for statistical significance which is not possible within the smaller sample sizes of individual studies.

Mind map A process of recording information in related groupings which is intended to assist lateral thinking. *See also* **cognitive map**.

Minimum datasets A group of statistics or other information that together comprise the minimum amount of information required to inform any management process, for example for contract monitoring.

Mission statement Statement of the overall purpose of an organisation.

Model Any representation of a real object or phenomenon, or template for the creation of an object or phenomenon.

Model-based reasoning Approach to the development of expert systems that uses formally defined models of systems, in contrast to more superficial rules of thumbs. *See also* **artificial intelligence** and **heuristic**.

Monitor An independent corporate body established under the Health and Social Care (Community Health and Standards) Act 2003. It is responsible for authorising, monitoring and regulating NHS foundation trusts.

Monitoring The systematic process of collecting information on clinical and non-clinical performance. Monitoring may be intermittent or continuous. It may also be undertaken in relation to specific incidents of concern or to check key performance areas. It is also used in respect of selection in recording data such as sex, ethnic origin and age, etc on applicants, short-listed candidates and appointees for retrospective review, to show whether an organisation's equal opportunities policies are being carried out successfully. Monitoring also includes analysing the information and data obtained to see if there are any discrepancies in treatment/success rates of different groups, identifying the reasons and taking remedial action where appropriate. Monitoring in respect of child care is where plans for a child, and the child's safety and wellbeing, are systematically appraised on a routine basis. Its function is to oversee the child's continued welfare and enable any necessary action or change to be instigated speedily, and, at a managerial level, to ensure that proper professional standards are being maintained.

Morbidity The incidence of a particular disease or group of diseases in a given population during a specified period of time.

Mortality The number of deaths in a given population during a specified period of time.

Motivators Factors leading to job satisfaction and high employee morale. *See* **Herzberg's two-factor theory**.

Movement The stage in a conciliation or mediation process during which the parties modify their views and their opinions become closer to each other's.

Multiprofessional A combination of several professions working towards a common aim.

National Service Framework Details about out how services should be organised to cater for patients with particular conditions; in particular it would detail the standards that services will have to meet to comply with the NSF. In all parts of the country, the NHS is required to organise its services to ensure the best quality and the fairest access. The National Service Frameworks, for example, may help decide which services are best provided in primary care, in hospitals and in specialist centres.

Natural team For example, a boss with direct subordinates.

Neonatal death rate The deaths of infants under four weeks of age per 1,000 live births. The early neonatal death rate is the deaths of infants under one week of age per 1,000 live births.

Neural computing *See* **connectionism**.

Neural network Computer program or system designed to mimic some aspects of neurone connections, including summation of action potentials, refractory periods and firing thresholds.

New outpatient A patient attending for an outpatient appointment for the first time for a particular ailment. If transferred to another department, the patient is also a new outpatient on their first attendance there.

Newsgroup A bulletin board service provided on a computer network like the internet, where messages can be sent by email and be viewed by those who have an interest in the contents of a particular newsgroup. *See also* **email** and **internet**.

Non-principals A generic term for doctors who wish to practice in general practice but who do not want the financial or time commitment of becoming a principal – includes retainers, returners, assistants and associates as well as the new salaried doctor opportunities available under primary care action pilots (PCAPs).

Non-recurrent expenditure 'One-off expenditure', e.g. provision of new buildings, major alterations and major pieces of equipment. Clearly capital expenditure is non-recurrent expenditure, but the purchase of minor pieces of equipment and the carrying out of maintenance work is non-recurrent, though chargeable to revenue.

Non-recurring measures These are one-off measures that affect the year of account only, e.g. raising capital through the sale of land or via a one-off payment or loan from an external source such as the Strategic Health Authority NHS Bank.

Objective A clearly identifiable and quantifiable target to be achieved in the future. A specific and measurable statement which also sets out how overall aims are to be achieved.

Office of Population Census and Surveys (OPCS) The central government office that collected information on the entire population; now the Office for National Statistics.

Official solicitor Officer of the Court. When representing a child, the official solicitor acts as a solicitor as well as a guardian ad litem (see CAFCASS).

Ombudsman Health Service Commissioner who investigates cases of maladministration in the health service.

Open-loop control Partially automated control method in which a part of the control system is given over to humans.

Open system Computer industry term for computer hardware and software that is built to common public standards, allowing purchasers to select components from a variety of vendors and to use them together.

Opinion A belief which is held but may not be based on provable fact.

Organisation A generic term used to describe an entire organisation as opposed to the term service which is used to describe one part of the organisation (see also **service**). Thus a hospital, a practice or a university or medical school may all be described as organisations.

Organisation and management development strategy A written document which sets out the strategy for developing the organisational processes and management skills needed by an organisation.

Organisational chart A graphical representation of the structure of the organisation, including areas of responsibility, relationships and formal lines of communication and accountability.

Organisational development (OD) An educational strategy aimed at changing the beliefs, attitudes, values and structures within an organisation so that it can better adapt to changing requirements. The emphasis is on interventions, rather than the objective assessment of services. A systematic process of improving organisational effectiveness and adaptiveness on the basis of behavioural science knowledge.

Originating capital debt The amount owed by an NHS trust to the consolidated fund. This is equal to the value of the net assets transferred to an NHS trust when it is set up. Assets donated to the NHS since 1948 are not included.

Outcome The effect on health status of a healthcare intervention or lack of intervention. The end result of care and treatment, that is the change in health, functional ability, symptoms or situation of a person, which can be used to measure the effectiveness of care and treatment.

Outpatient A patient attending for treatment, consultation, advice and so on, but not staying in a hospital.

Output (or programme) budgets A system of analysing expenditure by reference to objectives to be met (e.g. increased level of day care; more operations) instead of under input headings such as staff and running expenses, etc.

Out-turn prices The prices prevailing when the expenditure occurs, as distinct from the estimated prices.

Paramedics Ambulance personnel with extended qualifications in providing prehospital care according to protocols.

Paramount principle The principle that the welfare of the child is the paramount consideration in proceedings concerning children.

Parental responsibility Defined as all the rights, duties, powers, responsibilities and authority which by law a parent of a child has in relation to the child and his property.

Part III accommodation Residential care homes provided by local authorities under Part III of the National Assistance Act 1948.

Parties Parties to legal proceedings under the Children Act are entitled to attend the hearing, present their case and examine witnesses. The Act envisages that children will automatically be parties in care proceedings. Anyone with parental responsibility for the child will also be a party to such proceedings, as will the local authority. Others may be able to acquire party status.

Party A patient, carer, representative or NHS provider involved in a dispute.

Patient A person currently or previously under medical care.

Patient costing A system whereby costs are analysed in relation to specific patients or types of patient. This is the most complete analysis that can be undertaken, and enables different combinations of costs to be made to fulfil any requirement. It is particularly useful for evaluating proposed changes in service provision.

The Patient's Charter A list of required national standards and rights set by central government for the NHS.

Patients' council/forum/group This is a group led and determined by patients, meeting independently of staff with its own agenda and operations. There can be patient councils/forums/groups within inpatient services, day hospitals, residential or community-based services. These are different from users' groups that are separately funded and legal entities in their own right, for example charities such as the UK Advocacy Network.

Patterns of delivery The way in which services are delivered, their structure and relationship to each other. This does not relate to the content of services.

Payment by results A funding system for care provided to NHS patients, which pays healthcare providers on the basis of the work they do. It does this by paying a nationally set price or tariff for similar groups of treatments, known as healthcare resource groups (HRGs), which itself is based on the historic national average cost of providing services to those HRGs. The fixed tariffs for specified HRGs are set by the Department of Health and are intended to avoid price differentials across providers that could otherwise distort patient choice. Payment is on a 'per spell' basis, where a spell is defined as a continuous period of time spent as a patient within a trust, and may include more than one episode. The aim of payment by results is to provide a transparent, rules-based system for paying NHS trusts. It hopes to reward efficiency, support patient choice and diversity, and encourage strategies for achieving sustainable reductions in waiting times.

Percentage occupancy Occupied beds expressed as a percentage of the available beds during a given period.

Performance appraisal A process for assessing performance to assess training needs, job improvement plans and salary reviews, etc.

Performance indicators A standard of work that acts as a measurement of performance, for example response times to requests for work used to indicate the performance of the service. *See also* **quality indicator**.

Performance review A systematic check on the achievement of the organisation and individuals compared with set objectives.

Perinatal mortality rate Stillbirths and deaths of infants under one week of age per 1,000 total births.

Period of study leave (PSL) GPs can apply (in accordance with paragraph 50 of the Statement of Fees and Allowances) for financial assistance in connection with a period of study leave to undertake postgraduate education, which will result in benefit to the GP, primary care (in particular) and the NHS.

Permanency planning Deciding on the long-term future of children who have been moved from their families.

Personality The distinctive and identifiable characteristics of an individual human being.

Person specification Derived from the job description, it outlines the qualifications, skills and experience required to perform the job. It lists what is essential and what is desirable and it should be used for shortlisting and interviewing. Person specifications should be available and made known to all those considering applying for a post so that they are aware of the criteria that will be used to judge them.

Physician's workstation A computer system designed to support the clinical tasks of doctors. *See also* **electronic medical record**.

Planning The process by which the service determines how it will achieve its aims and objectives. This includes identifying the resources that will be needed to meet those aims and objectives.

Police protection The Children Act allows police to detain a child or prevent his/her removal for up to 72 hours if they believe that the child would otherwise suffer significant harm.

Policy An operation statement of intent in a given situation.

Portfolios Personal professional development tools, aimed at encouraging reflection and self-direction in identifying training needs. They record and monitor opportunities for learning, and provide tangible evidence of the outcomes. Content varies – for a job interview it will focus on practical skills, competencies and achievements, whereas for academic recognition it will reflect the ability to independently problem solve in the chosen field.

Positive action Measures by which people from particular racial groups are either encouraged to apply for jobs in which they have been under-represented, or are given training to help them develop their potential and so improve their chances when competing for particular work.

Postgraduate education allowance (PGEA) GPs are eligible if they maintain a balanced programme of education and training geared towards providing the best possible care for their patients. Courses are approved (in advance) by the regional directors of postgraduate general practice education (or their staff) and can be classified in the following three areas: health promotion and prevention, disease management and service management. GPs have to show that they have attended an average of five days' training a year. Any doctor who does not take part stands to lose financially as they will not be eligible for PGEA. The structure varies and approval may be given for, e.g.:

- lunchtime lecturettes (maybe a half or quarter session)

- in-house practice meetings on specific educational topics

- week-long courses at postgraduate centres (including at overseas resorts)

- national meetings

- reading (free) weekly medical magazines and answering multiple choice questions (MCQs) on the magazine content.

Postscript In computer technology the commercial language that describes a common format for electronic documents that can be understood by printing devices, and converted to paper documents or images on a screen.

Practice-based commissioning The term given to a form of practice level commissioning which enables practices (usually this refers to primary care teams led by GPs, although there are some exceptions) to commission care and other services that are directly tailored to the needs of their patients. Practices can keep up to 100% percent of any savings made by agreement with their local PCT.

Practice parameter *See* **clinical guideline**.

Preliminary hearing (children) Hearing to clarify matters in dispute, to agree evidence, and to give directions as to the timetable of the case and the disclosure of evidence.

Preventive maintenance and replacement programme A plan for the maintenance of machines to minimise the amount of time lost through breakdown by anticipating and preventing likely problems.

Primary care audit group (i.e. multidisciplinary) Groups of professionals and managers in health authorities whose remit is to encourage and facilitate the undertaking and implementation of audit in primary care – the cyclical reappraisal of structure process and outcome.

Primary care centre (PCC) Centre for out-of-hours treatment, allowed under changes to the GP contract in 1994.

Principals Doctors who have been established in general practice by the traditional route, i.e. by means of appointment to the health authorities' GMS Principal List.

Private bed (pay bed) A bed occupied by a patient who pays the whole cost of accommodation and medical and other services.

Private finance initiative (PFI) Provides a way of funding major capital investments as an alternative to the public procurement route which is funded directly by the Treasury. Private consortia, usually involving large construction firms, are contracted to design, build, and in some cases manage new projects. Contracts typically last for about 30 years, although some are longer, during which time the building is leased by a public authority. It remains a contentious issue, with many critics who state that it does not offer value for money and effectively transfers ownership of NHS hospitals out of the NHS. Others point to the relatively large number of new facilities built under the scheme that would not otherwise have been built.

Private patient A patient who pays the full cost of all the medical and other services.

Probation officer Welfare professional employed as an officer of the court and financed jointly by the local authority and the Home Office.

Procedure The steps taken to fulfil a policy; a particular and specified way of doing something.

Professional standards Professionally agreed levels of performance.

Prohibited steps order (children) Order that no step which could be taken by a parent in meeting his parental responsibility for a child, and which is of a kind specified in the order, shall be taken by any person without the consent of the court.

Project 2000 The system of nurse education which places increased emphasis on student-centred and research-based learning.

Protocol The adoption by all staff of local or national guidelines to meet local requirements in a specified way; an alternative word for procedure. *See also* **clinical guideline**.

Provider A healthcare organisation, such as an NHS trust, which provides healthcare and sells its services to purchasers.

Provider plurality This term refers to the use of a range of different organisations from NHS and independent, private, and 'not for profit' sectors in the delivery of services. In the context of NHS reforms, 'provider plurality' coupled with competition and patient choice is said to promote efficiency, effectiveness and value for money in the delivery of services.

Psychometric tests Standardised question and answer papers designed to measure personality.

Public dividend capital (PDC) A form of long-term government finance on which the NHS trust pays dividends to the government. PDC has no fixed remuneration or repayment obligations, but, in the long term, the overall return on PDC is expected to be no less than on an equivalent loan.

Patient and public involvement forums (PPI forums, PPIF) PPI forums were set up following the NHS Reform and Health Care Professions Act 2002. There are 572 forums – one for each trust in England. They are the local voice of the community on health matters and have a wide range of responsibilities.

Public private partnerships (PPP) The umbrella name given to a range of initiatives which involve the private sector in the operation of public services.

Purchaser A budget-holding body that buys health or social care services from a provider on behalf of its local population or service users.

Purchasing intelligence The knowledge purchasers need in order to make informed decisions when purchasing healthcare on behalf of their resident population. Includes demographic data, information on healthcare services, and the views of local people (local voices).

Qualitative reasoning A subspecialty of artificial intelligence concerned with inference and knowledge representation when knowledge is not precisely defined, e.g. 'back of the envelope' calculations.

Quality A specified standard of performance.

Quality assurance (QA) A generic term essentially meaning that one ensures not only that the right things get done, but also that none of the wrong things are done.

Quality improvement strategy A written statement of objectives relating to quality improvement and a plan for meeting those objectives. The strategy should be consistent with the business plan.

Quality indicator A standard of service which acts as a measurement of quality, for example incidence of infection used to indicate the quality of care. See also **performance indicators**.

Quango A quasi-autonomous non-governmental organisation. A body with virtual statutory power.

Read coding A hierarchically arranged thesaurus of clinical condition terms which provides a numeric coding system. The system was developed by Dr Read and is cross-referenced to other national and international classifications. It was developed initially for primary care medicine in the UK and subsequently enlarged and developed to capture medical concepts in a wide variety of situations. See also **terminology**.

Reasoning A method of thinking. See also **inference**.

Recovery order (children) Order which a court can make when there is reason to believe that a child in care, who is the subject of an emergency protection order or in police protection, has been unlawfully taken or kept away from the responsible person, or has run away, is staying away from the responsible person, or is missing.

Recurrent expenditure 'Ongoing expenditure' such as salaries and wages, travelling expenses, drugs and dressings, and provisions.

Reflection The process of returning verbal or body language communication to the original perpetrator to indicate agreement and acceptance.

Refuge (children) Enables 'safe houses' to legally provide care for children who have run away from home or local authority care. A recovery order can be obtained in relation to a child who has run away to a refuge.

Regular day admission A patient who attends electively and regularly for a course of treatment and care, but does not stay in hospital through the night.

Relate A voluntary body, formerly known as the Marriage Guidance Council, which assists couples to resolve differences that threaten their relationship.

Representation The method chosen to model a process or object. For example a building may be represented as a physical scale model, drawing or photograph. See also **reasoning** and **syntax**.

Representations (child care) See complaints procedure.

Research and development (R&D) Searching out knowledge and evidence about the relationship between different factors in the provision of services. Research does not require action in response to findings.

Residential care homes Residential accommodation, other than group homes, providing board and lodging and personal care to the residents. This includes homes for the elderly or physically disabled people.

Residential social worker (children) Provides day-to-day care, support and therapy for children living in residential settings, such as children's homes.

Resource assumptions Provisional estimates of cash resources (capital, revenue and joint finance) that may be made available over the next two to three years.

Resource management The different definitions of resource management all emphasise the involvement of doctors, nurses and other clinical staff in the continuing improvement of the quality and quantity of patient care through better use of resources and information.

Respite care Service giving family members or other carers short breaks from their caring responsibilities.

Responsibility The obligation that an individual assumes when undertaking delegated functions.

Responsible person (children) Any person who has parental responsibility for the child, and any other person which whom the child is living. With their consent, the responsible person can be required to comply with certain obligations.

Retainers Doctors appointed to practices under the Doctors' Retainer Scheme who are constrained from practising full-time or part-time, usually by virtue of domestic commitments, but who wish to keep in touch with medicine.

Returners Doctors wishing to return to clinical practice.

Revenue consequences of capital schemes (RCCS) Annual running costs of capital schemes.

Review The examination of a particular aspect of a service or care setting so that problem areas requiring corrective action can be identified.

Review (children) Local authorities have a duty to conduct regular reviews in order to monitor the progress of children they are looking after.

Review meetings The system whereby the NHSE regional offices monitor the performance of health authorities against planned objectives and set an action plan for further achievements.

Ringfencing The identification of funds to be used for a particular purpose only – usually applied to funds earmarked by central government for a particular use within the NHS or local government, e.g. the mental illness-specific grant.

Risk management A systematic approach to the management of risk to reduce loss of life, financial loss, loss of staff availability, loss of staff and patient safety, loss of availability of buildings or equipment, or loss of reputation.

Risk management strategy A written statement of objectives for the management of risk and a plan for meeting those objectives. The strategy should be consistent with the business plan.

Safe discharge of patients A procedure for the discharge of patients who require care in the community which complies with Department of Health guidelines.

Satisfaction survey Seeks the views of patients through responses to pre-prepared questions and is carried out through interview or self-completion questionnaires.

Section 8 orders (children) The four orders contained in the Children Act 1989 which, to varying degrees, regulate the exercise of parental responsibility.

Secure accommodation (children) Provides for the circumstances in which a child who is being looked after by the local authority can be placed in secure accommodation. Such accommodation is provided for the purpose of restricting the liberty of the child.

Seeding The process of 'planting' all or part of an idea or plan in the mind(s) of others such that those persons produce the plan as if it were their own original thought.

Semantics The meaning associated with a set of symbols in a given language, which is determined by the syntactic structure of the symbols, as well as knowledge captured in an interpretative model. *See also* **syntax**.

Seminar A session during which prepared papers are presented to the class by one or more students.

Service The term used to describe part of an organisation, as opposed to the entire organisation. *See also* **organisation**.

Service contract A legally binding contract between an organisation and an external supplier of goods or services. The contract sets out the agreed cost and quality for a given period.

Service level agreement The term used to describe a document, agreed between organisations or services that will provide and receive a service, which sets out in detail how the service will be provided.

Significant harm (children) 'Whether harm suffered by the child is significant turns on the child's health or development; his health or development shall be compared with that which could reasonably be expected of a similar child'.

Skill mix The balance of skill, qualifications and experience of nursing and other clinical staff employed in a particular area. The process of reassessing the skill mix required is known as reprofiling.

Slippage The shortfall compared with planned spending caused by delays in the planning or execution of expenditure. It can be expressed in terms of money or time.

Social worker Generic term applying to a wide range of staff who undertake different kinds of social welfare responsibilities. *See also* **education welfare officer**, **fieldworker**, **probation officer** and **residential social worker**.

Specialty costing The analysis of costs to clinical specialties, thus enabling comparisons to be made in the same institution over time or between different institutions.

Specific issue order (children) Order giving directions for the purpose of determining a specific question which has arisen, or which may arise, in connection with any aspect of parental responsibility for a child.

Staffed allocated beds Staffed beds allocated to particular specialties including those which are available and those which are temporarily not available.

Staff incident reporting system A standardised system for reporting incidents and near misses. The NHSE recommends that no more than two types of forms are used for this.

Standardised mortality ratio (SMR) The number of deaths in a given year as a percentage of those expected. The expected number is a standard sex/age mortality of a reference period.

Standing financial instructions Specific instructions issued by the board of a hospital or trust to regulate conduct of the organisation, its directors, managers and agents in relation to all financial matters.

Standing orders A series of established instructions governing the manner in which business will be conducted.

Standards Standards are a means of describing the level of quality that healthcare organisations are expected to meet or to aspire to. The performance of organisations can be assessed against this level of quality.

Strategy A long-term plan.

Suggestion The process of putting a thought, plan or desire to another person.

Supervision order (children) Order including, except where express contrary provision is made, an interim supervision order.

Supervisor (children) Person under whose supervision the child is placed by virtue of an order.

Supraregional services Specialist services for rarer conditions provided for a population significantly larger than that of an English region. They are specially funded.

Survey The collection of views from a sample of people in order to obtain a representative picture of the views of the total population being studied.

Synchronous communication A mode of communication when two parties exchange messages across a communication channel at the same time, e.g. telephones. *See also* **asynchronous communication**.

Synergy The extent to which investment of additional resources produces a return which is proportionally greater than the sum of the resources invested. Sometimes known as the '2 + 2 = 5' effect.

Syntax The rules of grammar that define the formal structure of a language. *See also* **semantics**.

Systematised Nomenclature of Human and Veterinary Medicine (SNOMED) A commercially available general medical terminology, initially developed for the classification of pathological specimens. *See also* **terminology**.

Targets Refer to a defined level of performance that is being aimed for, often with a numerical and time dimension. The purpose of a target is to incentivise improvement in the specific area covered by the target over a particular timeframe.

Target allocation National share of the resources available calculated by reference to established criteria of need.

Team Any group of people who must significantly relate with each other in order to accomplish shared objectives.

Teleconsultation Clinical consultation carried out using a telemedical service. *See also* **telemedicine**.

Telemedicine The delivery of healthcare services between geographically separated individuals, using telecommunication systems, e.g. video conferencing.

Temporarily closed beds Staffed allocated beds closed for less than one month.

Term In medical terminology an agreed name for a medical condition or treatment. *See also* **code** and **terminology**.

Terminal A screen and keyboard system that provides access to a shared computer system, e.g. a mainframe or mini-computer. In contrast to computers on a modern network, terminals are not computers in their own right.

Terminology A set of standard terms used to describe clinical activities. *See also* **term**.

T group Training group, refers to training in interpersonal awareness or sensitivity, where a group of people meet in an unstructured way to discuss the interplay of the relationships between them.

Theory X A theory about motivation expounded by McGregor, which suggests that people are lazy, selfish and unambitious, etc, and need to be treated accordingly. It contrasts with Theory Y, the optimistic view of people.

Theory Z An expression coined by Ouchi as a result of studying Japanese success in industry, to denote a process of organisational adaptation in which the management of the enterprise concentrates on co-ordinating people, not technology, in the pursuit of productivity.

Throughput The number of patients using each bed in a given period, such as a year. Also termed bed turnover.

Top slicing Usually used to refer to a proportional sum of money retained from budgets in a district or region to fund, e.g. region-wide initiatives, or supplement financial reserves.

Total quality management (TQM) Approach to management of organisations which aims to change organisational culture, so that continuous improvements in quality are achieved, by moving from a traditional command structure to one which encourages and empowers staff.

Training The process of modifying behaviour at work through instruction, example or practice.

Training and development strategy A written statement of objectives for the training and development of staff, and a plan for meeting these objectives. The strategy should be consistent with the business plan.

Training needs analysis An approach to assessing the training or development needs of groups of employees aimed at clarifying the needs of the job and the needs of the individuals in terms of the training required.

Treatment centre Centres are dedicated units that offer prebooked day and short-stay surgery and diagnostic procedures in specialties such as ophthalmology, orthopaedics, hernia repair and gallbladder and cataract removal, amongst others. Treatment centres can be run by the NHS or the independent sector, and exist mainly to provide additional capacity (including staff) to address waiting list targets.

Tribunal A court-like procedure for the resolution of disputes.

Turing test Proposed by Alan Turing, the test suggests that an artefact can be considered intelligent if its behaviour cannot be distinguished by humans from other humans in controlled circumstances. *See also* **artificial intelligence**.

Turnover interval The average number of days that beds are vacant between successive occupants.

Tutorial A discussion session, usually dealing with specified content, or a recent lecture or practical. Chaired by the teacher, it may have any number of students from one to 20 or so.

Unbundling and bundling Under the 'payment by results' system, trusts are reimbursed per spell, categorised by HRG (*see* **payment by results** definition p. 236). There are debates as to whether the HRG categories accurately reflect the cost of providing services, and whether they are flexible enough to incorporate varying treatment patterns. When people refer to 'unbundling' the tariff, they mean being able to clearly identify the individual elements which go to make up the cost of each component of the HRG. This would allow different organisations to carry out different parts of the treatment. For example, unbundling the tariff for an HRG that includes a hospital procedure and aftercare, means that the aftercare can be administered in the community, with both the hospital and community provider accurately reimbursed for the work that they do. Conversely, when people talk about 'bundling' the tariff, they mean budgeting for whole-patient pathways or treatment programmes, which allows the individual components to be negotiated locally.

Unusual medications Medications that are currently unlicensed or being used for an unlicensed indication. Patients must be informed before they receive such medications.

Underlying deficit This is the total amount of one-off measures the health economy has had to find to achieve a break-even position at year end, i.e. the overall position after ignoring 'in-year' non-recurrent measures.

Valid consent The legal principle by which a patient is informed about the nature, purpose and likely effects of any treatment proposed before being asked to consent to accepting it. *See also* **informed consent**.

Value analysis Also known as value engineering. Term used to describe an analytical approach to the function and costs of every part of a product with a view to reducing costs while retaining the functional ability.

Virement The transfer of resources from one budget heading to another. It is a means of using a planned and agreed saving in one area to finance expenditure in another area. Clear rules are needed about how virement operates so that, for instance, a budget for one-off purchases (e.g. purchase of equipment) is not spent on recurrent payments (e.g. employing staff).

Virtual reality Computer-simulated environment within which humans are able to interact in some manner that approximates interactions in the physical world.

Vital services In management terms those services that are essential to the normal operation of the organisation. Examples include electricity, water, medical gases and telecommunications.

Voicemail Computer-based telephone messaging system, capable of recording and storing messages, for later review or other processing, e.g. forwarding to other users. *See also* **email**.

Waiting list The number of people awaiting admission to hospital as inpatients.

Waiting time The time that elapses between (i) the request by a GP for an appointment and the attendance of the patient at the outpatients' department; or (ii) the date a patient's name is put on an inpatients' list and the date they are admitted.

Ward of court A child who, as the subject of wardship proceedings, is under the protection of the High Court. No important decision can be taken regarding the child while they are a ward of court, without the consent of the wardship court.

Wardship Legal process whereby control is exercised over the child in order to protect the child and safeguard his or her welfare.

Weighted capitation Sum of money provided for each resident in a particular locality. The three main factors reflected in the formula are: age structure of the population; its morbidity; and relative cost of providing services.

Welfare checklist (children) Refers to the innovatory checklist contained in the Children Act 1989.

Welfare report (children) The Children Act 1989 gives the court the power to request a report on any question in respect of a child under the Act.

Whole-time equivalents (WTEs) The total of whole-time staff, plus the whole-time equivalent of part-time staff, which is obtained by dividing the hours worked in a year by part-timers, by the number of hours in the whole-time working year.

Work in progress Waiting lists or queues waiting to be seen.

Work measurement A work study technique designed to establish the time for a qualified person to carry out a specified job to a defined level.

Work study Includes several techniques for examining work in all its contexts, in particular factors affecting economy and efficiency, with a view to making improvements.

Written agreement (children) Agreement arrived at between the local authority and the parents of children for whom it is providing services. These arrangements are part of the partnership model that is seen as good practice under the Children Act.

Further reading

Some useful sources of further information on these topics are to be found at the following websites:

- Department of Health – www.dh.gov.uk
- Healthcare Commission – www.healthcare commission.org.uk
- King's Fund – www.kingsfund.org.uk
- NHS Alliance – www.nhsalliance.org
- Royal College of Nursing – www.rcn.org.uk

Useful acronyms

The following list excludes virtually all clinical acronyms. Fortunately one doesn't need to know these acronyms but we felt a reference source might be useful. There has been a burgeoning of acronyms in recent years. We have removed some of the more obvious, such as degrees, diplomas and other medical qualifications and many very common clinical ones. Some have lapsed although they are still to be found referred to in literature and thus have been included. Interestingly some have appeared and disappeared in the interval between this and the previous edition! For interest's sake only, included are a handful of mildly amusing ones to be found, although you will need to look carefully for them. We hope that none cause offence, but the authors are only reporting those in current use or as reported in current literature.

AA	Attendance Allowance
AAA	annual accountability agreement *or* abdominal aortic aneurysm
AAO	American Academy of Ophthalmology
AAOS	American Academy of Orthopaedic Surgeons
AAOx3	awake, alert, oriented x 3 [person/place/time]
AAC	Advisory Appointments Committee
A&C	administrative and clerical
A&E	accident and emergency
AAGBI	Association of Anaesthetists of Great Britain and Ireland
AAMS	Association of Air Medical Services (US)
ABC	activity-based costing
ABG	arterial blood gases
ABI	area-based initiative
ABM	activity-based management
ABN	Association of British Neurologists
ABS	adult basic skills
ABHI	Association of British Healthcare Industries
ABM	activity-based management
ABPI	Association of the British Pharmaceutical Industry
AC	Audit Commission (comprises chair, deputy and 18 members all appointed by the Secretary of State from a wide range of fields)

ACA	area cost adjustment (part of the SSA)	ACP	American College of Physicians
ACAC	Area Clinical Audit Committee	ACRA	Advisory Committee on Resource Allocation (obsolete)
ACAD	Advice and Counselling on Alcohol and Drugs	ACPC	Area Child Protection Committee
ACAS	Advisory, Conciliation and Arbitration Service (set up by the UK government to assist in the resolution of disputes between employers and employees)	ACR	American College of Radiology
		ACRPI	Association of Clinical Research for the Pharmaceutical Industry
		ACT	assertive community treatment
		ACTAF	Association of Community Trusts and Foundations, now Community Foundation Network
ACBS	Advisory Committee on Borderline Substances	ACTR	additional cost of teaching and research (in Scotland)
ACC	adjusted credit ceiling (part of the Capital Control Framework)	ACTS	Agency for Community Team Support
ACCEA	Advisory Committee on Clinical Excellence Awards	ADA	Americans with Disabilities Act
ACDA	Advisory Committee on Distinction Awards (consultants)	ADC	automatic data capture
		ADCU	anti-drugs co-ordination unit
		ADD	attention deficit disorder
ACDC	Ambulatory Care and Diagnostic Centre	ADH	additional duty hours (junior doctors)
ACDM	Association of Clinical Data Managers	ADHD	attention deficit hyperactivity disorder
ACDP	Advisory Committee on Dangerous Pathogens	ADI	acceptable daily intake
		ADL	activities of daily living
ACEVO	Association of Chief Executives of Voluntary Organisations	ADMS	Assistant Director of Medical Services
ACF	Association of Charitable Foundations	ADNS	Assistant Director of Nursing Services
ACGT	Advisory Committee on Genetic Testing	ADP	automatic data processing
ACHCEW	Association of Community Health Councils for England and Wales (now obsolete)	ADQ	average daily quantity: average amount of a medication prescribed for an adult in England
ACHMS	Asian Community Mental Health Services	ADR	adverse drug reaction
		ADS	attribution dataset
ACIE	Association of Charity Independent Examiners	ADSS	Association of Directors of Social Services
ACIG	Academy of Medical Royal Colleges Information Group	ADSU	automatic distress signal unit
		AED	automatic external defibrillator
ACLS	advanced coronary life support	AEF	aggregate external finance
ACM	Assessment and Care Management – Social Services Community Care Purchaser Division	AELS	advanced endocrinological life support
		AEN	additional educational needs (part of SSA)
ACME	Advisory Committee on Medical Establishment (Scotland) *or* Alliance for Continuing Medical Education	A4A	Awards for All
		AFAIAA	as far as I am aware
		AFC	*Agenda for Change*
ACMHS	Asian Community Mental Health Services	AfC	*Agenda for Change*
		AFOM	Association of the Faculty of Occupational Medicine
ACMT	(European) Advisory Committee on Medical Training	AFPP	Association for Perioperative Practice
ACOST	(Cabinet) Advisory Committee on Science and Technology	AFR	annual financial return

AfS	Action for Sustainability		**ALS**	advanced life support
AFWG	Allocation Formula Working Group (part of Home Office)		**ALSOB**	alcohol-like substance on breath
AGH	Advisory Group on Hepatitis		**AMA**	Association of Metropolitan Authorities *or* American Medical Association *or* against medical advice
AGM	annual general meeting			
AGMETS	Advisory Group for Medical Education, Training and Staffing (an overarching body designed to co-ordinate all issues relating to staffing and educating doctors)		**AME**	annual managed expenditure
			AMEE	Association for Medical Education in Europe
			AMIA	American Medical Informatics Association
AGREE	Appraisal of Guidelines for Research and Evaluation in Europe		**AMP**	annual maintenance plan *or* asset management plan
AGUM	Association for Genitourinary Medicine		**AMPS**	assessment of motor skills
AHA	Associate of the Institute of Hospital Administrators (previously area health authority)		**AMQ**	average monthly quantities: the assumed maintenance dose per month for an adult of a drug
AHCPA	Association of Health Centre and Practice Administrators		**AMRA**	asset management revenue account
			AMRC	Association of Medical Research Charities *or* Academy of Medical Royal Colleges
AHHRM	Association of Healthcare Human Resource Management			
AHP	allied health professional		**AMS**	Army Medical Services
AHRQ	Agency for Healthcare Research and Quality		**AMSPAR**	Association of Medical Secretaries, Practice Administrators and Receptionists
AI	artificial intelligence			
AICD	automatic internal cardiac defibrillator		**ANDPB**	advisory non-departmental public bodies
AIDS	acquired immune deficiency syndrome		**ANH**	artificial nutrition and hydration
			AOB	alcohol on breath
AIF	Area Investment Framework		**AOC**	Adult Opportunity Centre
AIM	activity information mapping *or* advanced informatics in medicine		**AODP**	Association of Operating Department Practitioners, formerly BAODA British Association of Operating Department Assistants
AIMS	Association for Improvements in Maternity Services			
AIOPI	Association of Information Officers in the Pharmaceutical Industry		**AOMRC**	Academy of Medical Royal Colleges
AIP	approval in principle		**AOP**	Association of Optometrists
AIR	adverse incident report		**AOT**	Assertive Outreach Team
ALA	Association of Local Authorities		**APC**	Area Prescribing Committee *or* antigen-presenting cell
ALAC	Artificial Limb and Appliance Centre. Now known as the DSC			
			APD	advanced professional development
ALARM	Association of Litigation and Risk Managers		**APH**	aged persons home, also known as EPH or Association of Public Health – now turned into UKPHA
ALB	arm's length bodies			
ALD	adult with learning difficulties		**APHA**	American Public Health Association
ALF	activity-led funding			
ALI	Adult Learning Inspectorate		**APHI**	Association of Public Health Inspectors
ALM	Action Learning for Managers			
ALMO	Arm's Length Management Organisation		**APLS**	advanced paediatric life support
			APMS	alternative primary medical services
ALOS	average length of stay			
ALPHA	Access to Learning for the Public Health Agenda		**APROP**	Action for the Proper Regulation of Private Hospitals

APSE	Association for Public Service Excellence
AQH	Association for Quality in Healthcare
AQS	Air Quality Strategy
A/R	alert and orientated
ARC	Arthritis and Rheumatism Council
ARF	annual retention fee
ARM	Association of Radical Midwives
ARSH	Association of Royal Society of Health
ARVAC	Association for Research in the Voluntary and Community Sector
AS	associate specialist
ASA	Ambulance Service Association
ASAP	as soon as possible
ASB	antisocial behaviour
ASBAH	Association for Spina Bifida and Hydrocephalus
ASBO	Anti-Social Behaviour Order
ASC	Action for Sick Children
ASD	autistic spectrum disorder
ASEC	Associate Specialist Education Committee
ASH	Action on Smoking and Health
ASIM	American Society of Internal Medicine
ASIT	Association of Surgeons in Training
ASME	Association for the Study of Medical Education
ASPFA	Asylum Seekers and People From Abroad – a social services team that pays out cash to people who cannot get Social Security benefits
ASPIRE	Action to Support Practices Implementing Research Evidence
ASSIST	Association for Information Management and Technology Staff in the NHS
ASTC	Associate Specialist Training Committee
ASTRO-PU	age sex temporary resident-originated prescribing unit
ASW	approved social worker – a social worker approved to carry out Sections under the Mental Health Act.
ASWCS	Avon Somerset and Wiltshire Cancer Services
ATLS	advanced trauma life support
ATMD	Association of Trust Medical Directors

ATU	alcohol treatment unit
AUDGP	Association of University Departments of General Practice
AURE	Alliance of UK Health Regulators on Europe
AVG	ambulatory visit group
AVMA	Action for Victims of Medical Accidents
AWMEG	All-Wales Management Efficiency Group
BAAF	British Agencies for Adoption and Fostering
BACS	British Association for Chemical Specialities or Blood Alcohol Content
BACCH	British Association for Community Child Health
BACTS	British Association of Clinical Terminology
BACUP	British Association of Cancer United Patients
BAEM	British Association for Accident and Emergency Medicine
BAMM	British Association of Medical Managers for clinicians in or interested in, management
BAMS	Benefits Agency Medical Service
BAN	British Approved Name
BAO	British Association of Otolaryngologists
BAOT	British Association of Occupational Therapists
BAP	British Association for Psychopharmacology
BAPS	British Association of Paediatric Surgeons or British Association of Plastic Surgeons
BAPT	British Association of Physical Training
BARQA	British Association of Research Quality
BASH	British Association for the Study of Headache
BASICS	British Association of Immediate Care
BASRaT	British Association of Sports Rehabilitators and Trainers
BASSAC	British Association of Settlements and Social Action Centres
BASW	British Association of Social Workers
BAUS	British Association of Urological Surgeons

BBP	blood-borne pathogen
BBS	bulletin board system
BBV	blood-borne virus
BC	block contract(ing) *or* borough council
BCA	basic credit approval (part of the Capital Control Framework)
BCCCF	Black Community Care Consultative Forum
BCD	black and culturally diverse
BCF	boundary change factor (part of SSA)
BCHS	*Better Care Higher Standards*
BCODP	British Council of Disabled People
BCS	British Computer Society
BCSH	British Committee for Standards in Haematology
BDA	British Dental Association *or* British Diabetic Association now called Diabetes UK *or* British Dietetic Association *or* British Dyslexia Association
BDD	body dysmorphic disorder
BDH	British Drug Houses (no longer trading)
BEAM	Biomedical Equipment Assessment and Management
BEHAF	British Ethnic Health Awareness Foundation
BGM	board general manager (an NHS in Scotland term)
BGS	British Geriatrics Society for Health in Old Age
BHAF	Black HIV and AIDS Forum
BHF	British Heart Foundation
BHS	British Hypertension Society
BIBRA	British Industrial Biological Association
BILD	British Institute of Learning Disabilities
BIM	British Institute of Management
BioRes	Biological and Biomedical Sciences Research (internet resource)
BIR	British Institute of Radiology
BIVDA	British in Vitro Diagnostics Association
BLROA	British Laryngological, Rhinological and Otological Association
BLS	basic life support
BMA	British Medical Association
BMCIS	building maintenance cost information system
BME	black and minority ethnic
BMI	body mass index (kg/m^2)
BMIS	British Medical Informatics Society
BMJ	*British Medical Journal*
BMR	basal metabolic rate
BNF	*British National Formulary*: quarterly publication containing details of prescribed drugs
BNI	British Nursing Index
BOA	British Orthopaedic Association
BOPCAS	British Official Publications Current Awareness Service
BOS	British Orthodontic Society
BP	*British Pharmacopoeia*
BPA	British Paediatric Association
BPAS	British Pregnancy Advisory Service
BPC	British Pharmaceutical Codex
BPD	borderline personality disorder
BPMF	British Postgraduate Medical Federation
BPPV	benign paroxysmal positional vertigo
BPR	business process re-engineering
BPS	British Pharmacological Society
BPSU	British Paediatric Surveillance Unit
BR	budget requirement
BrAPP	British Association of Pharmaceutical Physicians
BRCS	British Red Cross Society
BSA	Basic Skills Agency
BSAD	British Sports Association for the Disabled
BSCC	British Society for Clinical Cytology
BSE	bovine spongiform encephalopathy *or* breast self-examination
BSEC	Basic Surgical Education Committee
BSH	British Society for Haematology
BSI	British Standards Institution or British Society for Immunology
BSL	British Sign Language
BSPED	British Society for Paediatric Endocrinology and Diabetes
BSR	British Society of Rheumatology
BST	basic surgical training *or* basic specialist training
BTEG	Black Training and Enterprise Group
BTS	British Thoracic Society *or* Blood Transfusion Service
BSVP	*Better Services for Vulnerable People*
BUPA	British United Provident Association

BVACoP	Best Value Accounting Code of Practice
BVPI	Best Value Performance Indicator
BVPP	Best Value Performance Plan
BWS	beached whale syndrome
CAB	Citizens' Advice Bureau
CABA	compressed air breathing apparatus
CABE	Commission for Architecture and the Built Environment
CABG	coronary artery bypass graft
CADO	Chief Administrative Dental Officer
CAEF	Clinical Audit and Effectiveness Forum
CAF	Charities Aid Foundation
CAFCASS	Children and Family Court Advisory Support Service
CAIT	Citizens Advocacy Information and Training
CAL	computer-assisted learning
CALL	Cancer Aid Listening Line
CAM	complementary and alternative medicine
CAMHS	Child and Adolescent Mental Health Services: joint local and health authority services to young people with mental health problems
CAMO	Chief Administrative Medical Officer
CAMS	computer-aided medical systems
CAN	Community Action Network
CANO	Chief Area Nursing Officer
CAOx4	Conscious, Alert, and Oriented x4
CAP	College of American Pathologists
CAPD	continuous ambulatory peritoneal dialysis for people with kidney failure
CAPM	Capital Asset Pricing Model
CAPO	Chief Administrative Pharmaceutical Officer
CARE	clinical audit and research evidence or Craniofacial Anomalies Register
CAS	controls assurance statement or Care Assessment Schedule or Chemical Abstracts or Community Accountancy Service
CASE	Centre for Analysis of Social Exclusion
CASH	Consensus Action on Salt and Health
CASP	Critical Appraisal Skills Programme
CASPE	Clinical Accountability Service

	Planning and Evaluation Specialist Healthcare Training Group
CAT	computerised axial tomography or critically appraised topic or Community Alcohol Team
CATS	Capture Assess Treat and Support Services or Credit Accumulated Transfer Scheme (a national scheme)
CAWG	Controls Assurance Working Group
CBA	cost–benefit analysis
CbD	case-based discussion
CBS	common basic specification
CBRN	chemical, biological, radioactive and nuclear
CBT	cognitive–behavioural therapy or computer-based training
CC	Charity Commission or county council or chief complaint or city council
CCA	cost–consequence analysis or current cost accounting
CCC	NHS Centre for Coding and Classification
CCCG	Cochrane Colorectal Cancer Group
CCDC	consultant in communicable disease control
CCE	completed consultant episode (see FCE)
CCEPP	Cochrane Collaboration on Effective Professional Practice – now called EPOC
CCETSW	Central Council for Education and Training in Social Work (abolished October 2001)
CCG	Community Care Grant
CCHR	Citizens' Commission on Human Rights
CCN	County Councils' Network or change control notice
CCP	community care plan or change control procedure
CCR	cross cutting review
CCrISP	care of the critically ill surgical patient
CCSC	Central Consultants and Specialists Committee (a committee of the BMA)
CCSI	Critical Care Skills Institute
CCSR	cross-cutting spending review
CCST	certificate of completion of specialist training for junior doctors
CCT	compulsory competitive tendering: a sort of Dutch auction of public services, now partly replaced by

	the Best Value process *or* certificate of completion of training
CCU	coronary care unit *or* critical care unit
CCTR	Cochrane Controlled Trials Register
CCTV	closed circuit television
CCU	coronary care unit
CD	clinical director *or* clinical directorate *or* controlled drug *or* civil defence or cluster of differentiation
CDC	Centers for Disease Control and Prevention (USA)
CDDS	Council of Deans of Dental Schools
CDER	Center for Drug Evaluation and Research
CDHN	Community Development and Health Network
CDM	chronic disease management *or* construction, design and management
CDO	Chief Dental Officer
CDS	contract dataset: a collection of information recorded by the NHS trust that identifies a patient and their treatment which is sent to the health authority or community dental service
CDSC	Communicable Disease Surveillance Centre
CDSR	Cochrane Database of Systematic Reviews
CDSM	Committee on Dental and Surgical Materials (abolished 1994)
CDU	child development unit *or* central delivery unit *or* colourflow duplex ultrasound
CDX	Community Development Exchange
CE	chief executive
CEA	cost–effectiveness analysis
CEDP	Chief Executive Development Programme
CEEU	Clinical Effectiveness and Evaluation Unit of the RCP
CEF	Community Empowerment Fund
CEFET	Central England Forum for European Training
CEN	Comité Européen de Normalisation (European Standards organisation)
CEMACH	Confidential Enquiry into Maternal and Child Health

CEMD	Confidential Enquiry into Maternal Deaths
CEMVO	Council of Ethnic Minority Voluntary Sector Organisations
CEN	Community Empowerment Network
CEO	chief executive officer
CEPOD	Confidential Enquiry into Perioperative Deaths (*see* NCEPOD)
CERA	capital expenditure, revenue account
CertHSM	Certificate in Health Services Management
CES	Charities Evaluation Services
CESDI	Confidential Enquiry into Stillbirths and Deaths in Infancy
CESH	National Confidential Inquiry into Suicide and Homicide by People With Mental Illness
CERES	Consumers for Ethics in Research
CEX	clinical evaluation exercise
CF	cystic fibrosis
CfH	Connecting For Health
CFI	community finance initiative
CFISSA	Centrally Funded Initiatives and Services and Special Allocations
CFN	Community Foundation Network
CFO	Chief Finance Officer *or* conventionally financed option *or* co-financing public sector intermediary organisation
CfPS	Centre for Public Scrutiny
CFR	Capital Financing Reserve
CFRC	Children and Family Resource Centre
CFS	chronic fatigue syndrome (closely associated with ME)
CFSMS	Counter Fraud and Security Management Service
CG	clinical governance
CGD	chronic granulomatous disease
CGF	Child Growth Foundation
CGRDU	Clinical Governance Research and Development Unit
CGST	Clinical Governance Support Team
CHAI	Commission for Healthcare Audit and Improvement
CHAIN	Contact Help Advice and Information Network
CHAOS	chief has arrived on the scene
CHART	Community Health Action Resource Team

CHC	Community Health Council (now only in Wales)		CINAHL	Cumulative Index to Nursing and Allied Health
CHD	coronary heart disease		CIO	Confederation of Indian Organisations *or* charitable incorporated organisation
CHDGP	collection of health data from general practice project			
CHEST	Combined Higher Education Software Team		CIPC	Centre for Innovation in Primary Care
CHEX	Community Health Exchange		CIP(s)	capital investment programme(s)
CHG	Community Hospitals Group (now taken over by BUPA)		CIPFA	Chartered institute of Public Finance and Accountancy
CHI	Commission for Health Improvement *or* community health index		CIS	clinical information system
			CISH	Confidential Inquiry into Suicide and Homicide by People with Mental Illness
CHIA	Comprehensive Health Impact Assessment			
CHIME	Centre for Health Informatics in Medical Education		CISP	community information systems project
CHiQ	Centre for Health Information Quality (patient information)		CJC	Commissioning Joint Committee
			CJD	Creutzfeldt–Jakob disease
CHIR	Canadian Institutes of Health Research		CKD	chronic kidney disease
			CLA	Commissioner for Local Administration (the ombudsman)
CHIRP	confidential human factors incident reporting procedure		CLAPA	Cleft Lip and Palate Association
CHMU	central health monitoring unit (DoH)		CLDT	community learning disability team
			CLGMS	cash-limited general medical services
CHOU	central health outcomes unit		CLib	Cochrane Library
CHRE	The Council of Healthcare Regulatory Excellence		CLIP	central–local information partnership *or* Clinical Improvements Database
CHS	child health surveillance			
CHSA	Chest, Heart and Stroke Association		CM	community midwife
			CMA	cost minimisation analysis
CHMS	Council for Heads of Medical Schools		*CMAJ*	*Canadian Medical Association Journal*
CHMU	central health monitoring unit (obsolete)		CMB	Central Midwives Board
			CMC	Central Manpower Committee (no longer exists)
CHOU	central health outcomes unit			
CHP	Community Health Partnership *or* combined heat and power		CMD	continuing medical development
			CMDS	contract/core minimum dataset
CHRC	community health and resource centres		CME	continuing medical education
			CMF	Capital Modernisation Fund
CHS	community health services *or* child health surveillance		CMHN	community mental handicap nurse (obsolete)
CI	clinical indicator		CMHSD	Centre for Mental Health Services Development, Kings College London
CIA	chief internal auditor			
CIC	common information core *or* charitable incorporated organisation			
			CMHT	community mental health team
CIM	capital investment manual *or* *Cumulative Index Medicus*		CML	chronic myeloid leukaemia
			CMMS	case mix management system
			CMO	Chief Medical Officer
CIMP	Clinical Investment Management Programme		CMP	civilian medical practitioner
			CMPS	Centre for Management and Policy Studies
CIMS	Coalition for Improving Maternity Services			
			CMR	computerised medical record

CMS	Community Midwifery Service *or* clinical management support *or* contract management system
CMT	corporate management team
CN	charge nurse
CNM	clinical nurse manager
CNO	Chief Nursing Officer
CNS	clinical nurse specialist *or* community nursing service or central nervous system
CNST	Clinical Negligence Scheme for Trusts
CO	Cabinet Office *or* course organiser *or* complains of *or* chief officer *or* capital out-turn
COAD	chronic obstructive airways disease – usually called COPD
COGIT	Chief Officers' Group of Information Technology
COGPED	Committee of General Practice Education Directors
COI	Central Office of Information
COIN	circulars on the internet: all the HSCs etc *or* Clinical Oncology Information Network
COMA	Committee on Medical Aspects of Food Policy (abolished 2000)
COMARE	Committee on Medical Aspects of Radiation in the Environment
COMEAP	Committee on the Medical Effects of Air Pollutants
COPC	community-oriented primary care
COPD	chronic obstructive pulmonary disease
COPDEND	Conference of Postgraduate Dental Deans and Directors of Education
COPE	Committee on Publication Ethics
COPMED	Conference of Postgraduate Medical Deans
COR	capital out-turn and receipts return
CORE	clinical outcomes research and effectiveness
COREC	Central Office for Research Ethics Committees
COSHH	Control of Substances Hazardous to Health Legislation (1994 Regulations)
COT	Committee on Toxicity
CP	community plan *or* cerebral palsy
CPA	Care Programme Approach: patients' needs for care are assessed on a four-point scale. Level 4 means that you are dangerously ill and need

	supervision. Level 1 means that you are not thought to need anything more than a bit of advice and counselling; *or* comprehensive performance assessment *or* clinical pathology accreditation *or* critical path analysis
CPAG	Child Poverty Action Group *or* Capital Prioritisation Advisory Group
CPAP	continuous positive airway pressure
CPC	cost per case
CPCCH	consultant paediatrician in community child health
CPCME	Centre for Postgraduate and Continuing Medical Education
CPCU	child protection co-ordination unit
CPD	continuing professional development
CPEP	Clinical Practice Evaluation Programme
CPFA	charted public finance accountant
CPH	Certificate in Public Health
CPHL	Central Public Health Laboratory
CPHM	Certified Professional in Healthcare Material Management
CPHMCH	Committee Public Health Medicine and Community Health
CPHVA	Community Practitioners and Health Visitors Association – part of AMICUS
CPMP	Committee for Proprietary Medical Products (EU)
CPN	community psychiatric nurse
CPNA	Community Psychiatric Nurses' Association – now the Mental Health Nursing Association
CPO	Chief Pharmaceutical Officer
CPOD	Centre for Professional and Organisational Development
CPPIH	Commission for Patient and Public Involvement in Health
CPR	Child Protection Register *or* cardiopulmonary resuscitation *or* capital payments and receipts return
CPSM	Council for Professions Supplementary to Medicine
CPU	contracts and purchasing unit *or* central processing unit
CPWP	Capital Programmes Working Party
CQI	continuous quality improvement
CQSW	Certificate of Qualification of Social Work abolished 1989

CRAG   Clinical Research and Audit Group *or* Charging for Residential Accommodation Guide – guidance for local authorities on community care financial assessment *or* Clinical Resource and Audit Group, the lead body within the Scottish Executive Health Department promoting clinical effectiveness in Scotland

CRAGPE/ CRAGPIE   Committee of Regional Advisers in General Practice Education

CRANE   Craniofacial Anomalies Register

CRB   Criminal Records Bureau

CRC   Clinical Research Centre *or* Cancer Research Campaign

CRCF   Conference of Royal Colleges and their Faculties

CRD   Centre for Reviews and Dissemination

CRDC   Central Research and Development Committee

CRE   Commission for Racial Equality (monitors the effects of the Race Relations Act 1976)

CRED   clinical governance/education and R&D subgroup

CRES   cash-releasing efficiency savings

CRHP   Council for the Regulation of Healthcare Professionals

CRIO   Chief Registration and Inspection Officer: responsible for the Health and Social Service Registration and Inspection Units and Guidance ad Litem service

CRIR   Committee for Regulating Information Requirements

CRMD   Cochrane Review Methodology Database

CRT   community rehabilitation team *or* cathode ray tube

CS   capital strategy

CSA   Child Support Agency *or* Common Services Agency

CSAG   Clinical Standards Advisory Group

CSASHS   Common Services Agency for the Scottish Health Service

CSBS   Clinical Standards Board for Scotland

CSC   Community Sector Coalition

CSCI   Commission for Social Care Inspection

CSD   carbonated soda drinks

CSEC   Corporate Specialist Education Committee

CSF   Community Support Framework *or* cerebrospinal fluid

CSM   Committee on Safety of Medicines *or* Christian Socialist Movement

CSMC   Civil Service Management Committee

CSO   Central Statistical Office *or* civil society organisation (or NGO)

CSP   Chartered Society of Physiotherapy *or* Children's Services Plan

CSPG   Central Support Protection Grant

CSR   comprehensive spending review

CSS   children's social services *or* certificate of satisfactory service *or* cascading style sheets

CSSD   central sterile services/supplies department *or* central support service department

CSTC   Corporate Specialist Training Committee

CSV   Community Service Volunteers

CT   computerised tomography

CTBSL   council tax benefit subsidy limitation

CTD   close to death *or* circling the drain

CTG   cardiotocography electronic measurement of foetal heart and uterine contractions

CTN   Charity Trustees Network

CTO   compulsory treatment order

CTPLD   Community Team for People with Learning Disabilities

CU   Casualties Union

CUA   cost–utility analysis

CUE   community unit for the elderly

CUV   current use value

CV   curriculum vitae

CVCP   Committee of Vice Chancellors and Principals

CVE   continuous vocational education

CVS   Council for Voluntary Service *or* cardiovascular system

CYA   cover your arse

CYPF   Children and Young People's Fund

CYPS   Children and Young People's Services

CYPU   Children and Young People's Unit

D&T   Drugs and Therapeutics

D&TP   *Drugs and Therapeutic Bulletin*

D/C   discontinue *or* discharge

DA   distributable amount *or* district audit

DAAT	drug and alcohol team	**DHA**	district health authority (obsolete April 2002)
DAN	Disabled People's Direct Action Network	**DHSC**	Directorate of Health and Social Care (obsolete)
DAN	duty assessment nurse	**DHSS**	Department of Health and Social Security later split into DoH and DSS
DAP	Dean's Advisory Panel		
DARE	Database of Abstracts of Reviews of Effectiveness	**DHSSPS**	Department of Health, Social Services and Public Safety
DART	drug and alcohol resistance training		
DASG	drugs- and alcohol-specific grant	**DHT**	district handicap team
DAT	drugs action team *or* Disability Appeal Tribunal (obsolete) *or* digital audio tape	**DI**	director of information
		DIA	Drug Information Association
		DIAL	disablement information and advice lines
DATA	Distress Awareness Training Agency		
DB	database	**DIC**	disseminated intravascular coagulation *or* dead in car
DBFO	design, build, finance and operate (*see also* DFBO)		
		DID	dissociative identity disorder
DCT	disabled children's team	**DIG**	disablement income group
DCFS	Directorate of Counter Fraud Services	**DIO**	district immunisation officer
		DIPEx	Database of Individual Patient Experiences
DDA	Disability Discrimination Act 1995 *or* The Disabled Drivers' Association		
		DIPG	Drug Information Pharmacists' Group
DDD	defined daily dose		
DDRB	Doctors' and Dentists' Review Body	**DIPHSM**	Diploma in Health Services Management
DDPHRCS	Diploma in Dental Public Health, Royal College of Surgeons of England	**DISP**	developing/development of information systems for purchasers
		DipSW	Diploma in Social Work
DDRB	Doctors' and Dentists' Review Body	**DIS**	departmental investment strategy
		DISP	developing information system for purchasers
DEB	Dental Estimates Board		
DEC	Development and Evaluation Committee replaced by NICE in 2000	**DISS**	Disability Information Service Surrey
		DisCASS	Disabled Citizens' Advice and Support Service
DEL	departmental expenditure limit		
DENS	doctor's educational needs	**DLA**	Disability Living Allowance
DFBO	design, finance, build and operate (less common version of DBFO)	**DLCV**	drugs of limited clinical value
		DLF	Disabled Living Foundation
DfEE	Department for Education and Employment (now renamed) DfES	**DMARD**	disease modifying anti-rheumatic drug
		DMC	district medical committee
DfES	Department for Education and Skills	**DMD**	Drug Misuse Database *or* Duchenne muscular dystrophy
DFT	distance from target (relating to HA's financial allocation)	**DMF**	Disabled Motorists' Federation
		DMFT	number of decayed, missing or filled teeth
DFFP	Diploma of Faculty of Family Planning		
		DMHE	Department of Mental Health for the Elderly
DFG	Disabled Facilities Grant		
DG5	The Public Health part of the European Union	**DMO**	district medical officer (obsolete)
		DMT	departmental management team
DGH	district general hospital	**DMU**	directly managed unit
DGM	district general manager	**DN**	district nurse
DH	Department of Health (England) (*see* DoH)	**DNA**	did not arrive *or* did not attend

DNAR	do not attempt resuscitation		**DTD**	document type definition
DNDRN	The Dementias and Neurodegenerative Disease Research Network		**DTF**	Diversity Task Force
			DTI	Department of Trade and Industry
DNGNet	Disability Network Group		**DTNI**	day time net inflow
DNI	do not intubate (similar to DNR)		**DTTO**	drug testing and treatment order
DNR	do not resuscitate		**DTP**	diphtheria tetanus pertussis: a vaccine
DNS	director of nursing services		**DUI**	driving under the influence
DNW	Drugs North West		**DV**	domiciliary visit (by consultant) or dependent variable or domestic violence or deo volente (God willing)
DOA	dead on arrival or date of accident (in A&E departments) or date of admission			
			DWA	Disability Working Allowanc: a benefit for people working at least 16 hours a week who have a disability affecting their working ability. Now replaced by DPTC
DOB	date of birth			
DoF	director of finance			
DOGPE	director of general practice education			
			DWM	dead white male
DoH	Department of Health		**DWP**	Department for Work and Pensions
DOPS	direct observation of procedural skills		**EAC**	estimated annual cost
DPB	Dental Practice Board		**EAG**	expert advisory group
DPC	data protection commissioner		**EAN**	European article number
DPGPE	director of postgraduate GP education		**EAPN**	European Anti-Poverty Network
			EASR	European age-standardised rate: a measure of the incidence of disease
DPH	director of public health			
DPI	Disabled Peoples' International			
DPR	data protection registrar or directorate performance review		**EBCP**	evidence-based clinical practice
			EBD	emotional and behavioural difficulties
DPTC	Disabled Person's Tax Credit (now abolished)			
			EBH	evidence-based healthcare
DRC	Disability Rights Commission or depreciated replacement cost		**EBL**	evidence-based learning
			EBM	evidence-based medicine
DRF	direct revenue funding		**EBMH**	evidence-based mental health
DRG	diagnosis-/diagnostic-related group		**eBNF**	the *BNF* on a CD ROM
DRS	Dental Reference Service		**EBOC**	evidence-based on call
DSC	Disablement Service Centre or Directory of Social Change		**EBP**	evidence-based practice
			EBS	Emergency Bed Service (London)
DSCA	Defence Secondary Care Agency		**EBV**	Epstein–Barr virus
DSCN	dataset change notice		**EC**	European Community or Experience Corps
DSD	decontamination services department			
			ECDL	European Computer Driving Licence
Dsh	deliberate self-harm			
DSL	doctors' support line		**ECG**	electrocardiogram
DSO	direct service organisation		**ECN**	emergency care network
DSON	detailed statement of need		**ECP**	emergency care practitioner
DSPD	dangerous and severe personality disorder		**ECR**	extra-contractual referral, now replaced by OAT
			ECTS	European credit transfer scheme
DSS	Department of Social Security, now the DWP or decision support systems		**ED**	enumeration district: the smallest unit for census data – about 200 homes or economic development
DSU	day surgery unit			
DTA	Development Trusts Association			
DTB	*Drug and Therapeutic Bulletin*			
DTC	Drug and Therapeutics Committee or day treatment centre or diagnostic and treatment centre		**EDA**	Erectile Dysfunction Association
			EDI	electronic data interchange: exchanging information electronically, not including faxing

EDIFACT	Electronic Data Interchange: a particular structure which complies with ISO 9735. This is the standard for EDI adopted by the NHS	**EMLC**	European Midwives' Liaison Committee
		EMO	examining medical officer
		EMR	electronic medical record
		EMS	emergency medical services
EDIT	elderly dementia intervention team	**EMW**	early morning wakening
EDP	emotionally disturbed person *or* education development plan	**EMWA**	European Medical Writers' Association
EDS	Ehlers–Danlos syndrome	**ENB**	English National Board for Nursing, Midwifery and Health Visiting (obsolete)
EDT	emergency duty team: social services departments		
EEA	European Economic Area	**ENHPA**	European Network of Health Promotion Agencies
EEC	European Economic Community		
EFGCP	European Forum for Good Clinical Practice	**ENDPB**	executive non-departmental public bodies
EFL	external financing limit	**ENIL**	European Network on Independent Living
EFM	electronic fetal monitoring		
EFMI	European Federation for Medical Informatics	**ENP**	emergency nurse practitioner
		EO	employers' organisation
EFQM	European Foundation for Quality Management	**EOC**	Equal Opportunities Commission (set up under the Sex Discrimination Act 1975 to monitor sex discrimination)
EGFR	epidermal growth factor receptor *or* estimated glomerular filtration rate		
EHMA	European Healthcare Management Association	**EP**	emergency planning *or* English partnerships
EHO	environmental health officer	**EPACT**	electronic prescribing analysis and costs
EHP	education and health partnership		
EHR	electronic health record	**EPCS**	environmental, protective and cultural services
EHS	extremely hazardous substance		
EHU	electronic health unit	**EPH**	elderly person's home
EIA	European Information Association	**EPHR**	electronic patient health record
EIS	early intervention service *or* executive information system	**EPICS**	elderly person's integrated care scheme
EL	Executive Letter (has year and number with it)	**EPO**	emergency planning officer
		EPP	Expert Patients' Programme
eLIB	Electronic Libraries Programme	**EPR**	electronic patient record
ELP	essential lifestyles planning: person-centred planning tool emphasising rhythms and routines of daily life used in learning disability services	**EQUIP**	Effectiveness and Quality in Practice Group (within DoH, chaired by CMO and CNO) *or* education and quality in primary care
ELS	Existing Liabilities Scheme	**ERA-ETDA**	European Renal Association-European Dialysis and Transplant Association
EM	electronic mail (email)		
EMA	emergency medical admission *or* Education Maintenance Allowance	**ERDIP**	Electronic Record Development Implementation Programme
EMAG	Ethnic Minority Achievement Grant	**ERG**	electroretinogram *or* external reference group
EMAS	Employment Medical Advisory Service		
EMEA	European Medicines Evaluation Agency	**ERI**	Edinburgh Research and Innovation Limited
EMG	electromyogram	**ERIC**	estates returns information collection
EMI	elderly mentally infirm *or* elderly mentally ill		
EMIS	Egton Medical Information System	**EROS**	electronic records in office systems

ERS	external reference group (relating to NSFs)
ES	educational supervisor *or* employment service
ESAT	emergency services action team (obsolete)
ESF	European Social Fund *or* education standards fund
ESMI	elderly severely mentally infirm *or* elderly severely mentally ill
ESOL	English for speakers of other languages
ESP	economic and social partnership
ESRA	European Society of Regulatory Affairs – now TOPRA
ESRC	Economic and Social Science Research Council
ESRI	Economic and Social Research Institute (Ireland)
ESV	employer-supported volunteering
ET	executive team *or* environmental technologies
ETA	estimated time of arrival
ETF	environment task force
ETP	employer training pilot
ETT	endotracheal tube
EU	European Union
EWC	expected week of confinement
EWO	educational welfare officer
EWTD	European Working Time Directive
EYDCP	early years development and childcare plan
EYDP	early years development partnership
EYPD	early years and play department
EZ	employment zone
FA	Friedreich's ataxia
FAB	Family Action Benchill
FAM	fraud awareness month – an annual event
FARR	fixed asset restatement reserve
FAWN	Funding Advice Workers Network
FBC	full business case
FC	fixed cost *or* factor cost *or* Family Credit, now replaced by Tax Credits
FCAS	Federation of Charity Advice Services
FCDL	Federation for Community Development Learning
FCE	finished consultant episode (*see* CCE)
FCS	financial control system

FDA	US Food and Drug Administration
FDIU	fetal death *in utero*
FDL	Finance Directorate Letter
FDTL	Fund for the Development of Teaching and Learning
FE	further education
FEC	further education college
FEFC	Further Education Funding Council, disbanded in 2001 and replaced by the Learning and Skills Council
FENTO	Further Education National Training Organisation
FES	Family Expenditure Survey
FFCE	first finished consultant episode
FFP	fresh-frozen plasma
FHom	faculty of homeopathy
FHR	fetal heart rate
FHS	family health services (the primary healthcare providers, including GPs, dentists, pharmacists and opticians)
FHSA	Family Health Service Authority – role now taken over by the health authority
FHSAA	Family Health Service Appeal Authority
FHSCU	family health services computer unit
FHT	fetal heart tones
FIAC	Federation of Independent Advice Centres
FIBD	found in bed dead
FIG	Food Initiatives Group
FIP	financial information project
FIPO	Federation of Independent Practitioner Organisations
FIS	Financial Information Service (run by IPF) *or* financial information system *or* Family Income Supplement (became WFTC)
FIT	focused individualised training
FITTA	fixed-term training appointment
FIU	fraud investigation unit
FM	facilities management
FMD	foot and mouth disease
FMIP	financial management information project
FMIS	financial management information systems
FMP	Financial Management Programme
FMR	functions and manpower review
FOM	Faculty of Occupational Medicine of Royal College of Physicians

FORD	found on road dead	**GAPS**	genetic information and patient services
FPA	Family Planning Association		
FP10	a prescription form	**GATB**	Global Alliance for TB Drug Development
FPC	family planning clinic *or* Family Practitioner Committee, which was replaced by the FHSA		
		GATS	general agreement on trade in services
FPharmM	faculty of pharmaceutical medicine	**GBP**	pounds sterling – for people who don't have a £ sign
FPHM	faculty of public health medicine		
FPS	family planning services *or* family practitioner services	**GBS**	Guillaine–Barré syndrome
		G-CAT	Government IT Catalogue
FR	financial regulation	**GCC**	General Chiropractic Council
FRED	financial reporting exposure draft (draft FRS)	**GCS**	Glasgow Coma Score
		GCSE	general certificate of secondary education
FRS	financial reporting standard *or* Fellow of the Royal Society		
		GDA	guideline daily amount
FRSH	Fellow of the Royal Society of Health	**GDC**	General Dental Council
FSA	Food Standards Agency *or* Financial Services Authority	**GDP**	general dental practitioner *or* gross domestic product
		GDS	general dental services
FSID	Foundation for the Study of Infant Deaths	**GENECIS**	General Clinical Information System
FSM	free school meals	**GHG**	general healthcare group
FSO	forum support organisations	**GHQ**	General Health Questionnaire
FSS	forensic science service	**GHS**	General Household Survey
FSU	family support unit – now know as family unit (FU)	**GIDA**	Government Intervention in Deprived Areas
FT	full-time *or* foundation trust	**GIGO**	garbage in garbage out
FTC	Federal Trade Commission	**GIS**	geographical information system: computers designed to create, manipulate, analyse and display geographical data
FTE	full-time equivalent		
FTP	fitness to practise		
FTPD	foundation training programme director		
FTTA	fixed-term training appointments	**GLACHC**	Greater London Association of Community Health Councils
FU	family unit: a mixture of residential and outreach work for children and young people and their families *or* follow-up	**GLAD**	Greater London Association of Disabled People
		GLADD	Gay and Lesbian Association of Doctors and Dentists
FWATAG	Flexible Working and Training Advisory Group	**GM**	general manager *or* Geiger–Müller
FWN	further work needed	**GMAS**	Greater Manchester Ambulance Service
FY	full year		
FY1	foundation year 1	**GMC**	General Medical Council
FY2	foundation year 2	**GMCDP**	Greater Manchester Coalition of Disabled People
FYC	full-year cost		
FYE	full-year equivalent *or* full-year effect	**GMO**	genetically modified organisms
GAAP	generally accepted accounting practice	**GMP**	general medical practitioner *or* *Good Medical Practice*
		GMS	general medical services
GAD	Government Actuary's Department	**GMSC**	General Medical Services Committee
GAG	getting ahead of the game		
GAL	guardian ad litem: usually an independent social worker	**GNP**	gross national product
		GNVQ	general national vocational qualifications
GALRO	guardian ad litem reporting officer: these are appointed to represent the best interests of the child	**GO**	Government Office for the Regions

GOC	General Optical Council *or* Gynaecological Oncology Centre
GOK	God only knows
GOMER	get out of my emergency room (US slang for an unwelcome patient)
GOP	General Optical Council
GOS	general ophthalmic service
GOSC	General Osteopathic Council
GOSH	Great Ormond Street Hospital for Children
GP	general practitioner *or* Green Paper
GPAS	General Practice Assessment Survey: produced by the NPCRDC
GPASS	General Practice Administration System Scotland
GPC	General Practitioners' Committee
GPCC	GP commissioning consultant
GPCG	GP commissioning group: *see* HSC 1998/030
GPEC	GP emergency centre
GPFC	General Practice Finance Corporation
GPFH	general practitioner fundholder (obsolete)
GPIAG	General Practice Airways Group
GPMSS	general practice minimum system specification
GPWA	GP Writers' Association
GPwSI	GPs with a special interest
GRE	grant-related expenditure (replaced by NRE)
GREA	grant-related expenditure assessment (replaced by SSA)
GRIPP	getting research into purchasing and practice
GSCC	General Social Care Council
GSI	Government Secure Intranet
GSL	general sales list: a medicine which can be sold anywhere
GSM	global system of mobility
GSOH	good sense of humour: as important in the Health Service as on the lonely hearts pages
GSW	gun shot wound
GTAC	Gene Therapy Advisory Committee
GTLRC	Gypsy and Traveller Law Reform Coalition
GTN	Government Telephone Network
GUCH	Grown Up Congenital Heart Patients' Association
GUI	graphical user interface
GUM	genitourinary medicine: where STDs are treated
GWC	General Whitley Council
H&S	health and safety
HA	health authority *or* housing association
HaCCRU	Health and Community Care Research Unit based in Liverpool University
HAG	housing association grant
HAI	hospital-acquired infection
HARP	Hulme Action Research Project: works with people with mental health problems
HAS	Health Advisory Service *or* human activity system
HASHD	hypertensive arteriosclerotic heart disease
HASSASSA	Health and Social Services and Social Security Adjudication Act
HAT	Housing Action Trust
HAWNHS	Health at Work in the NHS
HAZ	health action zone (obsolete)
HB	health board (in Scotland) *or* Housing Benefit
HBAI	households below average income
HBG	health benefit group
HC	Health Council *or* Health Circular *or* Healthcare Commission *or* Huntingdon's chorea
HCA	Hospital Caterers' Association *or* home care assistant – social care worker who provides domiciliary care, formerly known as home helps, *or* historic cost accounting
HCAG	Hospital Consultants' Advisory Group: a steering body for projects on work patterns for consultants
HCFA	Health Care Financing Administration, the federal agency that administers the Medicare, Medicaid and Child Health Insurance Programs in the USA
HCG	human chorionic gonadotrophin
HCHS	hospital community health service: hospital services, ambulances and certain community health services such as district nursing. These services are provided mostly by NHS trusts
HCIA	Health Care Information, an American company which analyses health data. Now part of Solucient
HCS	holiday care service
HCSP	healthcare service for prisoners

HCW	healthcare worker: provides nursing support in clinical areas; NVQ qualified
HAD	Health Development Agency (obsolete) *or* Huntingdon's Disease Association
HDL	high-density lipoprotein
HDM	house dust mite
HDU	high dependency unit, one step down from the ITU
HE	health education *or* higher education
HEA	Health Education Authority now replaced by the HAD or Health Equity Audit
HEASIG	High Ethnicity Authorities' Special Issues Group
HEBS	Health Education Board for Scotland
HEED	Health Economic Evaluations Database
HEFC	Higher Education Funding Council
HEFCE	Higher Education Funding Council for England
HEFM	Health Estates and Facilities Management Association
HEI	higher education institution
HEIF	Higher Education Innovation Fund
HELMIS	Health Management Information Service (Nuffield Institute, Leeds)
HEO	health education officer
HEP	Health Education Partnership
HEPA	high-efficiency particulate air
HERO	higher education and research opportunities in the UK
HEROINE	Health Electronic Resources Online In Northern England
HEVU	health education video unit
HES	hospital episode statistics *or* hospital eye service
HFEA	Human Fertilisation and Embryology Authority
HfHT	Help for Health Trust (obsolete)
HFMA	Healthcare Financial Management Association
HGAC	Human Genetics Advisory Commission
HGC	Human Genetics Commission
HHT	hand-held terminal
HIA	Health Impact Assessment *or* Housing Improvement Agency
HIBCC	Health Index Bar Code Council *or* Health Index Business Communications Council

HImP	Health Improvement Programme
HIMP	Health Improvement and Modernisation Programme
HIP	Health Investment Programme
HIPE	Hospital Inpatient Enquiry Scheme
HIS	hospital information system
HISN	high individual support needs
HISS	hospital information and support system
HIU	health inequalities unit
HIV	human immunodeficiency virus
HIYE	Health in Your Environment
HJSC	Hospital Junior Staff Committee (of BMA)
HL7	Health level 7 (a healthcare-specific communication standard for data exchange between computer applications)
HLC	healthy living centre
HLF	Heritage Lottery Fund
HLI	healthy living initiative
HLPI	high-level performance indicator
HMIC	Health Management Information Consortium
HMR	hospital medical record
HMO	health maintenance organisation (USA) *or* house in multiple occupation
HMR	hospital medical record
HNA	health needs assessment
HMRC	Her majesty's Revenue and Customs
HMSO	Her Majesty's Stationery Office (became TSO but now OPSI)
HNI	housing needs index
HO	house officer *or* Home Office
HoN	*Health of the Nation* White Paper on prevention
HoNOS	Health of the Nation Outcomes Scale
HOWIS	Health of Wales Information Service: the official website for NHS in Wales)
HP	health promotion
HPA	Health Protection Agency
HPC	Health Professions Council
HPE	higher professional education *or* Health Promotion England (obsolete)
HPERU	Health Policy and Economic Research Unit
HPH	Health Promoting Hospital
HPR	health process redesign

HPSS	health promotion specialist service *or* health and personal social services
HR	human resources – personnel
HRD	human resource development
HRD-MET	Human Resources Directorate-Medical Education and Development
HRG	healthcare resource group
HRQO	health-related quality of life
HSAC	Health Service Advisory Committee (of HSE)
HSC	Health and Safety Commission *or* health service commissioner *or* HSC Health Service Circular – management letters from the DoH replacing ELs, HSGs, FDLs and FHSLs
HSCIC	health and social care information centre
HSDU	hospital sterile and disinfection unit
HSE	Health and Safety Executive
HSG	health service guidance *or* health strategy group *or* housing support grant
HSI	health service indicators
HSJ	*Health Services Journal*
HSMC	Health Services Management Centre University of Birmingham
HSP	heart sink patient *or* Healthy Schools Programme
HSPI	health service prices index
HSPSCB	High Security Psychiatric Services Commissioning Board (obsolete)
HSSB	Health and Social Services Board (Northern Ireland)
HST	higher surgical training *or* trainee, a senior registrar in old-speak
HSTAT	Health Services/Technology Assessment Text
HSV	herpes simplex virus
HSW	health and safety at work
HSWA	Health and Safety at Work Act 1974
HTA	Health Technology Assessment
HTAI	Health Technology Assessment International
HTH	hope this helps
HTM	high-technology medicine
HV	health visitor *or* home visit
HVA	Health Visitors' Association
HVHSC	The Human and Veterinary Healthcare Sectoral Consultation (bringing together interested bodies in the public and private sectors to draw up key principles concerning

	biotechnology and genetically modified organisms)
HWI	Healthy Workplace Initiative
HWRC	household waste recycling centre
I4H	information for health
I&D	incision and drainage
IAGI	intended average gross income (of GPs) (the total money paid on average to GPs, i.e. inclusive of indirectly reimbursed expenses)
IAMRA	International Association of Medical Regulatory Authorities
IADL	instrumental activities of daily living
IAG	information age government
IAGI	intended average gross income
IANI	intended average net income (of GPs) (the total money paid on average to GPs, exclusive of indirectly reimbursed expenses)
IANR	intended average net remuneration
IAPO	International Alliance of Patients' Organisations
IAVI	International AIDS Vaccine Initiative
IBD	interest-bearing debt
IBMS	Institute of Biomedical Science
IBNR	incurred but not reported (clinical negligence liability)
ICA	Invalid Care Allowance now replaced by Carers' Allowance
ICAS	Independent Complaints Advocacy Service
ICATS	Integrated Clinical Assessment and Treatment Services
ICC	Integrated Child Credit
ICD	The World Health Organization's International Statistical Classification of Diseases and Related Health Problems (now on 10th revision)
ICES	Institute for Clinical Evaluative Sciences
ICFM	Institute of Charity Fundraising Managers' Trust
ICHS	International Centre for Health and Society
ICIDH	International Classification of Impairment, Activities and Participation
ICN	infection control nurse *or* integrated care network
ICP	integrated care pathway *or* intracranial pressure

ICRC	International Committee of the Red Cross	**ILSI**	International Life Sciences Institute
ICT	infection control team *or* information communication technology	**IMA**	Irish Medical Association
		IM&T	information management and technology
ICU	intensive care unit	**IMC**	information management centre
ICW	integrated clinical workstation *or* indigenous community worker	**IMD**	Index of Multiple Deprivations
		IMG	international medical graduates
ICWS	integrated clinical work station	**IMGE**	former Information Management Group of NHS Executive
ID2000	Indices of Deprivation 2000	**IMHO**	in my humble opinion
IDA	Improvement Development Agency	**IMLS**	Institute of Medical Laboratory Sciences
IDDM	insulin-dependent diabetes mellitus		
IdeA	Improvement and Development Agency	**IM**	infant mortality rate
		INASP	International Network for the Availability of Scientific Publications
IDF	International Diabetes Federation		
IELTS	international English language testing service	**INES**	International Network of Engineers and Scientists for Global Responsibility
IEMC	inter-Balkan European medical centre		
IFM	information for the management of healthcare	**INSET**	in-service training
		IOP	Institute of Psychiatry
IFPMA	International Federation of Pharmaceutical Manufacturers' Associations	**IoS**	item of service: something that GPs get paid for on a itemised basis under the terms of the *Red Book*
IHF	International Hospital Federation	**IP**	inpatient
IHM	Institute of Healthcare Management	**IPF**	Institute of Public Finance
IHRIM	Institute of Health Record Information and Management	**IPH**	Improvement Partnership for Hospitals
IHSM	Institute of Health Service Managers – now part of the IHM	**IPM**	Institute of Personnel Management
		IPPC	integrated pollution prevention control
IHA	Independent Healthcare Association of 600 independent hospitals and homes	**IPPF**	International Planned Parenthood Federation
IHCD	Institute of Health and Care Development	**IPPR**	Institute of Public Policy Research
		IPR	individual performance review *or* independent professional review *or* intellectual property rights
IHE	international health exchange *or* Institute of Hospital Engineering		
IHEEM	Institute of Healthcare Engineering and Estate Management	**IPS**	integrated personnel system *or* formerly the Indicative Prescribing Scheme
IHF	International Hospital Federation		
IHRIM	Institute of Health Record Information and Management	**IRL**	initial resource limit
		IRIS	interactive resource information system
IHSM	Institute of Health Services Management	**IRO**	industrial relations officer
IIP	Investors in People initiative	**IRP**	independent reconfiguration panel
ILA	individual learning account	**IRR**	internal rate of return
ILAF	independent local advisory forum	**IS**	Income Support, formerly Supplementary Benefit, before that National Assistance, before that the Poor Law
ILCOR	International Liaison Committee on Resuscitation		
ILD	Index of Local Deprivation (replaced by IMD)	**ISB**	Information Standards Board *or* invest to save budget
ILF	Independent Living Fund		
ILP	Independent Living Project	**ISBN**	International Standard Book Number

ISD	information and statistics division
ISDD	Institute for the Study of Drug Dependence
ISDN	integrated services digital network
ISE	individualised sensory environment
ISG	information services group
ISO	International Organization for Standardization *or* Infrastructure Support Organisation
ISPOR	International Society for Pharmacoeconomics and Outcomes Research
ISQua	International Society for Quality in Health Care
ISSM	Institute of Sterile Services Management
IS	intensive support team
ISTAHC	International Society of Technology Assessment in Health Care
ISTC	independent sector treatment centre
IT	information technology
ITC	independent treatment centre
ITN	invitation to negotiate
ITS	Independent Tribunal Service – now replaced by the Appeals Service
ITT	invitation to tender
ITU	intensive therapy/treatment unit
IUHPE	International Union for Health Promotion and Education
IV	independent variable *or*, of course, intravenous
IVF	*in vitro* fertilisation
IWL	*Improving Working Lives*
IYF	inter-year flexibility
J	judge (in law reports)
JAMA	*Journal of the American Medical Association*
JANET	joint academic network
JCB	Joint Commissioning Board
JCC	Joint Consultative Committee *or* Joint Consultants Committee
JCCO	Joint Council for Clinical Oncology
JCE	Joint Commissioning Executive
JCHMT	Joint Committee for Higher Medical Training
JCHST	Joint Committee for Higher Surgical Training
JCPTGP	Joint Committee on Postgraduate Training in General Practice
JCVI	Joint Committee on Vaccination and Immunisation
JDC	Junior Doctors' Committee
JE	job evaluation
JEWP	Job Evaluation Working Party
JEMS	*Journal of Emergency Medicine*
JFC	Joint Formulary Committee
JFSSG	Joint Food Safety and Standards Group
JHU	joint health unit
JIF	Joint Investment Fund (Scotland)
JIGSAW	project designed to reduce the need for hospital beds. Co-ordinated by GMAS
JIT	just in time (supplies delivery)
JIP	joint investment plan – what you have to write in your BSVP group
JISC	Joint Information Systems Committee
JLDS	Joint Learning Disability Service (runs CLDTs)
JNC(J)	Joint Negotiating Committee on Junior Doctors' Terms and Conditions of Service
JPAC	Joint Professional Advisory Committee or Joint Planning Advisory Committee (replaced by SWAG)
JRCT	Joseph Rowntree Charitable Trust
JRF	Joseph Rowntree Foundation
JSA	Job Seeker's Allowance
JSE	Joint Strategy Executive
JSG	joint strategy group
JSOG	joint senior officers' group
KF	King's Fund
KFOA	King's Fund Organisational Audit
KED	Kendrick extrication device
KI	key indicator (social services)
KIGS	key indicators, geographical system
KISS	keep it simple stupid
KSF	Knowledge and Skills Framework – part of Agenda for Change
KTD	Kendrick traction device
KTP	knowledge transfer partnership
KVO	keep veins open
LA	local authority
LAA	local authority association
LAC	looked after children *or* local authority circular *or* local authority company
LACOTS	Local Authorities' Co-ordinating Body on Food and Trading Standards
LAD	local authority district
LAF	local advisory forum
LAFS	local authority financial settlement
LAG	local advisory group

LAN	local area network	LGIB	local government international bureau
LAP	local area partnership *or* local action plan	LGIU	local government information unit
LAPIS	locality and practice information system	LGMB	local government management board
LARIA	Local Authorities Research and Intelligence Association	LGPS	local government pension scheme
		LHB	local health board (Wales)
LAS	locum appointment service *or* London Ambulance Service	LHCC	local healthcare co-operative Scottish – a sort of PCG
LASA	London Advice Services Alliance	LHG	local health group – a sort of Welsh PCG
LASFE	local authorities' self-financed expenditure	LIF	Local Initiatives Fund
LASS	local authority social services	LIFT	Local Improvement Finance Trust
LASSL	local authority social services letter	LIG	local implementation group
LAT	locum appointment for training	LIMS	laboratory information management systems
LATF	Local Asthma Taskforce	LINC	Library and Information Commission (obsolete)
LATS	London Academic Training Scheme (part of LIZEI)	LIO	local implementation officer *or* local infrastructure organisation
LAWDC	Local Authority Waste Disposal Company	LIP	local implementation plan
LCFS	local counter fraud specialist	LIS	local implementation strategy *or* library information system
LCMG	local communications user group	LISI	Low Income Scheme Index: a measure of deprivation based on claims for exemption from prescription charges on grounds of low income
LD	learning difficulties *or* local democracy *or* liberal democrat		
LDA	local development agency *or* London Development Agency		
LDAF	Learning Disabilities Award Framework		
LDC	Local Dental Committee – the statutory body of GDPs that represents dental practices in the local area	LIT	local implementation team
		LIZ	London Initiative Zone
		LIZEI	London Implementation Zone Education Initiative
LD/MH	learning difficulties/mental handicap	LLL	lifelong learning
		LLSC	Local Learning and Skills Council
LDP	local delivery plan	LLTI	limiting long-term illness
LDSAG	local diabetes service advisory group	LMC	local medical committee: statutory local committee for all GPs in the area covered by the health authority
LEA	local education authority		
LEC	local enterprise company		
LEI	local employment initiative		
LEL	lower explosive limit	LMCA	Long-term Medical Conditions Alliance
LEO	leading empowered organisations	LMWAG	local medical workforce advisory groups, formed in 1996 to co-ordinate postgraduate medical education between groups of trusts. There are around five or six in each NHS region
LETS	Local Exchange Trading Scheme		
LFS	Labour Force Survey		
LGA	Local Government Association		
LGBT	lesbian gay bisexual and transgender		
LGC	local government chronicle	LNC	local negotiating committee
LGFR	local government finance report	LNRS	local neighbourhood renewal strategy
LGFS	local government financial settlement *or* local government financial statistics	LOBNH	lights on but nobody home
		LOS	length of stay: a measure of activity in hospital wards
LGHA	Local Government and Housing Act 1989		

LNRS	local neighbourhood renewal strategy
LPC	Local Pharmaceutical Committee: a committee of pharmacists
LPI	labour productivity index
LPM	litres per minute
LREC	local research ethics committee
LPS	local pharmaceutical services
LPSA	local public service agreement
LRD	Labour Research Department
LREC	local research ethics committee
LRR	local reference rent
LSC	Legal Services Commission *or* Learning and Skills Council
LSCG	local specialised commissioning group
LSCS	lower segment Caesarean section
LSHTM	London School of Hygiene and Tropical Medicine
LSI	learning style inventory
LSP	local strategic partnership
LSVT	large-scale voluntary transfer
LTA	long-term agreement
LTC	long-term condition
LTM	learning to manage health information
LTP	local transport plan
LTPS	Liability to Third Parties Scheme
LTSA	long-term service agreement
LTVS	long-term ventilatory support
LTSA	long-term service agreement
LURG	local user representative group
LWPG	local winter planning group
LYS	life years saved
MA	Maternity Allowance
MAA	Medical Artists Association of Great Britain
MAAG	Medical Audit Advisory Group *or* Multidisciplinary Audit Advisory Group
MAAQ	Multidisciplinary Audit and Quality Group replaced by the ACTS
MAB	Metropolitan Asylums Board (obsolete)
MAC	Medical Advisory Committee
MACA	Mental After Care Association
MADEL	medical and dental education levy
MADEN	Medical and Dental Education Network
MAF	Management Accountancy Framework
MAGGOT	medically able, go get other transportation

MALDA	multi-agency learning disability assessment
MANCAS	Manchester Care Assessment Schedule
MAP	management action plan
MaPSaF	The Manchester Patient Safety Framework
MAR2C	Matching Resources to Care: this is a mental health information system for caseload monitoring devised to study cases of serious mental illness. MARC2 can compare data from social services, health services and the voluntary sector
MARMAP	multi-agency risk management assessment process
MARP	multi-agency risk assessment panel: decides whether mentally ill people are dangerous
MAS	minimal access surgery
MASC	medical academic staff committee *or* medical advisors' support centre
MAST	multi-agency support team
MASTA	Medical Advisory Services for Travellers Abroad
MAT	medical appeal tribunal
MAVIS	Mobility Advice and Vehicle Information Service
MBA	Master of Business Administration
MC	Medicines Commission
MCA	Medicines Control Agency *or* motorcycle accident
MCCD	medical certificate of cause of death
MCI	mass casualty incident
MCN	managed clinical network
MCO	managed care organisation
MCP	male chauvinist pig (obsolete?)
MCQ	multiple choice question
MCRG	medical career research group
MCSP	Member of the Chartered Society of Physiotherapy
MDA	Medical Devices Agency
MDAP	Multi-Deanery Appointment Process
MDD	Medical Devices Directorate
MDDUS	Medical and Dental Defence Union of Scotland
MDG	Management Development Group (Scotland) *or* muscular dystrophy group
MDI	metered dose inhaler
MDM	medical decision making

MDO	mentally disordered offender *or* medical defence organisation	**MIDIRS**	Midwife Information and Resource Service
MDR	multiple drug resistant	**MIE**	Medical Informatics Europe
MDS	minimum dataset	**MIG**	Medical Information Group
MDT	mobile data terminal *or* multi disciplinary team	***MIMS***	*Monthly Index of Medical Specialties*
MDU	Medical Defence Union	**MIMMS**	major incident medical management and support
ME	management executive *or* myalgic encephalitis	**MINAP**	Myocardial Infarction National Audit Project
MEC	management executive committee *or* management education for clinicians	**MIND**	organisation of mental health users
		MINI	Mental Illness Needs Index
MEDITEL	a GP information system	**Mini-CEX**	mini-clinical evaluation exercise
MEDLARS	Medical Literature Analysis and Retrieval System	**MIQUEST**	s method of extracting information from GP computer systems
MEDS	medical deputising service	**MISG**	Mental Illness Specific Grant: government subsidy to supplement spending by local authorities on social care for mentally ill people living in the community
MEL	Management Executive Letter (Scotland)		
MENCAP	Royal Society for Mentally Handicapped Children andAdults		
MEQ	modified examination question	**MIS**	management information systems
MeReC	*MeReC Bulletin* published by the National Prescribing Centre	**MIT**	minimally invasive therapy *or* Massachusetts Institute of Technology
MERV	medical emergency response vehicle	**MITAG**	Medical Information and Technology Advisory Group
MESB	Medical Education Standards Board		
MeSH	medical subject headings	**MIU**	minor injuries unit
MESOL	management education scheme by open learning	**MLA**	medical laboratory assistant *or* Museums, Libraries and Archives Council
MFF	market forces factor		
MFS	market forces supplement	**MLD**	mild learning disability
MGA	Myasthenia Gravis Association	**MLSO**	*Medical Laboratory Scientific Officer*
MGRG	Management Guidance Review Group	**MMC**	*Modernising Medical Careers*
MHA	Mental Health Act 1983	**MMS**	medical management services
MHAC	Mental Health Act Commission	**MMSAC**	Medical Manpower Standing Advisory Committee (representatives from BMA, Royal Colleges, Regional Manpower committees, Medical Research Council and Council of Deans)
MHC	major histocompatability complex		
MHE	mental health enquiry		
MHG	mental health grant		
MHIG	mental health information group		
MHMDS	mental health minimum dataset		
MHPAF	Mental Health Performance Assessment Framework	**MO**	medical officer
		MOD	Ministry of Defence
MHPSS	Manchester Health Promotion Specialist Service	**MOH**	Medical Officer of Health – a predecessor of the DPH
MHIS	Mental Health Information Strategy	**MOI**	mechanism of injury
MHRA	Medicines and Healthcare Products Regulatory Agency	**MOP**	mobile optical practice
		MOR	millennium operating regime
MHRT	mental health review tribunal convened to hear appeals against detention under the MHA	**MoU**	memorandum of understanding
		MPA	medical prescribing adviser *or* Masters in Public Administration
MHT	Mental Health Task Force	**MPC**	Medical Practices Committee (abolished 2002)
MIA	Medical Insurance Agency		

MPDS	medical priority dispatch system
MPET	Multi-Professional Education and Training Levy
MPIG	minimum practice income guarantee
MPS	Modernising Public Services Group *or* Medical Protection Society
MPT	maximum part time
MPU	Medical Practitioners' Union
MRC	Medical Research Council
MREC	Multicentre Research Ethics Committee
MRFIT	Multiple Risk Factor Intervention Trial
MRO	medical records officer
MRP	minimum revenue provision (part of Capital Control Framework)
MSAC	Maternity Services Advisory Committee
MSD	Merck Sharp and Dohme Ltd
MSDS	material safety data sheet
MSEB	Medical Standards Education Board replacing JCPTGP and STA
MSF	union for skilled and professional workers, including many NHS employees. Formerly ASTMS. Now joined into AMICUS *or* Médecins Sans Frontières *or* multisource feedback
MSGP-4	national study of morbidity in general practice
MSI	Marie Stopes International
MSLC	Maternity Services Liaison Committee: brings together professions involved in maternity services with lay people to agree procedures and monitor their effectiveness as they appear to individual women
MSP	Member of the Scottish Parliament
MSPCG	Most Sparsely Populated Councils Group
MSU	medium secure unit *or* short for MSSU
MTA	management team assistant
MTFP	medium-term financial plan
MTO	medical technical officer
MUSCLE	multistation clinical examination
MV	millennium volunteer
MWC	Mental Welfare Commission
MWCS	Mental Welfare Commission for Scotland
MWEP	Medical Workforce Expansion Programme

MWF	Women's Medical Federation
MWSAC	Medical Workforce Standing Advisory Committee (working for the education committee of the GMC on appraising doctors and dentists in training for SCOPME and on general clinical training during the pre-registration year)
MWSAG	Medical Workforce Standing Advisory Group
NA	nursing auxiliary
NAAS	National Association of Air Ambulance Services
NAB	National Assistance Board (1948–1966)
NAC	National Abortion Campaign
NACAB	National Association of Citizens Advice Bureaux
NACC	National Association for Colitis and Crohn's Disease
NACEPD	National Advisory Council on Employment of People with Disabilities
NACGP	National Association of Commissioning GPs
NACPME	National Advice Centre for Postgraduate Medical Education
NACRO	National Association for the Care and Resettlement of Offenders
NACT	National Association of Clinical Tutors
NACVS	National Association of Councils for Voluntary Service
NAFHP	National Association of Fundholding Practices (obsolete)
NAGST	National Advisory Group for Scientists and Technicians
NAGPT	National Association of GP Tutors
NAGS	NICE Appraisal Groups
NAHAT	former National Association of Health Authorities and Trusts (obsolete)
NAHCSM	National Association of Health Care Supplies Managers
NAHSSO	National Association of Health Service Security Officers
NAHWT	National Association of Health Workers and Travellers
NALHF	National Association of Leagues of Hospital Friends
NANOS	North American Neuro-Ophthalmology Society
NANP	National Association of Non-Principals (now NASGP)

NANT	National Appraisal of New Technologies	**NCB**	National Children's Bureau
NAO	National Audit Office	**NCC**	National Consumer Council
NAPC	National Association of Primary Care formed from the embers of the Fundholding National Association to represent the interests of PCGs	**NCBV**	National Coalition for Black Volunteering
		NCC	National Consumer Council
		NCCA	National Centre for Clinical Audit, now absorbed into NICE or National Community Care Alliance
NAPMECA	National Association of Postgraduate Medical Education Centre Administration	**NCCG**	non-consultant career grade
NAPP	National Association for Patient Participation	**NCCHTA**	National Co-ordinating Centre for Health Technology Assessment
NAPS	National Anti-Poverty Strategy (Ireland)	**NCCSD**	National Co-ordinating Centre for NHS Service Delivery and Organisation Research and Development at the London School of Hygience and Tropical Medicine
NAS	National Autistic Society		
NASEN	National Association for Special Educational Needs	**NCE**	net current expenditure
NASGP	National Association of Sessional GPs representing locums, freelance GPs and Salaried GPs (i.e. non-principals)	**NCEPOD**	National Confidential Enquiry into Patient Outcome and Death (formerly CEPOD)
		NCH	National Children's Home – Action For Children
NASS	National Asylum Support Service	**NCI**	National Captioning Institute
NATN	National Association of Theatre Nurses or National Association of Training Nurses	**NCIL**	National Centre for Independent Living
		NCIS	National Criminal Intelligence Service
NatPaCT	National Primary and Care Trust Development Programme	**NCISH**	National Confidential Enquiry into Suicide and Homicide by People with Mental Illness
N&MC	Nursing and Midwifery Council		
NAVB	National Association of Volunteer Bureaux	**NCL**	National Civic League
		NCMO	National Case Mix Office
NAVHO	National Association of Voluntary Help Organisations	**NCSC**	National Care Standards Commission (abolished 2004)
NAWO	National Alliance of Women's Organisations	**NCSSD**	National Counselling Service for Sick Doctors
NBA	National Blood Authority (England)	**NCT**	National Childbirth Trust
NBAP	National Booked Admissions Programme	**NCV**	National Centre for Volunteering (obsolete)
NBS	National Board for Nursing, Midwifery and Health Visiting for Scotland	**NCVO**	National Council for Voluntary Organisations
NBG	lacking evidence of effectiveness	**NCVCCO**	National Council of Voluntary Child Care Organisations
NBI	National Beds Inquiry		
NBS	National Board for Nursing, Midwifery and Health Visiting for Scotland (obsolete)	**NCVQ**	National Council for Vocational Qualifications
		NCVYS	National Council for Voluntary Youth Services
NBTS	National Blood Transfusion Service (obsolete)	**ND**	New Deal
NB	net book value	**NDC**	National Disability Council or New Deal for Communities
NCAS	National Clinical Assessment Service (formerly NCAA National Clinical Assessment Authority)	**NDPB**	non-departmental public body
		NDPHS	National Disabled Persons' Housing Service
NCASP	National Clinical Audit Support Programme		

NDT	National Development Team for People with Learning Disabilities
NDTMS	National Drug Treatment Monitoring System
NDU	nurse development unit
NDYP	New Deal for Young People
NEAT	new and emerging applications of technology
NED	non-executive director
NEET	not in education employment or training
NEJM	*New England Journal of Medicine*
NeLH	National electronic Library for Health
NERC	Natural Environment Research Council
NESTA	National Endowment for Science Technology and the Arts
NET	new and emerging technologies
NF	Nuffield Foundation
NFA	no fixed address
NFAP	National Framework for Assessing Performance
NFI	National Fraud Initiative
NFP	not for profit
NFR	not for resuscitation
NFW	no further work
NGfL	National Grid for Learning
NGO	non-governmental organisation
NHAIS	National Health Authority Information Systems
NHD	notional half day (consultants)
NHF	National Heart Forum
NHFA	Nursing Homes Fees Agency
NHIS	National Health Intelligence Service
NHLI	National Heart and Lung Institute, Imperial College
NHS	National Health Service
NHS(S)	National Health Service in Scotland
NHSAR	National Health Service Administrative Register
NHSBSP	NHS Breast Screening Programme
NHSCA	NHS Consultants Association
NHSCCA	NHS and Community Care Act (1990)
NHSCCC	NHS Centre for Coding and Classification
NHSCSF	NHS Counter Fraud Service
NHSCSFMS	NHS Counter Fraud and Security Management Service
NHSCR	NHS Central Register
NHS CRS	NHS Care Records Service
NHSCTA	NHS clinical trials advisor
NHSE	NHS Executive (abolished 2002) *or* NHS estates
NHSEED	NHS Economic Evaluation Database
NHSEHU	NHS ethnical health unit
NHS FAM	NHS fraud awareness month
NHSFT	NHS foundation trust
NHSIA	NHS Information Authority (abolished 2005)
NHSIII	NHS Institute for Innovation and Improvement
NHS IMC	NHS information centre
NHS KSF	NHS Knowledge and Skills Framework
NHSL	NHS logistics
NHSLA	NHS Litigation Authority
NHSME	NHS Management Executive (in England) now called the NHSE
NHSME	NHS Management Executive (Scotland)
NHSOE	NHS Overseas Enterprises
NHS(S)	National Health Service in Scotland
NHSS	National Health Service Supplies, *or* NHS Scotland
NHSSMS	NHS Security Management Service
NHST	NHS trust
NHSTD	NHS Service Training Directorate/ Division
NHSTF	NHS trust federation
NHSTU	NHS training unit
NHSP	NHS partners
NHSS	NHS supplies *or* national healthy schools standard
NHST	NHS trust
NHSTD	NHS training directorate
NHSTF	NHS Trust Federation
NHSTU	NHS training unit
NHSU	NHS University (obsolete)
NHSnet	intranet for the NHS
NI	National Insurance
NIACE	National Institute of Adult and Continuing Education
NIAS	Northern Ireland Ambulance Service
NIC	net ingredient cost – the basic price of a drug *or* National Insurance Contribution
NICARE	Northern Ireland Centre for Health Care Co-operation and Development

NICE	National Institute for Health and Clinical Excellence *or* Northern Institute for Continuing Education	**NPFIT**	National Programme for IT in the NHS
NICEC	National Institute for Carers and Educational Counselling	**NPG**	*Modernising Health and Social Services*: National Priorities Guidance HSC 1998/159
NICON	NHS Confederation in Northern Ireland	**NPHT**	Nuffield Provincial Hospitals Trust
NICS	Northern Ireland Civil Service	**NPIS**	National Poisons Information Service
NICU	neonatal intensive care unit	**NPL**	National Physical Laboratory
NICVA	Northern Ireland Council for Voluntary Action	**NPRB**	Nurses' Pay Review Body
		NPSA	National Patient Safety Agency
NIH	National Institute of Health *or* Nuffield Institute for Health (Leeds)	**NPT**	near patient testing
		NPV	net present value
NIHSS	Nosocomial Infection National Surveillance Scheme	**NRC**	National Regionalisation Consortium
NILO	National Investment and Loans Office	**NRCI**	national reference cost index
NIMHE	National Institute for Mental Health in England	**NRE**	non-recurring expenditure
		NRLS	National Reporting and Learning System
NINo	National Insurance number	**NRPB**	National Radiological Protection Board
NISW	National Institute of Social Work (obsolete)	**NRR**	National Research Register
NJC	National Joint Council	**NRS**	neighbourhood renewal strategy
NLM	National Library of Medicine	**NRT**	nicotine replacement therapy
NOS	national occupation standards	**NSC**	National Screening Committee (UK)
NOMIS	National Online Manpower Information Service	**NSCAG**	National Specialist Commissioning Advisory Group
NOP	national opinion polls	**NSEC**	National Smoking Education Campaign
NMAC	National Medical Advisory Committee	**NSF**	National Service Framework *or* National Schizophrenia Fellowship (now called Rethink)
NMAP	Nursing Midwifery and Allied Health Professionals (internet resource)		
		NSFMH	National Service Framework – Mental Health
NMC	Nursing and Midwifery Council	**NSMI**	National Sports Medicine Institute UK
NMDS	nursing minimum dataset		
NMET	non-medical education and training	**NSPCC**	National Society for the Prevention of Cruelty to Children
NMIS	nurse management information system	**NSRC**	National Schedule of Reference Costs
NNH	number needed to harm	**NSTS**	NHS Strategic Tracing Service
NNT	number needed to treat	**NSU**	non-specific urethritis – a common STD
NOF	National Opportunities Fund		
NP	non-principal	**NSV**	national supplies vocabulary
NPA	National Pharmaceutical Association	**NTA**	National Treatment Agency
		NTN	national training number
NPAT	National Patients' Access Team	**NTO**	national training organisation
NPC	National Prescribing Centre – based in Liverpool. Formerly known as MASC. Publishes *MeReC Bulletin* which is distributed to all GPs on request *or* net present cost	**NTT**	nuchal translucency thickness: screening method for Down's sydrome
		NTTRL	National Tissue Typing Reference Laboratory
NPCRDC	National Primary Care Research and Development Centre – based in the University of Manchester		

NVP	newly vulnerable person
NVQ	National Vocational Qualification
NWCS	nationwide clearing service: all trusts must submit data about admitted patient care which is then forwarded to HAs.
NWIPP	National Workforce Information and Planning Programme
NWN	NHS-wide networking
NWSI	nurse with a special interest
NYCD-OHMH	New York City Department of Health and Mental Hygiene
O&M	organisation and methods
OAT	out of area treatment (the replacement for ECR)
OBC	outline business case
OBD	occupied bed day
OBS	output-based specification
OCD	obsessive–compulsive disorder
OCN	Open College Network
OCPA	Office of the Commissioner for Public Appointments
OCR	optical character recognition *or* optical character reader
OCS	order communication system *or* organisational codes service
OD	organisational development *or* overdose *or* once daily *or* outside diameter
ODA	Overseas Development Agency *or* Overseas Doctors Agency *or* operating department assistant
ODP	operating department practitioner
ODPM	Office of the Deputy Prime Minister
ODTS	Overseas Doctors' Training Scheme of appropriate Royal College
ODO	operating department orderly
OECD	Organisation for Economic Co-operation and Development
OEL	occupational exposure limit
OH	occupational health
OHAG	Oral Health Advisory Group
OHE	Office of Health Economics (London)
OHN	*Our Healthier Nation* (Cm3852)
OHS	occupational health service
OIC	officer in charge
OIE	Office International des Epizooties
OIHCP	Office for Information on Health Care Performance
OISC	Office of the Immigration Services Commissioner
OJEC	*Official Journal of the European Community*

OME	Office of Manpower Economics
OMNI	Organising Medical Networked Information
OMP	ophthalmic medical practitioner
OMV	open market value
OMVEU	open market value in existing use
ONS	Office for National Statistics: the result of a merger in April 1996 of the Central Statistical Office and the Office of Population Censuses and Surveys
OOH	out of hours
OP	outpatient
OPAC	Online Public Access Catalogue
OPCS	former Office of Population, Census and Surveys (system for classifying disease and treatment), now Office for National Statistics (ONS)
OPD	outpatient department
OPHIS	Office for Public Health in Scotland
OPM	Office of Public Management
OPSI	Office of Public Sector Information (was TSO and, prior to that, HMSO)
OR	operation research: a scientific method which uses models of a system to evaluate alternative courses of action with a view to improving decision making
OSB	other services block (now replaced by EPCS)
OSC	Overview and Scrutiny Committee
OSCE	observed structured clinical examination
OSDLS	Open Source Digital Library System
OST	Office of Science and Technology
OT	occupational therapist/therapy
OTC	over the counter – medicines not requiring a prescription
OU	Open University
OVE	occlusive vascular event
OWAM	*Organisation with a Memory*
OWW	One World Week
OXERA	Oxford Economic Research Associates
PA	patients' association – patients' mechanism to communicate with medical services *or* police authority *or* personal assistant
PABX	public area branch exchange
PAC	Public Accounts Committee
PACE	promoting action on clinical effectiveness *or* Property Advisers to the Civil Estate or Police & Criminal Evidence Act 1984

PACS picture archiving and communication system: a replacement for X-ray film

PACT prescribing analysis and costs: GPs get regular PACT reports from the PPA giving details of their recent prescribing, comparing them with local and national averages *or* placing, assessment and counselling team

PAD peripheral arterial disease

PAF Performance Assessment Framework *or* public audit forum

PAGB Proprietary Association of Great Britain

PALS patient advice and liaison service

PAMIS Parliamentary Monitoring and Intelligence Service

PAMP pathogen-associated molecular pattern

PAMs professions allied to medicine – e.g. physiotherapists, OTs etc

PAR programme analysis and review

PARN Professional Associations Research Network

PAS patient administration system : a main hospital database *or* physician-assisted suicide

PASA purchasing and supply agency

PASG pneumatic anti-shock garment

PAT personnel accountability tag *or* policy action team *or* peer assessment tool

P&T professional and technical

PAYE Pay As You Earn

PBC public benefit corporation

PBL problem-based learning

PBR pre-budget report *or* payment by results

PBRS public benefit recording system

PBx private branch exchange: type of internal telephone network

PC primary care *or* patients' council *or* personal computer *or* politically correct *or* parish council *or* public convenience

PCA patient-controlled analgesia – usually a morphine pump

PCAG primary care audit group – i.e. multidisciplinary

PCAPs primary care act pilots: the NHS (Primary Care) Act 1997 allowed NHS trusts, NHS employees, qualified bodies and suitably experienced medical practitioners to submit proposals to provide general medical services under a contract with the health authority

PCC primary care centre

PCG primary care group (obsolete *see* HSC 1998/230)

PCIP primary care investment plan

PCHR personal child health record

PCL provision for credit liabilities

PCMCN Peninsula Cardiac Managed Clinical Network

PCO primary care organisation: generic term for PCT in England, health and social services board in Northern Ireland, local health board in Wales and primary care division within area health board in Scotland

PCP personal communication profile *or* person-centred planning

PCRC primary care resource centre

PCRTA primary care research team assessment

PCS public and commercial services union

PCS/E Patient Classification System/Europe

PCT primary care trust

PDC public dividend capital: a form of long-term government finance on which the NHS trust pays dividends to the government. PDC has no fixed remuneration or repayment obligations, but in the long term the overall return on PDC is expected to be no less than on an equivalent loan

PDD prescribed daily dose: the average daily dose which is actually prescribed *or* pervasive development disorder

PDF Partnership Development Fund

PDO property damage only

PDP personal development plan *or* practice development plan

PDR personal development review

PDS personal dental services *or* Parkinson's Disease Society

PDSA plan, do, study, act

PE physical examination *or* pulmonary embolism

PEA pulseless electrical activity

PEAT	patient environment action team		**PHeL**	Public Health electronic Library
PEC	professional executive committee		**PHIS**	Public Health Institute of Scotland
PECS	picture exchange communication system		**PHL**	public health laboratory
			PHLS	public health laboratory service
PEDC	potential elderly domiciliary clients (part of SSA)		**PHO**	public health observatory
			PHOENIX	primary healthcare organisations exchanging new ideas for excellence
PEDW	Patient Episode Database Wales		**PHP**	public health practitioner
PEG	percutaneous endoscopic gastrostomy		**PHPU**	public health policy unit
PEM	prescription event monitoring		**PHR**	personal health record
PES	public expenditure survey *or* Property Expenses Scheme		**PHRRC**	Public Health Research and Resource Centre at the University of Salford
PESC	Public Expenditure Survey Committee (obsolete)		**PHSS**	personal health summary system
PESR	potential elderly supported residents (part of SSA)		**PI**	performance indicator *or* parallel imports
PET	positron emission tomography		**PIA**	partnership in action *or* personal injury accident *or* patient impact assessment
PETA	People for the Ethical Treatment of Animals			
PETS	paediatric emergency transfer service		**PICKUP**	professional, industrial and commercial updating
PEWP	Public Expenditure White Paper		**PICS**	platform for internet content selection
PF	patients' forum		**PICU**	paediatric or psychiatric ICU
PFC	patient-focused care *or* Professional Fees Committee		**PIDA**	Public Interest Disclosure Act
			PIF	patient information forum
PFI	private finance initiative, now replaced by PPP		**PIG**	policy implementation group *or* promoting independence grant *or* professional interest group
PFMA	practice fund management allowance: allowance given to GP fundholders to manage their allocation. The allowance is primarily spent upon staff and equipment		**PIL**	patient information leaflet
			PIMS	product information management system
			PIN	personal identification number *or* prior identification notice
PFU	private finance unit		**PIU**	performance and innovation unit
PGCME	postgraduate and continuing medical education		**PLAB**	professional and linguistic assessment board
PGD	postgraduate dean *or* patient group directions		**PLOS**	Public Library of Science
			PLP	personal learning plan
PGEA	postgraduate education allowance		**PLPI**	product licence parallel import
PGMDE	postgraduate medical and dental education		**PLT**	protected learning time
			PM	project management
PHA	Public Health Alliance, now part of UKPHA		**PMCPA**	Prescription Medicines Code of Practice Authority
PHAB	physically disabled and able-bodied		**PMD**	performance management directorate
PHANYC	Public Health Association of New York City		**PMETB**	Postgraduate Medical Education and Training Board
PHC	primary health care		**PMI**	private medical insurance
PHCDS	public health common dataset		**PMR**	physical medicine and rehabilitation
PHCSG	primary healthcare specialist group			
PHCT	primary healthcare team		**PMA**	personal medical attendant: what insurance companies etc call a doctor who writes a report for them
PHCSG	Primary Health Care Specialist Group of the British Computer Society			

PMD	prescribing monitoring document	PPG	principal police grant *or* planning policy guidance
PMETB	Postgraduate Medical Education and Training Board	PPI	patient and public involvement *or* proton pump inhibitor
PMF	Performance Management Framework	PPIF	patient and public involvement forum
PMI	private medical insurance	PPM	planned preventative maintenance
PMLD	profound and multiple learning disabilities	PPO	preferred provider organisation
PMR	physical medicine and rehabilitation *or* progressive muscle relaxation	PPP	private patients' plan *or* public private partnership
		PPPFC	Private Practice and Professionals Fees Committee
PMS	personal medical service *or* post-marketing surveillance	PPPP	Public–Private Partnership Programme (also known as '4Ps')
PND	postnatal depression	PPRS	Pharmaceutical Price Regulation Scheme
PNL	prior notification list (of patients for screening)	PPU	private patients' unit
POC	point of care	PQ	parliamentary question *or* post-qualification
POCT	point of care testing		
PODS	patient's own drugs	PQASSO	Practical Quality Assurance System for Small Organisations
POINT	publications on the internet (Department of Health)	PR	public relations *or* per rectum (no known connection?)
POISE	procurement of information systems effectively: the standard procedure followed for procurement of information systems	PRA	preventing and responding to aggression
		PRB	pay review body
POLIS	Parliamentary Online Indexing Service	PREPP	post registration education and preparation for practice (nurses)
POLST	physician's orders for life-sustaining treatment	PRHO	pre-registration house officer
		PRIAE	Policy Research Institute on Ageing and Ethnicity
POM	prescription-only medicine	PRIMIS	primary care information services
POMR	problem-oriented medical records	PRINCE	Projects in Controlled Environments: a standard project management methodology used in all NHS information systems projects
POPUMET	Protection of Persons Undergoing Medical Examination (regulations)		
POSIX	portable operating system interface		
POU	pulmonary oncology unit – chest cancers		
POVA	protection of vulnerable adults from abuse	PRO	Public Record Office
		PRODIGY	Prescribing RatiOnally with Decision-support In General-practice studY
PPA	Prescription Pricing Authority: costs all prescriptions dispensed in England in order to pay chemists for the costs of the drugs etc they dispense		
		PRP	performance-related pay
		PRT	personal risk training
		PRU	police resources unit (part of Home Office)
PPBS	planning, programming and budgeting system	PSA	public service agreement *or* prostate-specific antigen
PPC	promoting patient choice		
PPDP	practice professional development plan	PSBR	public sector borrowing requirement
PPDR	practice profession development and revalidation	PSC	public sector comparator
		PSFD	public sector financing deficit
PPE	personal protective equipment	PSG	prescribing strategy group
PPF	Priorities and Planning Framework	PSHE	personal social and health education

PSI	Policy Studies Institute (London)
PSL	period of study leave: GPs can apply in accordance with paragraph 50 of the Statement of Fees and Allowances for financial assistance in connection with a period of study leave to undertake postgraduate education, which will result in benefit to the GP, primary care in particular and the NHS
PSM	professions supplementary to medicine
PSNC	Pharmaceutical Services Negotiating Committee: represents chemists in negotiations with the DoH
PSNCR	public sector net cash requirement
PSND	public sector net deficit
PSRCS	police standard radio communication system
PSS	personal social services
PSSRU	personal social services research unit
PSU	prescribing support unit
PSX	public service expenditure
PT	part-time
PTCA	percutaneous transluminal coronary angioplasty
PTL	patient-targeting list
PTS	patient transport services
PTSD	post-traumatic stress disorder
PU	prescribing unit: developed to take account of elderly patients' greater need for medication. Patients over 65 years count as three PUs and those under 65 years as one
PUNs	patient's unmet needs
PVC	prime vendor contract
PVS	persistent vegetative state
PWLB	Public Works Loans Board
PYE	part-year effect
QA	quality assurance
QAA	Quality Assurance Authority
QALY	quality-adjusted life year
QABME	Quality Assurance of Basic Medical Education
QC	Quality Control or Quick Connect
QCA	Qualifications and Curriculum Authority
QOF	Quality and Outcomes Framework
QOL	quality of life
QR	quick release
QSW	qualified social worker

QUANGO	quasi-autonomous non-governmental organisation
R&D	research and development
RA	regional advisor or research associate or revenue account or regional assembly or rheumatoid arthritis
RADAR	Royal Association for Disability and Rehabilitation
RADTS	Referral Assessment, Diagnostics and Treatment Service
RAE	research assessment exercise
RAG	research allocation group (NHS Executive)
RAGE	radiotherapy action group exposure
RAM	risk allocation matrix
RAO	referral and advice officer: first point of contact for enquiries about social services
RAP	referrals, assessments and packages of care in adult personal social services
RAPt	rehabilitation for addicted prisoners trust
RARM	remote and rural medicine
RA(SG)	revenue account (specific grants)
R&S	recruitment and selection
RASP	resource allocation and service planning
RAWP	Resource Allocation Working Party: the working party devised a method of distributing resources to health authorities equitably in relation to need, which was used from 1977–1989. The system has been superseded by weighted capitation payments
RB	representative body (BMA)
RBE	relative biological effectiveness
RBMS	referral booking and management system
RCA	Royal College of Anaesthetists or root cause analysis
RCC	rural community council
RCCS	revenue consequences of capital schemes or Reid clinical classification system
RCCO	revenue contributions to capital outlay
RCGP	Royal College of General Practitioners
RCH	residential care home
RCM	Royal College of Midwives
RCN	Royal College of Nursing

RCO	refugee community organisation
RCOG	Royal College of Obstetricians and Gynaecologists
RCOphth	Royal College of Ophthalmologists
RCP	Royal College of Physicians
RCPath	Royal College of Pathologists
RCPCH	Royal College of Paediatrics and Child Health
RCPHIU	Royal College of Physicians Health Informatics Unit
RCPiLab	Royal College of Physicians Information Laboratory
RCPsych	Royal College of Psychiatrists
RCR	Royal College of Radiologists
RCS	Royal College of Surgeons
RCSLT	Royal College of Speech and Language Therapists
RCT	randomised control trial
RCU	regional co-ordination unit
RDA	regional development agency *or* rural development area
RDBMS	relational database management system
RDC	rural district council (obsolete except in former UK colonies) *or* Rural Development Commission
RDF	Resource Description Framework
RDN	Resource Discovery Network
RDPGPE	regional director of postgraduate general practice education
RDRD	regional director of research and development
RDS	respiratory distress syndrome
RDSU	research and development support unit
RDU	regional dialysis unit
REA	regional education advisor
REACH	research and education for children in asthma *or* retired executives action clearing house
REAL	research, education, audit, libraries
REC	research ethics committee *or* Racial Equality Council
REDG	regional education and development group
RES	regional economic strategy
RFA	requirements for accreditation (GP computers)
RFC	request for comment
RFDS	Royal Flying Doctor Service
RG	registrar-general
RGD	revenue grants distribution

RGD(RG)	revenue grants distribution (review group)
RGPEC	regional general practice education committee
RGN	registered general nurse
RHA	regional health authority (obsolete)
RHB	regional hospital board (obsolete)
RHI	regional head of information
RHV	registered health visitor
RIDDOR	reporting of injuries, diseases and dangerous occurrences regulations
RINN	recommended international non-proprietary name
RIPA	Royal Institute of Public Administration
RIPHH	Royal Institute of Public Health and Hygiene
RIS	radiology information system
RITA	record of individual (in-training) training assessment
RIU	regulatory impact unit
RJDC	regional junior doctors' committee
RLG	NHS regional librarians group
RLQ	right lower quadrant
RLS	restless legs syndrome
RM	resource management
RMA	refuse(s) medical assistance
RMC	Regional Manpower Committee (now gone)
RMI	resource management initiative
RMN	registered mental nurse
RMO	resident medical officer *or* responsible medical officer
RN	registered nurse
RNCC	registered nursing care contribution
RNHA	Registered Nursing Home Association
RNIB	Royal National Institute for the Blind
RNID	Royal National Institute for Deaf People
RNMH	registered nurse for the mentally handicapped
RO NHS	regional office *or* revenue out-turn
ROC	return on capital *or* Retained Organs Commission (obsolete)
ROCE	return on capital employed
ROCR	review of central returns
ROE	Regional Office for Europe (WHO)
ROS	return on sale
ROSPA	Royal Society for the Prevention of Accidents
RoW	rights of women
RP	reporting party

RPA	Review of Public Administration	SALT	speech and language therapist
RPC	Regional Planning Conference (often now part of Regional Assembly)	SAMH	Scottish Association of Mental Health
		SAMM	safety assessment of marketed medicines (guidelines)
RPGD	regional postgraduate dean	SAP	single assessment process
RPHTF	Regional Prison Health Task Force	SAPHE	Self-Assessment in Professional and Higher Education 1996–9
RPPG	regional policy planning guidance		
RPSGB	Royal Pharmaceutical Society of Great Britain	SAR	subjective analysis return or search and rescue
RPST	Risk Pooling Scheme for Trusts	SARS	severe acute respiratory syndrome
RR	relative risk	SAS	staff and associate specialists or standard accounting system or Scottish Ambulance Service
RRMS	relaxing and remitting multiple sclerosis		
RS	rescue squad	SAT	service action team
RSC	Royal Society of Chemistry	SAZ	sport action zone
RSCG	regional specialised commissioning group	SBS	small business service
		SBU	Swedish Council on Technology Assessment in Health Care
RSCN	registered sick children's nurse		
RSH	Royal Society of Health	SCA	Supplementary Credit Approval (part of Capital Control Framework)
RSI	repetitive strain injury or rapid sequence induction or rough sleepers' initiative		
		SCBA	self-contained breathing apparatus
		SCBU	special care baby unit
RSIN	rural stress information network	SCCD	Standing Conference on Community Development
RSM	Royal Society of Medicine		
RSS	Royal Statistical Society	SCD	sickle cell disease
RSU	regional secure unit or rough sleepers' unit	SCF	Save the Children Fund or Scottish Council Foundation or Safer Communities Fund
RSVP	Retired and Senior Volunteers' Programme		
		SCG	specialised commissioning group
RSW	residential social work	ScHARR	School of Health and Related Research, University of Sheffield
RTF	regional task force		
RTA	road traffic accident	SCHIN	Sowerby Centre for Health Informatics at Newcastle
RTIA	receipts taken into account (part of Capital Control Framework)		
		SCI	self-certificate for first week of an illness
RVSN	regional voluntary sector network		
RxList	internet drug index	SCID	severe combined immune deficiency
SABA	supplied air breathing apparatus	SCIE	Social Care Institute for Excellence
SAC	specialist advisory committee (of the Royal Colleges): oversees higher medical training	SCIEH	Scottish Centre for Infection and Environmental Health
		SCM	specialist in community medicine
SACN	Scientific Advisory Committee on Nutrition	SCMH	Sainsbury Centre for Mental Health
		SCMO	senior clinical medical officer
SAD	seasonal affective disorder	SCODA	Standing Conference on Drug Abuse
SAED	semi-automatic external defibrillator		
		SCOPE	Society for people with Cerebral Palsy
SaFF	Service and Finance Framework: document setting out commissioning intentions for the following year.		
		SCOPME	Standing Committee on Postgraduate Medical and Dental Education
SAGNIS	Strategic Advisory Group for Nursing Information Systems	SCORPME	Standing Committee on Regional Postgraduate Medical Education
SAHC	Scottish Association of Health Councils	SCOTH	Scientific Committee on Tobacco and Health

SCP	Society of Chiropodists and Podiatrists *or* single capital pot *or* spinal column point (position on pay-scale) *or* shared care protocol *or* short course programme
SCPMDE	Scottish Council for Postgraduate Medical and Dental Education
SCR	social care region
SCS	Senior Civil Service
SCT	Society of County Treasurers
SCVO	Scottish Council for Voluntary Organisations
SCVS	CVS Scotland
SDA	Severe Disability Allowance (obsolete) *or* service delivery agreement *or* Sex Discrimination Act
SDO	service delivery organisation
SDP	service delivery practice (NHS web database) *or* subdivisional partnership *or* severe disability premium
SDU	service delivery unit
SEA	significant event audit
SEAC	Spongiform Encephalopathy Committee: advises HMG on BSE
SEACAG	South East Ambulance Clinical Audit Group
SEAP	South East Advocacy Project
SEC	specialist education committee *or* standards and ethics committee
SEG	socio-economic group
SEHD	Scottish Executive Health Department
SEMI	severe and enduring mental illness
SEN	special educational needs *or* state enrolled nurse
SEO	Society of Education Officers
SEPHO	South East Public Health Observatory
SERNIP	Safety and Efficiency Register of New Interventional Procedures run by the Medical Royal Colleges
SERPS	State Earnings-Related Pension Scheme
SEU	social exclusion unit *or* sentence enforcement unit
SFA	statement of fees and allowances: the GP's *Red Book*
SFDF	Scottish Food and Drink Federation
SFF	Service and Finance Framework: document setting out commissioning intentions for the following year

SFI	standing financial instructions: financial procedures and framework for the health authority *or* social fund inspector
SG	staff grade
SG1 (2 or 3)	Sector Group 1 etc (part of CLP covering best value)
SGHT	Standing Group on Health Technology
SGML	standard general mark-up language
SGPC	Scottish General Practitioners' Committee: part of the BMA
SGR	Scientists for Global Responsibility
SGUMDER	Standing Group on Undergraduate Medical and Dental Education and Research
SHA	special health authority *or* strategic health authority *or* Socialist Health Association
SHARE	Scottish Health Authorities Revenue Equalisation
SHAS	Scottish Health Advisory Service
SHEPS	Society of Health Education and Health Promotion Specialists
SHIFT	substitution of hospital and other institutional-focused technology
SHMO	senior hospital medical officer
SHO	senior house officer
SHOT	serious hazards of transfusion
SHOW	Scottish Health on the Web
SHRINE	Strategic Human Resources Information Network
SHTAC	Scottish Health Technology Assessment Centre
SI	statutory instrument
SIA	Spinal Injuries Association
SIDS	sudden infant death syndrome
SIFT	service increment for teaching: cash to hospitals for training medical students
SIFTR	service increment for teaching and research: the costs of undergraduate medical (and dental) education and research in teaching hospitals is met through SIFTR It is intended to prevent some NHS trusts being at a disadvantage in cost terms by having to include these elements in contract prices
SIG	special interest group
SIGN	Scottish Intercollegiate Guidelines Network

SIMS	standardised incident management system
SING	Sexuality Issues Network Group
SIS	Supplies Information Service *or* Statistical Information Service (run by IPF)
SITF	Social Investment Task Force
SLA	service level agreement
SLS	selected list scheme for drugs which are restricted to particular conditions
SMA	spinal muscular atrophy
SMAC	Standing Medical Advisory Committee
SMART	specific, measurable, attainable, relevant, timed (of objectives)
SMAS	substance misuse advisory service
SMC	Scottish Medicines Consortium (a sort of Scottish NICE)
SMI	severe mental impairment: people with SMI do not have to pay Council Tax
SMO	senior medical officer
SMP	Statutory Maternity Pay
SMR	standardised mortality ratio *or* standardised morbidity ratio
SN	staff nurse
SNAFU	situation normal, all fouled up
SNMAC	Standing Nursing and Midwifery Advisory Committee
SNOMED	systematised nomenclature of human (and veterinary) medicine
SNP	single nucleotide polymorphism: a marker of genetic difference *or* Scottish Nationalist Party
SNTN	Scottish national training number
SO	standing orders
SOAP	Shipley Ophthalmic Assessment Service
SOCITM	Society of Information Technology Managers
SODoH	Scottish Department of Health (obsolete)
SOHHD	Scottish Home Office and Health Department (obsolete)
SON	statement of need
SOP	standard operational procedure
SoS/SofS	Secretary of State
SOSIG	Social Science Information Gateway
SP	strategic plan
SPA	Scottish Prescribing Analysis *or* Small Practices Association
SPAIN	Social Policy Ageing Information Network
SPC	summary of product characteristics
SPG	(NHS) security policy group
SPIN	Sandwell Public Information Network
SPP	statutory paternity pay
SPS	standard payroll system
SPV	special purpose vehicle
SQP	suitably qualified person
SR	Society of Radiographers *or* senior registrar (obsolete) *or* spending review or sister
SRD	state-registered dietician
SRE	sex and relationship education
SRSAG	supra-regional services advisory group
SS	spreadsheet
SSA	standard spending assessment
SSAP	statement of standard accounting practice (now being replaced by FRS)
SSARG	Standard Spending Assessment Reduction Grant
SSAT	Social Security Appeal Tribunal
SSC	shared services centre *or* Sector Skills Council
SSCF	Safer and Stronger Communities Fund
SSD	social services department
SSDP	Strategic Service Development Plan
SSHA	Society of Sexual Health Advisers
SSI	Social Services Inspectorate: transferred to Commission for Social Care Inspection 2004 or Standard Spending Indicator (part of SSA)
SSIP	Strategic Service Implementation Plan
SSIS	Social Services Information System
SSM	special study module *or* system status management
SSP	Statutory Sick Pay *or* subregional strategic partnership
SSR	service strategy and regulation
SSRADU	social services research and development unit
SSRG	social services research group
SSSI	Site of special scientific interest
STA	specialist training authority of Royal Colleges
STAR	short-term assessment and rehabilitation team: social services

	teams which provide up to four weeks of care for people leaving hospital and residential homes and returning home
STAR-PU	specific therapeutic group age–sex related prescribing unit
StBOP	*Shifting the Balance of Power*
STC	specialty training committee (of local postgraduate dean)
STD	sexually transmitted disease
STEIS	strategic executive information system
STG	special transitional grant: Department of Health money given to social services to change to community care (now defunct)
StN	student nurse
STP	short-term programme
STSS	short-term support services: planned residential respite care for people with learning disabilities.
SU	strategy unit (Cabinet Office) *or* students' union
SUI	serious untoward incident
SURE	Service User Research Enterprise
SWAG	Specialist Workforce Advisory Group: a group focused on the number of doctors required to provide the service
SWG	Specialty Working Group *or* Settlement Working Group *or* Service Working Group
SWOT	an analysis of strengths, weakness, opportunities and threats (usually relates to organisations but could apply equally to an individual)
TAB	team assessment behaviour
T&CS	Terms and conditions of service (*see also* TCS)
TAG	Technical Advisory Group
TALOBIA	there's a lot of it about
T&O	trauma and orthopaedics
TAP	trainee assistant practitioner
TATT	tired all the time
TBA	to be announced *or* to be arranged
TC	town council *or* total communication
TCBL	temporary capital borrowing limit (part of Capital Control Framework)
TCI	to come in
TCP	Total Commissioning Project
TCS	terms and conditions of service (*see also* T&CS)

TDHC	The Doctors' Healthcare Company
TEACCH	treatment and education of autistic and related communication handicapped children
TEC	Training and Enterprise Council (now abolished)
TEETH	tried everything else, try homoeopathy
TEL	Trust Executive Letter
TICK	teamwork, integrity, courage, knowledge
TIE	theatre in education
TIP	Trust Implementation Plan (Scotland)
TIS	technical information services
TLA	three letter abbreviation or acronym like this one
TME	trust management executive
TMB	too many birthdays
TME	total managed expenditure
TNA	training needs analysis
TOD	took own discharge
TOIL	time off in lieu
TOPRA	The Organisation for Professionals in Regulatory Affairs
TOPS	Termination of Pregnancy Service
TOPSS	Training Organisation for Personal Social Services
TPC	teenage pregnancy co-ordinator
TPD	training programme director
TPP	Total Purchasing Project
TPQ	threshold planning quantity
TPU	teenage pregnancy unit
TQM	total quality management
TR	technical release (term used by Audit Commission)
TRB	temporary revenue borrowing limit (part of Capital Control Framework)
TRiP	turning research into practice
TRIPS	trade-related intellectual property rights
TRO	time ran out
TSE	transmissible spongiform encephalopathies
TSC	technical subcommittee
TSG	Transport Supplementary Grant
TSO	The Stationery Office (formerly HMSO and now OPSI)
TSP	Training Support Programme
TSS	total standard spending
TSSU	theatre sterile supplies unit
TUBE	totally unnecessary breast examination

TUPE	Transfer of Undertakings (Protection of Employment) Regulations 1981
TV	transfer value
TWG	technical working group
UA	unitary authority: a council which carries out all the functions in its area
UASC	unaccompanied asylum-seeking children
UASSG	Unlinked Anonymous Surveys Steering Group
UB	Unemployment Benefit (now JSA)
UCAS	Universities College Admission Service
UEL	upper explosive limit
UEMS	European Union of Medical Specialists
UGM	unit general manager
UK	unit labour cost: staff cost required to provide a given unit of activity
UKADCU	UK Anti-Drugs Co-ordination Unit (formerly Drugs Co-ordination Unit)
UKAN	United Kingdom Advocacy Network
UKCC	United Kingdom Central Council for Nursing, Midwifery and Health Visiting (abolished 2002) or UK Cochrane Centre
UKCHHO	United Kingdom Clearing House on Health Outcomes (Leeds)
UKCNR	UK Clinical Research Network
UKDIPG	United Kingdom Drug Information Pharmacists' Group
UKHFAN	United Kingdom Health for All Network
UKOLN	UK Office for Library and Information Networking
UKPHA	United Kingdom Public Health Alliance
UKTSSA	United Kingdom Transplant Support Service Authority
ULTRA	Unrelated Live Transplant Regulatory Authority
UMLS	unified medical language system
UNICEF	United Nations Children's Fund
UNISON	trades union for public sector workers, incorporating COHSE, NALGO and NUPE
UPA	underprivileged area: a measure of deprivation – 0 is the mean for England
URL	universal (or uniform) resource locator (on internet)

UTD	unit training director
UTG	unified training grade (now SpR)
UTH	university teaching hospital
VA	voluntary action or voluntary-aided or vote account
VAMP	a GP information system supplier user group
VAT	value added tax
VB	volunteer bureau
VC	voluntary-controlled or variable cost
VCO(s)	voluntary and community organisation(s)
VCS	voluntary and community sector
VCT	voluntary competitive tendering
VDRFAMP	vascular disease risk factor assessment and management process
VFM	value for money
VFMU	value for money unit
VHI	Voluntary Health Insurance (Ireland)
VOCOSE	voluntary, community and social economy
VPE	virtual private exchange (type of internal telephone network)
VSA	volatile substance abuse
VSC	voluntary service co-ordinator
VSNTO	Voluntary Sector National Training Organisation
VSpR	visiting specialist registrar
VSO	voluntary sector option (New Deal) or voluntary service overseas
VSPG	voluntary sector policy and grants
VTE	venous thromboembolism
VTN	visiting training number
VTR	vocational training record
VTS	vocational training scheme (the mandatory scheme of structured experience and training in hospitals and the community for doctors planning a career in general practice)
WAA	Working Age Agency
WADEM	World Association for Disaster and Emergency Medicine
WAHAT	Welsh Association of Health Authorities and Trusts
WAIS	wide area information server
WA	wide area network
WAT	workforce action team
WCVA	Wales Council for Voluntary Action
WeBNF	web-accessible *BNF*

WEST	winter and emergency services team	**WO**	Welsh Office
WF	Work Foundation (formerly Industrial Society)	**WONCA**	World Organization of National Colleges Academies and Academic Associations of General Practitioners/Family Physicians
WFP	*Working for Patients*	**WP**	White Paper *or* word processor
WFTC	Working Families' Tax Credit now replaced by Tax Credits	**WP10**	Working Paper 10 (now NMET)
WGSMT	Working Group on Specialist Medical Training	**WPA**	Western Provident Association
		WRC	women's resource centre
WHCSA	Welsh Health Common Services Agency (obsolete) now part of Welsh Health Estates	**WRT**	workforce review team
		WRVS	Women's Royal Voluntary Service
		WTC	working tax credit
WHDI	Welsh Health Development International	**WTD**	Working Time Directive
		WTE	whole-time equivalents (the total of whole-time staff, plus the whole time equivalent of part-time staff, which is obtained by dividing the hours worked in a year by part-timers by the number of hours in the whole-time working year)
WH	Welsh Health Estates		
WHO	World Health Organization		
WIC	walk in centre		
WIGS	women in grey suits		
WIH	work in hand		
WIMS	works information management system		
		WTEP	whole-time equivalent posts
WIST	women in surgical training scheme	**WTI**	Waiting Time Initiative
WM	workload measure (e.g. OBD, LOS, FCE)	**WU**	women's unit
		YCS	young chronic sick
WMA	World Medical Association	**YDU**	young disabled unit
WNAB	Workforce Numbers Advisory Board	**YOT**	youth offender team
		ZBB	zero-base budgeting
WNC	Womens' National Commission		

Abbreviations

Latin abbreviations continue to be found in textbooks and learned journals. It is useful to know their meaning and indeed they may be used, albeit cautiously, in writing. We would suggest for clarity it is often better to write 'see above' and 'see below' rather than 'v. sup.' and 'v. inf'.

- c. (circa): about, used of uncertain dates

- cf. (confer): compare; used to suggest that another work might usefully be consulted in relation to the subject under discussion.

- et al. (at alii): and others; used in multi-author references although it is customary to include all the authors in the first citation and/or in the bibliography.

- ibid. (ibidem): in the same place; relates to the immediately prior source.

- loc. cit. (loco citato): in the place already mentioned; relates to sources before the immediately prior citation.

- op. cit. (opere citato): in the work already mentioned; relates to sources before the immediately prior citation (loc. cit and op. cit. are more or less identical).

- q.v. (quod vide): which see; used to cross-refer to material that can be found elsewhere within a piece of writing. Note cf. refers to external material.

- sc. or scil. (scilicet = scire licet); that is to say, namely.

- s.v. (sub voce): under the word; used in connection with alphabetically arranged reference works.

- v. (vide): see, look up.

- v. inf. (vide infra): see below.

- viz (abbreviation for videlicet): that is to say, namely.

- v.sup. (vide supra): see above.

Index

Page numbers in *italic* refer to tables or figures. Acronyms and abbreviations can be found on pp. 244–82.